The GABA Receptors

The Receptors

Series Editor

David B. Bylund

University of Nebraska Medical Center, Omaha, NE

Board of Editors

S. J. Enna
University of Kansas
Kansas City, Kansas

Bruce S. McEwen
Rockefeller University
New York, New York

Morley D. Hollenberg
University of Calgary
Calgary, Alberta, Canada

Solomon H. Snyder
Johns Hopkins University
Baltimore, Maryland

The GABA Receptors

SECOND EDITION

Edited by

S. J. Enna

University of Kansas Medical School, Kansas City, KS

Norman G. Bowery

The Medical School Edgbaston, University of Birmingham, UK

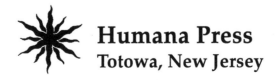

Humana Press
Totowa, New Jersey

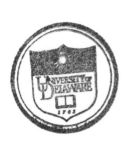

QP
563
G32
G324
1997

For additional copies, pricing for bulk purchases, and/or information about other Humana titles, contact Humana at the above address or at any of the following numbers: Tel.: 201-256-1699; Fax: 201-256-8341; E-mail: humana@interramp.com

Cover illustration: Fig. 1 from Chapter 4, "Pharmacology of Mammalian GABA$_A$ Receptors," by Neil Upton and Thomas Blackburn.

Cover design by Patricia F. Cleary.

Photocopy Authorization Policy:

Printed in the United States of America. 10 9 8 7 6 5 4 3 2 1

ISBN 0-89603-458-5 (alk. paper)

Preface

Thirteen years have passed since publication of the first edition of *The GABA Receptors*. During that time dramatic advances have been made in defining further the properties of this neurotransmitter system. Thus, in 1983 evidence indicating pharmacologically distinct subtypes of GABA receptors was just emerging and work had commenced on the purification and isolation of these sites. Two broad categories of receptors were proposed, $GABA_A$ and $GABA_B$, based primarily on differential sensitivities to antagonists and their distinctive electrophysiological properties. Though only a few classes of drugs known to interact with the GABA system were marketed, preclinical and clinical studies were underway to identify additional agents. Given the growing appreciation of the importance of the GABAergic system as a target for drugs, it was predicted that the area was ripe for exploitation. The present monograph is a testament to the accuracy of that prophecy.

Detailed in this second edition of *The GABA Receptors* are the wealth of recent data accumulated on the fundamental properties of GABA receptors. With respect to the $GABA_A$ site, molecular cloning experiments have demonstrated unequivocally the multiplicity of these receptors, all of which form neuronal membrane-bound chloride ion channels. Given the number of different subunits that can join to form the heteropentameric construct, there is a potential for several thousand molecularly distinct $GABA_A$ receptors, although only a few are thought to be present in mammalian brain. Elegant genetic engineering studies have produced animal models used to examine the biological and pharmacological importance of individual $GABA_A$ receptor subunits. It has also been discovered that the sensitivity of the $GABA_A$ receptor is modulated by certain steroids, revealing yet another approach to the manipulation of this system. Such information has provided a more precise characterization of the mechanism of action of established drugs and has been used to design novel and more selective therapeutics.

As for the $GABA_B$ receptor, the synthesis of highly potent and specific antagonists has provided tools to define its properties. Although the genes responsible for expressing $GABA_B$ receptors have yet to be isolated, it appears certain there are multiple, pharmacologically distinct subtypes of this G-protein coupled site.

v

The discovery of a third broad category of GABA receptors, the GABA$_C$ site, suggests that the classification of this receptor system is far from complete, indicating further the therapeutic potential that remains in developing additional agents capable of regulating GABA receptor function.

The past decade has also witnessed the cloning and expression of the GABA transporter. Inasmuch as this protein plays a crucial role in regulating the synaptic activity of GABA, it is a prime target for modifying GABAergic function.

Included among the new agents developed during the past decade are agonists, antagonists, and partial agonists for the benzodiazepine component of the GABA$_A$ site, as well as drugs that modify GABA reuptake or metabolism. Some of these are already available for human use, while others are awaiting approval, or are still in clinical trials. Thus, as anticipated, the accumulating data on the molecular, biochemical, and physiological properties of GABA receptors and related proteins have, since the first edition of this volume, expanded significantly the list of drugs that interact with this neurotransmitter system and have spurred the synthesis of additional agents.

These and related issues are detailed in the various chapters of *The GABA Receptors.* Besides providing an overview of the topic, this timely volume should serve as a guide to the direction of future research in the area. The information provided will be of interest to nuerobiologists in general, and to pharmacologists, medicinal chemists, and neurophysiologists in particular.

S. J. Enna
Norman G. Bowery

Contents

Contributors

DELIA BELELLI • *Neurosciences Institute, Department of Pharmacology and Clinical Pharmacology, Ninwells Hospital and Medical School, University of Dundee, Scotland*

D. BENKE • *Institute of Pharmacology, University of Zurich, Switzerland*

J. BENSON • *Institute of Pharmacology, University of Zurich, Switzerland*

THOMAS BLACKBURN • *SmithKline Beecham, Harlow, UK*

NORMAN G. BOWERY • *Department of Pharmacology, The Medical School Edgbaston, University of Birmingham, UK*

MARTIN CUNNINGHAM • *Molecular Devices Corporation, Sunnyvale, CA*

RUDOLF A. DEISZ • *Max-Planck Institute of Psychiatry, Munich, Germany*

BJARKE EBERT • *Department of Medicinal Chemistry, PharmaBiotec Research Center, The Royal Danish School of Pharmacy, Copenhagen, Denmark*

S. J. ENNA • *Department of Pharmacology, Toxicology, and Therapeutics, University of Kansas Medical School, Kansas City, KS*

J. M. FRITSCHY • *Institute of Pharmacology, University of Zurich, Switzerland*

WOLFGANG FROESTL • *Research and Development Department, Pharmaceuticals Division, CIBA-GEIGY, Basel, Switzerland*

BENTE FRØLUND • *Department of Medicinal Chemistry, PharmaBiotec Research Center, The Royal Danish School of Pharmacy, Copenhagen, Denmark*

CLAIRE HILL-VENNING • *Neurosciences Institute, Department of Pharmacology and Clinical Pharmacology, Ninwells Hospital and Medical School, University of Dundee, Scotland*

MASAAKI HIROUCHI • *Department of Pharmacology, Kyoto Prefectural University of Medicine, Kyoto, Japan*

GRAHAM A. R. JOHNSTON • *Adrien Albert Laboratory of Medicinal Chemistry, Department of Pharmacology, University of Sydney, Australia*

BARUCH I. KANNER • *Department of Biochemistry, Hadassah Medical School, The Hebrew University, Jerusalem, Israel*

POVL KROGSGAARD-LARSEN • *Department of Medicinal Chemistry, PharmaBiotec Research Center, The Royal Danish School of Pharmacy, Copenhagen, Denmark*

KINYA KURIYAMA • *Department of Pharmacology, Kyoto Prefectural University of Medicine, Kyoto, Japan*

JEREMY LAMBERT • *Neurosciences Institute, Department of Pharmacology and Clinical Pharmacology, Ninwells Hospital and Medical School, University of Dundee, Scotland*

B. LÜSCHER • *Institute of Pharmacology, University of Zurich, Switzerland*

STUART J. MICKEL • *Research and Development Department, Pharmaceuticals Division, CIBA-GEIGY, Basel, Switzerland*

H. MÖHLER • *Institute of Pharmacology, University of Zurich, Switzerland*

JOHN A. PETERS • *Neurosciences Institute, Department of Pharmacology and Clinical Pharmacology, Ninwells Hospital and Medical School, University of Dundee, Scotland*

MARCO PISTIS • *Neurosciences Institute, Department of Pharmacology and Clinical Pharmacology, Ninwells Hospital and Medical School, University of Dundee, Scotland*

U. RUDOLPH • *Institute of Pharmacology, University of Zurich, Switzerland*

NEIL UPTON • *SmithKline Beecham, Harlow, UK*

CHAPTER 1

Structure and Function of GABA Reuptake Systems

Baruch I. Kanner

1. Introduction

High affinity sodium-coupled transport systems are responsible for the reuptake of neurotransmitters from the synaptic cleft. They appear to play an important role in the overall process of synaptic transmission, namely in its termination (Iversen, 1971, 1973). The process is catalyzed by sodium-coupled neurotransmitter transport systems located in plasma membranes of nerve endings and glial cells (Kanner, 1983, 1989; Kanner and Schuldiner, 1987). These transport systems have been investigated in detail by using plasma membranes obtained upon osmotic shock of synaptosomes. It appears that these transporters are coupled not only to sodium, but also to additional ions like potassium or chloride.

The most abundant and well-characterized of these uptake systems in rat brain are those for GABA and L-glutamate, two major neurotransmitters in the central nervous system (Kanner, 1983, 1989; Kanner and Schuldiner, 1987). Multiple GABA transporter species have been detected in membrane vesicles and reconstituted preparations from rat brain, suggesting diversity of these systems (Mabjeesh and Kanner, 1989; Kanner and Bendahan, 1990). The application of molecular cloning techniques to this area has revealed that this diversity is larger than expected *(see* Section 5.*)*. In this review, emphasis will be placed on the GABA transporter and those related to it. The properties of the L-glutamate transporter, which is structurally and functionally different, have been reviewed recently (Kanner, 1993).

2. Mechanistic Studies

GABA is accumulated by electrogenic cotransport with sodium and chloride. The electrogenicity of the process has recently been shown directly

The GABA Receptors Eds.: S. J. Enna and N. G. Bowery
Humana Press Inc., Totowa, NJ

(Kavanaugh et al., 1992; Mager et al., 1993). We have been able to demonstrate directly that both sodium and chloride ions are cotransported with GABA by the transporter. This has been accomplished using a partly purified transporter preparation that was reconstituted into liposomes and by the use of Dowex columns (Aldrich, Milwaukee, WI) to terminate the reactions. These proteoliposomes catalyzed GABA- and chloride-dependent ^{22}[Na+] transport, as well as GABA- and sodium-dependent ^{36}[Cl-] translocation (Keynan and Kanner, 1988). Using this system, the stoichiometry has also been determined kinetically, i.e., by comparing the initial rate of the fluxes of [^{3}H]-GABA, ^{22}[Na+], and ^{36}[Cl-]. The results are similar to those found using the thermodynamic method, yielding an apparent stoichiometry of 2.5 Na$^+$: 1 Cl$^-$: 1 GABA (Radian and Kanner, 1983; Keynan and Kanner, 1988). This is in harmony with the predicted restrictions; if GABA is translocated in the zwitterionic form—the predominant one at physiological pH—an electrogenic co-transport of the three species requires a stoichiometry of nNa$^+$:mCl$^-$: GABA with $n > m$. Many other neurotransmitter transporters, including those for norepinephrine, dopamine, serotonin, choline, and glycine, require chloride in addition to sodium for optimal activity (Kuhar and Zarbin, 1978).

3. Reconstitution and Purification

Using methodology that enables reconstitution of many samples simultaneously and rapidly, one of the subtypes of the GABA transporter has been purified to apparent homogeneity (Radian and Kanner, 1985; Radian et al., 1986). It is a glycoprotein and has an apparent molecular weight of 70–80 kDa. The transporter retains all the properties observed in membrane vesicles.

4. Biochemical Characterization of the GABA Transporter

The effect of proteolysis on the function of the transporter was examined. It was purified using all steps except for lectin chromatography (Radian et al., 1986). After papain treatment and lectin chromatography, GABA transport activity was eluted with N-acetyl glucosamine. The characteristics of transport were the same as that of the pure transporter (Kanner et al., 1989).

In order to define which regions of the transporter were cleaved, antibodies were raised against synthetic peptides corresponding to several regions of the rat brain GABA transporter. According to our model (*see* Section 6.), this glycoprotein has 12 transmembrane α-helices with both amino and carboxyl termini located in the cytoplasm. The antibodies recognized the intact transporter on Western blots. The papainized transporter runs on sodium dodecyl sulfate-polyacrylamide gels as a broad band with an apparent molecular mass between about 58 and 68 kDa, compared to 80 kDa for the untreated transporter. The transporter fragment was recognized by all the antibodies, except for that raised against the amino terminus. Pronase cleaves the transporter to a relatively sharp 60 kDa band, which reacts with the antibodies against the internal loops but not with antibodies directed against either the amino- or the carboxyl-terminal. This pronase-treated transporter, upon isolation by lectin chromatography, was reconstituted. It exhibits full GABA transport activity. This activity exhibits the same features as the intact system, including an absolute dependence on sodium and chloride as well as electrogenicity. The amino- and carboxyl-terminal parts of the transporter are not required for functionality (Mabjeesh and Kanner, 1992).

Fragments of the (Na^+ + Cl^-)-coupled $GABA_A$ transporter were produced by proteolysis of membrane vesicles and reconstituted preparations from rat brain (Mabjeesh and Kanner, 1993). The former were digested with pronase, the latter with trypsin. Fragments with different apparent molecular masses were recognized by sequence-directed antibodies raised against this transporter. When GABA was present in the digestion medium, the generation of these fragments was almost entirely blocked (Mabjeesh and Kanner, 1993). At the same time, the neurotransmitter largely prevented the loss of activity caused by the protease. The effect was specific for GABA; protection was not afforded by other neurotransmitters. It was only observed when the two cosubstrates, sodium and chloride, were present on the same side of the membrane as GABA (Mabjeesh and Kanner, 1993). The results indicate that the transporter may exist in two conformations. In the absence of one or more of the substrates, multiple sites located throughout the transporter are accessible to the proteases. In the presence of all three substrates, conditions favoring the formation of the translocation complex, the conformation is changed so that these sites become inaccessible to protease action.

5. A New Superfamily of Na-Dependent Neurotransmitter Transporters

Partial sequencing of the purified $GABA_A$ transporter allowed the cloning of the first member of the new family of Na-dependent neurotransmitter transporters (Guastella et al., 1990). After expression cloning of the noradrenaline transporter, it became clear that it had significant homology with the GABA transporter (Pacholczyk et al., 1991). The use of functional cDNA expression assays and amplification of related sequences by polymerase chain reaction (PCR) resulted in the cloning of additional transporters that belong to this family, such as the dopamine and serotonin transporters, additional GABA transporters, transporters of glycine, proline, taurine, betaine, and two orphan transporters, whose substrates are still unknown (Blakely et al., 1991; Hoffman et al., 1991; Kilty et al., 1991; Shimada et al., 1991; Usdin et al., 1991; Borden et al., 1992; Clark et al., 1992; Fremeau et al., 1992; Guastella et al., 1992; Liu et al., 1992a,b; Liu et al., 1993a,b; Lopez-Corcuera et al., 1992; Smith et al., 1992; Uchida et al., 1992; Uhl et al., 1992; Yamauchi et al., 1992). In addition, another family member, which was originally thought to be a choline transporter, probably is a creatine transporter (Mayser et al., 1992; Guimbal and Kilimann, 1993). A novel glycine transporter cDNA encoding for a 799 amino acid protein has recently been isolated. This is significantly longer than most members of the superfamily. If we take into account that part of the mass of these transporters is constituted by sugar, it could encode for the 100 kDa glycine transporter which was purified and reconstituted (Lopez-Corcuera et al., 1991).

6. Shared Features of Family Members

The deduced amino acid sequences of these proteins reveal 30–65% identity between different members of the family. Based on these differences in homology, the family can be divided into four subgroups: transporters of biogenic amines (noradrenaline, dopamine, and serotonin); various GABA transporters, as well as transporters of taurine and creatine; transporters of proline and glycine; and orphan transporters. These proteins share some features of a common secondary structure. Each transporter is composed of 12 hydrophobic putative transmembrane α-helices. The lack of a signal peptide suggests that both amino- and carboxy-termini face the cytoplasm. These regions contain putative phosphorylation sites that may be involved in regulation of the transport process. The second extracellular loop between helices 3 and 4 is the largest, and it contains putative glycosylation sites.

Alignment of the deduced amino acid sequences of 13 different members of this superfamily, whose substrates are known (subgroups A–C) revealed that some segments within these proteins share a higher degree of homology than others. The most highly conserved regions (>50% homology) are helix 1 together with the extracellular loop connecting it with helix 2, and helix 5, together with a short intracellular loop connecting it with helix 4, and a larger extracellular loop connecting it with helix 6. These domains may be involved in stabilizing a tertiary structure that is essential for the function of these transporters. Alternatively, they may be related to a common function of these transporters, such as the translocation of sodium ions. The region stretching from helix 9 is far less conserved than the segment containing the first 8 helices. Possibly this domain contains some residues that are involved in translocating the different substrates. The least conserved segments are the amino- and carboxy-termini. As mentioned above, these areas may be involved in the regulation of the transport process. The orphan transporters differ from all other members of the family in three regions. They contain much larger extracellular loops between helices 7–8 and helices 11–12.

7. Structure-Function Relationships

It has been shown previously that parts of amino- and carboxyl-termini of the GABA transporter are not required for function (Mabjeesh and Kanner, 1992). In order to define these domains, a series of deletion mutants was studied in the GABA transporter (Bendahan and Kanner, 1993). Transporters truncated at either end until just a few amino acids distant from the beginning of helix 1 and the end of helix 12 retained their ability to catalyze sodium- and chloride-dependent GABA transport. These deleted segments did not contain any residues conserved among the different members of the superfamily. Once the truncated segment included part of these conserved residues, the transporter's activity was severely reduced. However, the functional damage was not caused by impaired turnover or impaired targeting of the truncated proteins (Bendahan and Kanner, 1993).

The substrate translocation performed by the various members of the superfamily is sodium- and chloride-dependent. In addition, some of the substrates contain charged groups as well. Therefore, charged amino acids in the membrane domain of the transporters may be essential for their normal function. This was tested using the GABA transporter (Pantanowitz et al., 1993). Out of five charged amino acids within its membrane domain, only one, arginine$_{69}$ in helix 1, is absolutely essential for activity. It is not merely the positive charge that is important, since even its substitution to other positively charged amino acids does not restore activity. The functional damage is not caused by impaired turnover or impaired targeting of the mutated protein. The three other positively charged amino acids and the only negatively charged one are not critical (Pantanowitz et al, 1993).

The transporters of biogenic amines contain an additional negatively charged residue in helix 1. Replacement of aspartate$_{79}$ in the dopamine transporter with alanine, glycine, or glutamate significantly reduced the uptake of dopamine and MPP$^+$ (parkinsonism-inducing neurotoxin), and binding of CFT (cocaine analog) without affecting B_{max}. Apparently, aspartate$_{79}$ in helix 1 interacts with dopamine's amino group during the transport process. Serine$_{356}$ and serine$_{359}$ in helix 7 are also involved in dopamine binding and translocation, perhaps by interacting with the hydroxyls on the catechol (Kitayama et al., 1992).

Studies of other proteins indicate that in addition to charged amino acids, aromatic amino acids containing π-electrons are also involved in maintaining the structure and function of these proteins (Sussman and Silman, 1992). Therefore, tryptophan residues in the membrane domain of the GABA transporter were mutated into serine and leucine (Kleinberger-Doron and Kanner, 1994). Mutations at the 68 and 222 position (in helix 1 and helix 4, respectively) led to a decrease of over 90% of the GABA uptake. The available data indicate the importance of helices 1, 4, and 7 in the function of the different transporters, but the nature of their contribution to the overall translocation process remains unclear.

We have explored the role of the hydrophilic loops connecting the putative transmembrane domains. Deletions of randomly picked nonconserved single amino acids in the loops connecting helices 7 and 8 or 8 and 9 result in inactive transport upon expression in HeLa cells. However, transporters where these amino acids are replaced with glycine retain significant activity. The expression levels of the inactive mutant transporters was similar to that of the wild-type, but one of these, ΔVal-348, appears to be defectively targeted to the plasma membrane. Our data are compatible with the idea that a minimal length of the loops is required, presumably to enable the transmembrane domains to interact optimally with each other (Kanner et al., 1994).

8. Conclusions

Recent breakthroughs, including the purification of some of the sodium-coupled neurotransmitter transporters, followed by the cloning of their cDNAs, have considerably improved our understanding of the structure of these transporters. Studies using site-directed mutagenesis revealed the importance of specific residues in the function of these transporters. Additional mutations and further functional characterization of all the mutated transporters should help to define the functional contribution of different segments of these proteins to the overall transport process. Applying independent structural approaches will complement and extend our knowledge of the structure and function of these transporters.

References

Bendahan, A. and Kanner, B. I. (1993) Identification of domains of a cloned rat brain GABA transporter which are not required for its functional expression. *FEBS Lett.* **318,** 41–44.

Blakely, R. D., Benson, H. E., Fremeau, R. T., Jr., Caron, M. G., Peek, M. M., Prince, H. K., and Bradley, C. C. (1991) Cloning and expression of a functional serotonin transporter from rat brain. *Nature* **353,** 66–70.

Borden, L. A., Smith, K. E., Hartig, P. R., Branchek, T. A., and Weinshank, R. L. (1992) Molecular heterogeneity of the GABA transport system. *J. Biol. Chem.* **267,** 21,098–21,104.

Clark, J. A., Deutch, A. Y., Gallipoli, P. Z., and Amara, S. G. (1992) Functional expression and CNS distribution of β-alanine sensitive neuronal GABA transporter. *Neuron* **9,** 337–348.

Fremeau, R. T., Jr., Caron, M. G., and Blakely, R. D. (1992) Molecular cloning and expression of a high affinity l-proline transporter expressed in putative glutamatergic pathways of rat brain. *Neuron* **8,** 915–926.

Guastella, J., Brecha, N., Weigmann, C., and Lester, H. A. (1992) Cloning, expression and localization of a rat brain high affinity glycine transporter. *Proc. Natl. Acad. Sci. USA* **89,** 7189–7193.

Guastella, J., Nelson, N., Nelson, H., Czyzyk, L., Keynan, S., Miedel, M. C., Davidson, N. C., Lester, H. A., and Kanner, B. I. (1990) Cloning and expression of a rat brain GABA transporter. *Science* **249,** 1303–1306.

Guimbal, C. and Kilimann, M. W. (1993) A Na^+ dependent creatine transporter in rabbit brain, muscle, heart and kidney. cDNA cloning and functional expression. *J. Biol. Chem.* **268,** 8418–8421.

Hoffman, B. J., Mezey, E., and Brownstein, M. J. (1991) Cloning of a serotonin transporter affected by antidepressants. *Science* **254,** 579–580.

Iversen, L. L. (1971) Role of transmitter uptake mechanism in synaptic neurotransmission. *Br. J. Pharmacol.* **41,** 571–591.

Kanner, B. I. (1983) Bioenergetics of neurotransmitter transport. *Biochim. Biophys. Acta* **726,** 293–316.

Kanner, B. I. (1989) Ion-coupled neurotransmitter transporter. *Curr. Opin. Cell Biol.* **1,** 735–738.

Kanner, B. I. (1993) Glutamate transporters from brain: a novel neurotransmitter transporter family. *FEBS Lett.* **325,** 95–99.

Kanner, B. I. and Bendahan, A. (1990) Two pharmacologically distinct sodium- and chloride-coupled high-affinity γ-aminobutyric acid transporters are present in plasma membrane vesicles and reconstituted preparations from rat brain. *Proc. Natl. Acad. Sci. USA* **87,** 2550–2554.

Kanner, B. I., Bendahan, A., Pantanowitz, S., and Su, H. (1994) The number of amino acid residues in hydrophilic loops connecting transmembrane domains of the GABA transporter GAT-1 is critical for its function. *FEBS Lett.* **356,** 191–194.

Kanner, B. I., Keynan, S., and Radian, R. (1989) Structural and functional studies on the sodium and chloride-coupled γ-aminobutyric acid transporter. Deglycosylation and limited proteolysis. *Biochemistry* **28,** 3722–3727.

Kanner, B. I. and Schuldiner, S. (1987) Mechanism of transport and storage of neurotransmitters. *CRC Crit. Rev. Biochem.* **22,** 1–39.

Kavanaugh, M. P., Arriza, J. L., North, R. A., and Amara, S. G. (1992) Electrogenic uptake of γ-aminobutyric acid by a cloned transporter expressed in oocytes. *J. Biol. Chem.* **267,** 22,007–22,009.

Keynan, S. and Kanner, B. I. (1988) γ-Aminobutyric acid transport in reconstituted preparations from rat brain: coupled sodium and chloride fluxes. *Biochemistry* **27,** 12–17.

Kilty, J. E., Lorang, D., and Amara, S. G. (1991) Cloning and expression of a cocaine-sensitive rat dopamine transporter. *Science* **254,** 578,579.

Kitayama, S., Shimada, S., Xu, H., Markham, L., Donovan, D. M., and Uhl, G. R. (1992)

Dopamine transporter site-directed mutations differentially alter substrate transport and cocaine binding. *Proc. Natl. Acad. Sci. USA* **89,** 7782–7785.

Kleinberger-Doron, N., and Kanner, B. I. (1994) Identification of tryptophan residues critical for the function and targeting of the γ-aminobutyric acid transporter (subtype A). *J. Biol. Chem.* **269,** 3063–3067.

Kuhar, M. J. (1973) Neurotransmitter uptake: a tool in identifying neurotransmitter- specific pathways. *Life Sci.* **13,** 1623–1634.

Kuhar, M. J. and Zarbin, M. A. (1978) Synaptosomal transport: a chloride dependence for choline, GABA, glycine and several other compounds. *J. Neurochem.* **31,** 251–256.

Liu, Q. R., Lopez-Corcuera, B., Nelson, H., Mandiyan, S., and Nelson, N. (1992a) Cloning and expression of a cDNA encoding the transporter of taurine and β-alanine in mouse brain. *Proc. Natl. Acad. Sci. USA* **89,** 12,145–12,149.

Liu, Q. R., Nelson, H., Mandiyan, S., Lopez-Corcuera, B., and Nelson, N. (1992b) Cloning and expression of a glycine transporter from mouse brain. *FEBS Lett.* **305,** 110–114.

Liu, Q. R., Lopez-Corcuera, B., Mandiyan, S., Nelson, H., and Nelson, N. (1993a) Molecular characterization of four pharmacologically distinct γ-aminobutyric acid transporters in mouse brain. *J. Biol. Chem.* **268,** 2104–2112.

Liu, Q. R., Mandiyan, S., Lopez-Corcuera, B., Nelson, H., and Nelson, N. (1993b) A rat brain cDNA encoding the neurotransmitter transporter with an unusual structure. *FEBS Lett.* **315,** 114–118.

Lopez-Corcuera, B., Liu, Q. R., Mandiyan, S., Nelson, H., and Nelson, N. (1992) Expression of a mouse brain cDNA encoding novel γ-aminobutyric acid transporter. *J. Biol. Chem.* **267,** 17,491–17,493.

Lopez-Corcuera, B., Vazquez, J., and Aragon, C. (1991) Purification of the sodium- and chloride-coupled glycine transporter from central nervous system. *J. Biol. Chem.* **266,** 24,809–24,814.

Mabjeesh, N. J. and Kanner, B. I. (1989) Low affinity γ-aminobutyric acid transport in rat brain. *Biochemistry* **28,** 7694–7699.

Mabjeesh, N. J. and Kanner, B. I. (1992) Neither amino nor carboxyl termini are required for function of the sodium- and chloride-coupled γ-aminobutyric acid transporter from rat brain. *J. Biol. Chem.* **267,** 2563–2568.

Mabjeesh, N. J. and Kanner, B. I. (1993) The substrates of a sodium- and chloride-coupled γ-aminobutyric acid transporter protect multiple sites throughout the protein against proteolytic cleavage. *Biochemistry* **32,** 8540–8546.

Mager, S., Naeve, J., Quick, M., Labarca, C., Davidson, N., and. Lester, H. A. (1993) Steady states, charge movements and rates for a cloned GABA transporter expressed in *Xenopus* oocytes. *Neuron* **10,** 177–188.

Mayser, W., Schloss, P., and Betz, H. (1992) Primary structure and functional expression of a choline transporter expressed in the rat nervous system. *FEBS Lett.* **305,** 31–36.

Pacholczyk, T., Blakely, R. D., and Amara, S. G. (1991) Expression cloning of a cocaine and antidepressant-sensitive human noradrenaline transporter. *Nature* **350,** 350–354.

Pantanowitz, S., Bendahan, A., and Kanner, E. I. (1993) Only one of the charged amino acids located in the transmembrane α helices of the γ-aminobutyric acid transporter (subtype A) is essential for its activity. *J. Biol. Chem.* **268,** 3222–3225.

Radian, R., Bendahan, A., and Kanner, B. I. (1986) Purification and identification of the functional sodium- and chloride-coupled γ-aminobutyric acid transport glycoprotein from rat brain. *J. Biol. Chem.* **261,** 15,437–15,441.

Radian, R. and Kanner, B. I. (1983) Stoichiometry of sodium- and chloride-coupled γ-aminobutyric acid transport by synaptic plasma membrane vesicles isolated from rat brain. *Biochemistry* **22,** 1236–1241.

Radian, R. and Kanner, B. I. (1985) Reconstitution and purification of the sodium- and chloride-coupled γ-aminobutyric acid transporter from rat brain. *J. Biol. Chem.* **260,** 11,859–11,865.

Shimada, S., Kitayama, S., Lin, C. L., Patel, A., Nanthakumar, E., Gregor, P., Kuhar, M., Uhl, G. (1991) Cloning and expression of a cocaine-sensitive dopamine transporter complementary DNA. *Science* **254,** 576–578.

Smith, K. E., Borden, L. A., Hartig, P. A., Branchek, T., and Weinshank, R. L. (1992) Cloning and expression of a glycine transporter reveal colocalization with NMDA receptors. *Neuron* **8,** 927–935.

Sussman, J. L. and Silman, I. (1992) Acetylcholinesterase: structure and use as a model for specific cation-protein interactions. *Curr. Opin. Struc. Biol.* **2,** 721–729.

Uchida, S., Kwon, H. M., Yamauchi, A., Preston, A. S., Marumo, F., and Handler, J. S. (1992) Molecular cloning of the cDNA for an MDCK cell Na^+- and Cl^--dependent taurine transporter that is regulated by hypertonicity. *Proc. Natl. Acad. Sci. USA* **89,** 8230–8234.

Uhl, G. R., Kitayama, S., Gregor, P., Nanthakumer, E., Persico, A., and Shimada, S. (1992) Neurotransmitter transporter family cDNAs in a rat midbrain library: 'orphan transporters' suggest sizable structural variations. *Mol. Brain Res.* **16,** 353–359.

Usdin, T. B., Mezey, E., Chen, C., Brownstein, M. J., and Hoffman, B. J. (1991) Cloning of the cocaine sensitive bovine dopamine transporter. *Proc. Natl. Acad. Sci. USA* **88,** 11,168–11,171.

Yamauchi, A., Uchida, S., Kwon, H. M., Preston, A. S., Robey, R. B., Garcia-Perez, A., Burg, M. B., and Handler, J. S. (1992) Cloning of a Na^+ and Cl^- dependent betaine transporter that is regulated by hypertonicity. *J. Biol. Chem.* **267,** 649–652.

CHAPTER 2

Diversity in Structure, Pharmacology, and Regulation of GABA$_A$ Receptors

H. Möhler, D. Benke, J. Benson, B. Lüscher, U. Rudolph, and J. M. Fritschy

1. Introduction

As the main inhibitory neurotransmitter in the brain, GABA is essential for the overall balance between neuronal excitation and inhibition. By acting on GABA$_A$ receptors, which are ligand-gated chloride channels, GABA mediates the principal fast inhibitory synaptic transmission. GABA exerts a ubiquitous influence largely by local feedback and feedforward circuits affecting a multitude of CNS functions. Adaptation of GABA-ergic transmission to various biological requirements, in particular to developmental maturation and cell-type specific signal transmission, is achieved by the expression of a multitude of structurally distinct GABA$_A$ receptors in the vertebrate brain. Receptor heterogeneity arises from a repertoire of at least 17 subunits, which can be grouped by the degree of sequence homology into 6α, 4β, 4γ, 1δ, and 2ρ subunits. The combinatorial assembly of these subunits (and splice variants of several of them) into a presumably pentameric heterooligomeric structure results in diverse receptor subtypes (for review, *see* Barnard, 1995; Luddens et al., 1995; Möhler et al., 1995a,b; Sieghart, 1995; Smith and Olsen, 1995). The most prevalent types of GABA$_A$ receptors have recently been identified and allocated to particular neuronal circuits. Apart from the physiological role in neuron-specific signal transduction (Table 1), GABA$_A$ receptor heterogeneity is of major pharmacological relevance. Many neuroactive drugs act on GABA$_A$ receptors, in particular ligands of the benzodiazepine (BZ) site, which are in clinical use for the treatment of anxiety, insomnia, muscle spasms, and epilepsy. By targeting receptor subtypes, the specificity and the side effect profile of these drugs are expected to be im-

The GABA Receptors Eds.: S. J. Enna and N. G. Bowery
Humana Press Inc., Totowa, NJ

Table 1
Functional Implications of GABA$_A$ Receptor Heterogeneity

Differential GABA-sensitivity of neurons
Affinity
Signal transduction
Differential allosteric modulation
Affinity
Efficacy
Differential subcellular localization
Synaptic, nonsynaptic, dendritic, somatic
Differential receptor regulation
Susceptibility to chemical modification
Alteration of subunit composition

proved. GABA also affects brain development by activating GABA$_A$ receptors. In embryonic and early postnatal brain, GABA exerts trophic actions possibly linked to the regulation of growth factor expression (Berninger et al., 1995). In this article, an overview is given on the structure and localization of the major GABA$_A$ receptors, their mutational analysis in vivo, the pharmacology of receptor subtypes, the pathophysiological role of GABA$_A$ receptors in disease, and the regulation of receptor function.

2. Molecular Structure of GABA$_A$ Receptors

As members of the transmitter-gated ion channel superfamily, GABA$_A$ receptors share structural and functional similarities with the nicotinic acetylcholine receptor, the glycine receptor, and the 5-HT$_3$ receptor, which include a pentameric pseudosymmetrical transmembrane subunit structure with a central pore. Each subunit is composed of a large N-terminal putatively extracellular domain, thought to mediate ligand-channel interactions, and four putative transmembrane domains with a large intracellular loop containing consensus sites for phosphorylation in most subunits (Betz, 1990; Galzi and Changeux, 1994; Macdonald and Olsen, 1994; Barnard, 1995; Möhler et al., 1995a). In vivo, fully functional GABA$_A$ receptors generally are assembled from a combination of α-, β-, and γ2-subunits (Benke et al., 1991, 1994; Duggan et al., 1991; Pollard et al., 1991; Mertens et al., 1993; Fritschy and Möhler, 1995; Bohlhalter et al., 1996). The subunit stoichiometry has been proposed to be two α-subunits, one β-subunit, and two γ-subunits (Backus et al., 1993; Barnard, 1995), based on electrophysiological evidence and on the possible co-occurrence of two variants of the α- and γ-subunits in one receptor (Duggan et al., 1991; Backus et al., 1993; Endo and Olsen, 1993; Mertens et al., 1993).

Putative functional domains for ligand binding sites have been proposed, based on mutagenesis experiments and photoaffinity labeling (Smith and Olsen, 1995). The GABA binding domain comprises parts of both the α- and β-subunits (Amin and Weiss, 1993; Smith and Olsen, 1995). The site of action of the convulsant picrotoxinin is located in the channel pore (ffrench-Constant et al., 1993). The binding domains of barbiturates and neurosteroids are molecularly less well defined (Lambert et al., 1995; Olsen and Snapp, 1995). Of particular pharmacological relevance is the formation of classical BZ binding sites when α- and β-subunits are co-expressed with the γ2-subunit, suggesting that the conformation of the α-subunit is rendered BZ sensitive by interaction with the γ2-subunit. However, this holds true only when the α-subunit is α1, α2, α3, or α5 (Pritchett et al., 1989; Pritchett and Seeburg, 1990), while the α4- and α6-subunits are BZ-insensitive, because of a single amino acid substitution (Luddens et al., 1990; Wisden et al., 1991; Wieland et al., 1992). A weak BZ-sensitivity is conveyed to GABA_A receptors by the γ1- and γ3-subunits (Ymer et al., 1990; Knoflach et al., 1991; Herb et al., 1992; Luddens et al., 1994), although these γ-subunits are very rare in vivo (Togel et al., 1994), in contrast to the almost ubiquitous γ2-subunit.

3. Major GABA_A Receptor Subtypes In Vivo

GABA_A receptor subtypes appear to be tailor-made for the specific functional requirements of distinct neuronal circuits. By double- and triple-immunofluorescence staining with antibodies to receptor subunits, a cell type-specific expression pattern of subunit combinations has been visualized in rat brain and spinal cord (Fritschy et al., 1992; Benke et al., 1994; Fritschy and Möhler, 1995; Bohlhalter et al., 1996). Subcellularly, staining is frequently localized in aggregates on the plasma membrane and no distinction of subunit expression was apparent at the light microscopic level. Therefore, the subunit pattern expressed in a neuron has been taken as an indication of the composition of its receptor. They are best distinguished by the type of α-subunit, which displays the highest number of variants. For example, serotonergic and basal forebrain cholinergic neurons express the α3-subunit, neighboring GABA neurons of similar size and morphology are characterized by the α1-subunit (Gao et al., 1993, 1995). The cell type-specificity also extends to the β-subunits. In the basal forebrain, cholinergic neurons express the β3-subunit; and GABA-ergic neurons express the β2-subunit (Gao et al., 1995). These two cell populations possess GABA_A receptors differing in both α- and β-subunit variants. The subtype-specific expression of GABA_A recep-

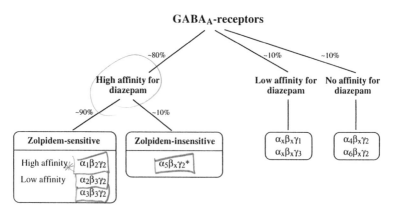

Fig. 1. Classification of native GABA$_A$ receptor subtypes.

tors is closely linked to the different functional properties of individual neurons and appears to reflect their integration in distinct neuronal circuits. In the following, the localization and subunit structure of the major GABA$_A$ receptor subtypes is described, grouped according to their BZ sensitivity (Fig. 1).

3.1. Benzodiazepine-Sensitive GABA$_A$ Receptors

About 80% of all GABA$_A$ receptors contain the classical BZ binding sites, and are of major pharmacological relevance. The BZ-sensitive receptor subtypes are characterized largely by the subunit combinations α1β2γ2, α2β3γ2, and α3β3γ2. In addition, receptors containing the combinations α5βxγ2 and αxβxγ2δ display classical BZ binding sites but are considerably less abundant.

3.1.1. GABA$_A$ Receptors Containing α1β2γ2 Subunits

The subunit combination α1β2γ2 constitutes the major GABA$_A$ receptor subtype in the brain. It amounts to at least 60% of the BZ-sensitive GABA$_A$ receptors, as demonstrated by immunoprecipitation and immuno-histochemical localization of the three subunits in the same neurons (Duggan et al., 1992; Benke et al., 1994; Ruano et al., 1994; Fritschy and Möhler, 1995; Bohlhalter et al., 1996). This receptor type is not only the main component in GABA-ergic signal transduction, but also mediates the basic pharmacological spectrum of the classical, high affinity BZ site ligands (Table 2) because of their high nanomolar affinities, except CL 218872 (Mertens et al., 1993; Benke et al., 1994).

Regarding identified neurons, α1β2γ2 receptors are expressed in numerous populations of GABA-ergic neurons at all levels of the neuraxis. In

Table 2
Summary of Drug Binding Profiles of Native GABA$_A$-Receptor Subtypes

	K_i [nM]; [³H]Flumazenil binding; Receptor population immunoprecipitated by subunit-specific antisera							
	α1β2γ2[a]	α2β3γ2[a]	α3β3γ2[a]	α4βxγ2[b]	α5[c]	γ1[d]	γ3[d]	δ[e]
Flumazenil	0.6⁺	1.2⁺	1.1⁺	130	0.6⁺	>10,000	1.1⁺	0.5⁺
Flunitrazepam	7	7	8	>10,000	3	38⁺	854	2
Diazepam	20	25	20	>10,000	20	—	—	5
Ro 15-4513	—	—	—	16⁺	1	> 10,000	6.9	0.4
βCCM	2	6	7	—	3	1550	11	0.2
Zolpidem	12	100	83	>10,000	30[c]	>10,000	>10,000	43
CL 218'872	195	960	670	>10,000	280	400	227	400

Displacement potencies of various benzodiazepine receptor ligands were determined for receptor populations immunoprecipitated from whole rat brain with the respective α-, β-, γ-, or δ-subunit-specific antiserum. ⁺, K_D-values derived from Scatchard analysis; —, not determined.

[a]For the α1β2γ2, α2β3γ2, and α3β3γ2 subunit combinations, which represent major GABA$_A$-receptor subtypes, the mean K_i-values for receptors immunoprecipitated with the respective α- and β-subunit antisera are given. The K_i-values for the individual α- and β-receptor populations were very similar (Benke et al., 1994). The presence of the γ2-subunit in the native receptors is inferred from the drug-binding profile of the respective recombinant receptors, from the subunits associated in immunopurified receptors and from the cellular coexpression of the respective three subunits. The presence of receptor subtypes with an additional type of α-subunit is possible, e.g., α1α2, α1α3, α2α3 (Marksitzer et al., 1993; Mertens et al., 1993; Benke et al., 1994; Fritschy et al., 1992; Fritschy and Mohler, 1995; reviewed by Stephenson, 1995; McKernan and Whiting, 1996).

[b]K_i-values for receptors immunoprecipitated with the α4-subunit-specific antiserum using [³H]Ro 15-4513 as radioligand. The drug binding profile corresponds to the α4β2γ2 recombinant receptor. The presence of β2 or β3 and γ2 is inferred from the subunits identified in α4-immunopurified receptors (no γ1 or γ3, β1 not tested; Benke et al., in preparation).

[c]K_i-values for receptors immunoprecipitated with the α5-subunit specific antiserum are given. The α5-subunit is frequently associated with a β-, the γ2-subunit and possibly an additional α-subunit. The heterogeneity of the α5-receptor population is documented by the regional difference of the K_i-value for zolpidem (hippocampus: K_i = 1220 nM, cortex: 270 nM, striatum: 19 nM; Mertens et al., 1993; the K_i-value in hippocampus corresponds to that of α5β2γ2 recombinant receptors). The K_i-value of 30 nM observed in whole brain points to an additional population of high affinity α5-receptors.

[d]K_i-values were taken from Benke et al. (1996) with [³H]flunitrazepam and [³H]flumazenil as radioligand for the γ1- and γ3-receptors, respectively.

[e]K_i-values are given for receptors immunoprecipitated with the δ-subunit specific antiserum (Mertens et al., 1993). The δ-receptor population is heterogeneous in that it can be associated with different α- and β-subunits and the γ2-subunit (e.g., αβδγ2). Receptors lacking the γ2-subunit do not respond to ligands of the benzodiazepine site (e.g., α1β1δ, Saxena and Macdonald, 1994).

particular, GABA-ergic neurons in the cerebellum, brainstem reticular formation, pallidum, substantia nigra, and basal forebrain, as well as interneurons in cerebral cortex and hippocampus, are intensely immunoreactive for the α1-subunit (Fritschy et al., 1992; Gao et al., 1993, 1995; Gao and Fritschy, 1994). The α1β2γ2 subunit combination has also been allocated to non-GABA-ergic neurons, such as olfactory bulb mitral cells, in association with the α3-subunit, and relay neurons in the thalamus, in combination with the δ-subunit. Only a few regions appear devoid of α1-subunit staining, notably the striatal complex, the granule cell layer of the olfactory bulb, and the reticular nucleus of the thalamus (Fritschy and Möhler, 1995).

3.1.2. GABA$_A$ Receptors Containing α2β3γ2 or α3β3γ2 Subunits

Receptors containing the α2- or α3-subunits represent about 25% of the BZ-sensitive GABA$_A$ receptors and are most abundant in regions where the α1-subunit is absent or expressed at low levels (Marksitzer et al., 1993; Benke et al., 1994; Fritschy and Möhler, 1995). This concerns particularly the striatum, hippocampal formation, and olfactory bulb for the α2-subunit, and the lateral septum, reticular nucleus of the thalamus, and several brainstem nuclei for the α3-subunit (Gao et al., 1993; Benke et al., 1994; Fritschy and Möhler, 1995). The co-expression of α2- or α3-subunits with the β3- and γ2-subunits is evident on the cellular level (Benke et al., 1994; Gao et al., 1995), for example, in hippocampal pyramidal cells (α2β3γ2) and in cholinergic neurons of the basal forebrain (α3β3γ2). The profile of BZ site ligands interacting with these receptors differs from that of the α1β2γ2 receptors, in that βCCM displays a slightly lower displacing potency (four- to fivefold) and zolpidem and CL 218872, a considerably lower displacing potency (9-14 fold) (Möhler et al., 1995a; Table 2). The neuronal circuits expressing α2β3γ2 and α3β3γ2 receptors are expected to be less prominently involved in the pharmacological responses to the latter drugs.

3.1.3. GABA$_A$ Receptors Containing the α5-Subunit

Receptors containing the α5-subunit are of minor abundance in the brain and are concentrated mainly in the hippocampus, olfactory bulb, hypothalamus, and trigeminal sensory nucleus (Fritschy and Möhler, 1995). They comprise various subtypes differentiated by their affinity for zolpidem (Table 2). For example, in the hippocampus and spinal cord, the receptor population immunoprecipitated by the α5-antiserum displays micromolar affinity for zolpidem (Mertens et al., 1993). In contrast, in brain areas where native α5 receptors display nanomolar affinities for zolpidem, the α5-subunit might be associated with an additional α-subunit, the α1- and α3-subunits being the prime candidates (Mertens et al., 1993).

3.1.4. GABA_A Receptors Containing the δ-Subunit

Receptors containing the δ-subunit display an enhanced GABA response, as demonstrated by comparative electrophysiological analysis of the subunit combination $\alpha1\beta2\gamma2$ and $\alpha1\beta2\gamma2\delta$ (Saxena and Macdonald, 1994). The δ-subunit is potentially associated with the subunits $\alpha1$, $\alpha3$, $\beta2,3$, and $\gamma2$ (Mertens et al., 1993). Pharmacologically, the presence of the δ-subunit results in a particularly high affinity for certain BZ site ligands (βCCM, diazepam), as shown for native receptors (Mertens et al., 1993; Table 2) and recombinant receptors ($\alpha1\beta1\gamma2\delta$) (Saxena and Macdonald, 1994). The δ-subunit is expressed mainly in granule cells of the cerebellum and, to a minor extent, in a few other brain regions, notably thalamus and olfactory bulb (Fritschy and Möhler, 1995).

3.2. Benzodiazepine-Insensitive GABA_A Receptors

GABA_A receptors that are insensitive to classical benzodiazepine ligands are not very prevalent in the brain, although they can be highly expressed in particular neurons. They consist largely of receptors containing the subunits $\alpha4$, $\alpha6$, or ρ (Table 2). Receptors containing the $\alpha4$-subunit are present at low abundance in numerous brain regions, while receptors containing the $\alpha6$-subunit are expressed almost exclusively in cerebellar granule cells (Laurie et al., 1992; Thompson et al., 1992; Fritschy et al., 1993; Varecka et al., 1994). The $\alpha4$- and $\alpha6$-receptors are diazepam-insensitive, but respond to certain nonclassical BZ ligands, such as Ro 15-4513 or bretazenil (Wong and Skolnik, 1992; Knoflach et al., 1996). Highly unusual receptors are formed from ρ-subunits, found mainly in retina. They form homomeric GABA-gated ion channels that are sensitive to picrotoxinin but insensitive to bicuculline, benzodiazepines, steroids, and barbiturates (Shimada et al., 1992; Kusama et al., 1993; Enz et al., 1995). Because of their unusual pharmacology, they have also been termed GABA_C receptors (for review, Johnston, 1994; *see also* Chapter 11 of this volume).

4. Mutational Analysis
of Receptor Function In Vivo

GABA_A receptor function in vivo can be analyzed by the targeted disruption of specific subunit genes. This has recently been accomplished for the $\gamma2$-subunit (Gunther et al., 1995), which, in combination with α- and β-subunits, occurs in most GABA_A receptors and is required for the presence of the BZ site. The physiological relevance of the BZ sites for brain development and function is unresolved. This is particularly striking, since the BZ site is an evolutionarily conserved modulatory element of GABA_A receptors.

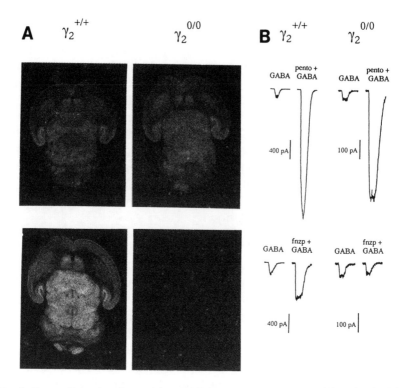

Fig. 2. Benzodiazepine-insensitive GABA$_A$ receptors generated in mice lacking the γ2-subunit. **(A)** Distribution of binding sites for GABA (top) and benzodiazepines (bottom) in newborn γ2$^{+/+}$ and γ2$^{0/0}$ mice depicted in autoradiographs of brain sections incubated with [^{3}H] SR 95531 (top) and [^{3}H] flumazenil (bottom) (×4.5). The distribution of GABA-binding sites is almost unaltered, but there is a nearly complete loss of benzodiazepine-binding sites in the mutant mice. **(B)** GABA-evoked whole cell currents in dorsal root ganglion neurons of newborn γ2$^{+/+}$ and γ2$^{0/0}$ mice. Current traces show the potentiation of the GABA response (GABA pulses 2s, 5 μ*M*) by pentobarbital (pento, 100 μ*M*), but not by flunitrazepam (fnzp, 1 μ*M*). Adapted from Gunther et al. (1995).

Following targeted disruption of the γ2-subunit gene, homozygous mutant mice were generated, which lack the γ2-subunit protein. In neonatal brain, the number and distribution of GABA binding sites was practically unaltered, and the BZ sites were almost entirely absent (Fig. 2). Correspondingly, diazepam was inactive behaviorally in neonates. Functional GABA$_A$ receptors had been formed from the remaining α- and β-subunits. The Hill coefficient and the single channel conductance of the GABA response corresponded to those of recombinant receptors composed of α- and β-subunits. In keeping with this subunit composition, the GABA response was potentiated by pentobarbital, but not by flunitrazepam (Fig. 2). These results demonstrate that functional $GABA_A$ receptors are formed in vivo in the absence of the γ2-subunit. Thus, the γ2-subunit serves no essential function for the assembly, transport, and insertion into the cell membrane of $GABA_A$ receptors. However, the γ2-subunit is essential for the establishment of normal signal transduction characteristics, as shown for the single channel conductance and the Hill coefficient. In addition, the γ2-subunit is required for the formation of BZ sites of the normal receptor (Gunther et al., 1995).

There was no indication of an essential role for an endogenous BZ-site ligand in governing embryonic development of the γ2-subunit homozygous mutant mice. At birth, their body weight and histology of the brain and various other organs were normal, and no impairment in feeding or lack of anterior pituitary hormones for endocrine control was apparent. Postnatally, however, the impaired $GABA_A$ receptor function was associated with retarded growth, sensorimotor dysfunction, and drastically reduced life span. The time by which most GABA-ergic synapses are expected to become operative coincides with the maximal life-span of the mutant mice. Most likely, the γ2-deficient $GABA_A$ receptors do not provide the precise control of GABA-ergic tone required in synaptic transmission. The lack of $GABA_A$ receptor regulation by a postnatally relevant endogenous BZ-site ligand might contribute to this phenotype. Mice heterozygous for the γ2-subunit gene develop normally and only a small population of their $GABA_A$ receptors is impaired. The heterozygous mutant animals will permit an analysis of a limited GABAergic deficit in behavioral terms. The animals will be of particular interest as potential models of anxiety disorders.

5. Pharmacology
of GABA_A Receptor Subtypes

$GABA_A$ receptors are the site of action of a variety of pharmacologically important drugs, including barbiturates, neurosteroids, ethanol, and benzodiazepines (Richards et al., 1991; Sieghart, 1992; Haefely, 1994; Möhler et al., 1995b; Lambert et al., 1995; Olsen and Sapp, 1995). Of particular clinical relevance are ligands acting at the BZ-site. By allosterically enhancing $GABA_A$ receptor function, they induce anxiolytic, anticonvulsant, muscle-relaxant, and sedative-hypnotic effects. Of major impact in $GABA_A$ receptor research was the recognition that the affinity, as well as the modulatory efficacy, of BZ-site ligands can change with receptor composition.

5.1. Benzodiazepine Site Ligands

Novel ligands of the BZ site are being developed with the aim of retaining the therapeutic effectiveness of classical benzodiazepines while reducing unwanted side-effects, such as tolerance, dependence liability, memory impairment, and ataxia. Two strategies are being followed to achieve this goal: reduction in efficacy and selectivity in receptor affinity.

5.1.1. Reduction in Efficacy

Although there are individual variations (Ducic et al., 1993), classical benzodiazepines, such as diazepam, interact with nearly all BZ sites with high affinity and high efficacy (full agonists), as demonstrated for both native and recombinant receptors. In contrast, partial agonists, typified by bretazenil or imidazenil, display high affinity at most, if not all, receptors; but compared to classical BZ agonists they act with reduced efficacy (Haefely et al., 1990; Puia et al., 1992; Wafford et al., 1993; Auta et al., 1994). It is important to note that a partial agonist does not simply mimic the profile of action of a full agonist. Partial agonists rather are expected to fail to cause those activities that are achieved by full agonists at a high receptor occupancy, such as ataxia, development of tolerance, ethanol potentiation, and other side effects of classical benzodiazepines. Therefore, partial agonists should provide anxiolytic drugs with a favorable side effect profile (Haefely et al., 1990; Haefely, 1994; Costa et al., 1995).

Pharmacologically, bretazenil and imidazenil exhibit strong anxiolytic activity, but only a low tolerance and dependence liability in animal tests, and a very weak potential to induce sedation, ataxia, locomotor impairment, or ethanol potentiation (Haefely et al., 1990; Ducic et al., 1993; Schoch et al., 1993; Costa et al., 1995). In humans the dependence liability was much reduce for bretazenil compared to alprazolam and diazepam (Busto et al., 1994). Partial agonism has thus been established as a successful strategy for the development of novel BZ site ligands with promising clinical potential. Partial agonist activity is also exerted by the ligands DN 2327 (Yasumatsu et al., 1994) and Y 23684 (Wada and Fukuda, 1991), of which the latter is currently undergoing clinical trials as an anxiolytic.

Apart from ligands that act as partial agonists at practically all BZ-sensitive $GABA_A$ receptors, there are BZ site ligands that display efficacies that vary depending on the $GABA_A$ receptor subtype. The best studied example is abecarnil, which acts as a partial agonist on recombinant receptors containing $\alpha2$- and $\alpha5$-subunits but acts as a full agonist on receptors containing the $\alpha1$- and $\alpha3$-subunits (Knoflach et al., 1993; Pribilla et al., 1993). It is therefore considered to be a selective partial agonist. Pharmacologically, abecarnil displays a favorable side-effect profile and is currently undergoing clinical trials as an anxiolytic (Duka et al., 1993). Finally, it appears that novel pharmaceutical profiles can be generated by further subtype-specific variations in modulatory efficacy. The novel BZ site ligand U 101017 displays prominent antistress activity but low anticonflict activity by acting with reduced efficacy at receptors containing α1-, α2-, or α5-subunits (von Voigtländer, in preparation).

5.1.2. Selective Affinity

Distinct GABA$_A$ receptor subtypes are expressed in different populations of neurons. Based on a selective-affinity profile, a ligand can be targeted to subsets of GABA-ergic brain circuits. Such ligands are expected to display pharmacological profiles that differ from classical benzodiazepines. The most prominent example is the hypnotic zolpidem. It shows high affinity for receptors containing the α1-subunit, which represent the majority of all GABA$_A$ receptors, while displaying lower affinity for receptors containing the α2- and α3-subunits, and even lower affinity for most receptors containing the α5-subunit (Table 2) (Pritchett and Seeburg, 1990; McKernan et al., 1991; Mertens et al., 1993). Zolpidem is reported to display fewer side effects than classical benzodiazepines in the treatment of insomnia (Scharf et al., 1991).

These examples indicate that favorable profiles of BZ site ligands can be achieved by reducing the efficacy of a ligand at all receptors (bretazenil, imidazenil) or, alternatively, by avoiding full activation of certain receptor subtypes. The latter can be achieved by ligands with subtype-selective efficacy (e.g., abecarnil) or subtype-selective affinity (e.g., zolpidem). The findings concerning abecarnil and zolpidem are of particular interest regarding receptor heterogeneity. In both cases, receptors containing α2- and α5-subunits are not fully activated. These receptors might therefore be located in neuronal circuits that are involved in mediating unwanted, rather than desirable, drug effects. Indeed, it is conspicuous that receptors containing the α2-subunit are strongly expressed in brain areas mediating reward (e.g., nucleus accumbens), and receptors containing the α5-subunit are concentrated in certain areas linked to memory functions (e.g., hippocampus) (Fritschy and Möhler, 1995).

5.2. Novel Modulatory Drug Target Sites

Recently, two novel modulatory drug binding sites located on GABA$_A$ receptors have been identified. Pyrrolopyrimidines, such as U 89843A, act at a site distinct from the sites for benzodiazepines, barbiturates, neurosteroids, or loreclezole. U 89843A enhances the GABA-induced currents of recombinant receptors in a flumazenil-insensitive fashion, irrespective of the types of α-subunit ($\alpha 1\beta 2\gamma 2$, $\alpha 3\beta 3\gamma 2$, and $\alpha 6\beta 2\gamma 2$ receptors, but not $\alpha 1\beta 2$ and $\alpha 1\gamma 2$ receptors). U 89843A induces sedation without loss of righting reflex in mice (Im et al., 1995). Furthermore, pyrazinones, such as U 92813, appear to interact with yet another drug modulatory site of $GABA_A$ receptors. The GABA-potentiating response of U 92813 is not flumazenil-sensitive, does not require the γ2-subunit in recombinant receptors. Since its binding site is present on an αβ-subunit combination ($\alpha 1\beta 2$) but not on $\alpha 1\gamma 2$ and $\beta 2\gamma 2$, it appears to be distinct from that of the pyrrolopyrimidines, barbituates, and neurosteroids (Im et al., 1993). These novel modulatory sites may hold the potential for further therapeutic advances.

6. $GABA_A$ Receptors in Disease

In view of the ubiquitous presence of GABA-ergic circuits in the brain, various neurologic and mental disorders might be expected to be related to alterations of $GABA_A$ receptors. However, so far only a few tentative links have been established to human diseases, such as epilepsy, Huntington's disease, craniofacial abnormalities, and Angelman's syndrome.

6.1. Epilepsy

The GABA hypothesis of seizure disorders (Meldrum, 1979; Gale, 1992; Olsen et al., 1992) suggests that deficits in GABA-ergic inhibitory synaptic transmission contribute to the synchronous epileptiform neuronal activity and the spread of focal seizure activity. In support of this hypothesis, compounds that block the synthesis, synaptic release, or postsynaptic action of GABA induce convulsions, and compounds with the reverse action are anticonvulsants. However, a primary alteration of the GABA system in the pathophysiology of epilepsy is not well defined, particularly concerning the role of $GABA_A$ receptors. In positron emission tomography (PET) studies of idiopathic partial epilepsy, binding of ^{11}C-flumazenil was found to be significantly lower in epileptic foci than in the contralateral homotopic reference region and in the remaining neocortex (Savic et al., 1988). This reduction in $GABA_A$ receptor binding was detectable in the absence of overt cell loss. In tissue samples of surgical resections from patients with focal epilepsies, a loss of $GABA_A$ receptors, as well as a lack of receptor alterations, have been described (reviewed by Olsen et al., 1990, 1992). At least in some of the cases, the $GABA_A$ receptor reduction was caused by major cell loss (Olsen et al., 1990; McDonald et al., 1991; Wolf et al., 1994). Thus, $GABA_A$ receptors do not appear to play a primary pathophysiological role in temporal lobe epilepsy.

In animal models of epilepsy, a reduction in receptor binding has been found in seizure-susceptible gerbils (Olsen et al., 1985). Following kindling-induced seizures in rats, an increased $GABA_A$ receptor binding confined largely to the dentate gyrus of the hippocampus has been found (Nobrega et al., 1990; Titulaer et al., 1994, 1995), in line with selective alterations of subunit mRNA levels restricted to the dentate gyrus granule cells (Clark et al., 1994; Kamphuis et al., 1994, 1995; Kokaia et al., 1994). An initial reduction of the β3- and γ2- subunit mRNA was followed by an increase of the α1- and γ2-subunit mRNAs, but the β-subunit mRNA was not significantly altered. Five days after the kindling, the mRNA levels had returned to normal, indicating that the maintenance of the kindled state is not caused by alterations of $GABA_A$ receptor subunit expression (Kokaia et al., 1994). From microdialysis studies in patients, impaired GABA release has recently been proposed to contribute to epileptic pathophysiology (During and Spencer, 1993), possibly linked to alterations of GABA transporters (During et al., 1995; Meldrum, 1995).

6.2. Huntington's Disease

Huntington's disease is an inherited neurodegenerative disorder characterized by progressive involuntary choreiform movements, psychopathological changes, and dementia (Hayden, 1981). Though a candidate gene for involvement in this disease has been identified (Huntington's Disease Collaborative Research Group, 1993), the pathogenesis is still unknown. Neuropathologically, the hallmark of Huntington's disease is a profound loss of striatal projection neurons, leading to atrophy of the caudate nucleus and putamen. At early stages of the disease, a decrease in $GABA_A$ receptor binding occurs in the caudate nucleus, as shown by PET (Holthoff et al., 1993), immunohistochemistry, and autoradiography (Faull et al., 1993). The loss of receptors occurs in the absence of overt neuropathological alterations. At late stages of Huntington's disease there is a further decrease of $GABA_A$ receptors in the atrophied striatum accompanied by a pronounced up-regulation in the globus pallidus, pointing to hypo- and hypersensitivity of the GABA system in the respective regions (Whitehouse et al., 1985; Faull et al., 1993). The loss of $GABA_A$ receptors as one of the earliest neuropathological changes in Huntington's disease is a strong indication for their pathophysiological implication.

6.3. Craniofacial Abnormalities

In the search for genetic causes of neurological defects, various animal mutants have been studied. Concerning $GABA_A$ receptor subunit genes, p^{cp} mice with a 95% penetrant, recessive, neonatally lethal cleft palate, are of particular interest. They contain a deletion of the cleft palate 1 *(cp1)* locus on chromosome 7, which is closely linked to the pink-eyed dilution *(p)* locus

(Lyon et al., 1992). This deletion has recently been found to include the genes encoding the GABA$_A$ receptor subunits α5, γ3, and β3 (Culiat et al., 1993, 1994; Nakatsu et al., 1993). The mutant mice display a corresponding loss of GABA$_A$ receptor subtypes, particularly in hippocampus, where receptors containing the α5-subunit are prevalent (Nakatsu et al., 1993). The *cp1* locus was localized to an interval beginning distally to the α5-subunit gene and ending within the coding region of the β3-subunit gene. Since mice containing a deletion that includes the α5- and the γ3-subunit genes, but not the β3-subunit gene, develop a normal palate (Culiat et al., 1994), it was proposed that deletion of the β3-subunit gene, and not another gene in the deletion interval, causes cleft palate. This has recently been verified by introducing a β3-subunit transgene under the control of a β-actin promoter into mice homozygous for the cleft palate deletion. The rescued animals displayed no obvious neurological defects (Culiat et al., 1995). Thus, the lack of GABA$_A$ receptors that normally contain the β-subunit contribute to the cleft palate phenotype in *p^{cp}* mice. This result is consistent with earlier teratological observations that GABA or diazepam can interfere with normal palate development in mice (Wee and Zimmerman, 1983). The human counterpart of the region deleted in *p^{cp}* is the locus 15q11-q13. Aberrations in this locus, especially those with a deletion or mutation of the β3-subunit gene, might contribute to familial or sporadic craniofacial abnormalities in man.

6.4. Angelman Syndrome

Alterations in chromosome 15q11-q13 are associated with Angelman syndrome, a genetic disorder characterized by severe mental retardation, microencephaly, ataxia, craniofacial abnormalities, and hypopigmentation (Angelman, 1965). The smallest known maternal deletion resulting in Angelman syndrome includes the β3-subunit gene (Saitoh et al., 1992; Knoll et al., 1993; Sinnett et al., 1993), although a single patient bearing a translocation contained an apparently intact β3-subunit gene (Reis et al., 1993). Although located in the same cluster of genes as the β3-subunit (Culiat et al., 1993; Nakatsu et al., 1993), the GABA$_A$ receptor α5-subunit gene is not involved in Angelman syndrome (Knoll et al., 1993; Sinnett et al., 1993). Paternal imprinting observed in Angelman syndrome has not been detected for the corresponding region of the mouse chromosome 7 (Nicholls et al., 1993). It remains to be determined what role, if any, GABA$_A$ receptor subunit genes play in the etiology of Angelman syndrome.

6.5. X-Linked Manic Depression

A possible relationship to human disease has been proposed for the α3-subunit gene. Its locus was mapped to a site on the X chromosome, Xq28, a location that makes it a potential candidate gene for the X-linked form of manic depression (Bell et al., 1989; Buckle et al., 1989). However, a detailed analysis of this gene locus has not yet been performed.

7. Regulation of GABA$_A$ Receptors

Adaptation to changing functional requirements is a key property of neuronal circuits. As part of the adaptation mechanism in the GABA system, neurons are able to modify GABA$_A$ receptor function by at least four different mechanisms: switch in receptor subtype, regulation of the number of receptors, covalent modification, and conformational alterations.

7.1. Regulation by Subunit Exchange

A switch in subunit gene expression is particularly evident during ontogeny, as shown in rat and marmoset monkey forebrain during late embryonic and early postnatal development. Embryonic GABA$_A$ receptors are characterized mainly by the presence of the α2-subunit, but lack the α1-subunit. Beginning shortly before birth, these receptors are replaced by the adult pattern, in which the α1-subunit predominates and only minor receptor populations with the α2-subunit remain (Fritschy et al., 1994; Hornung and Fritschy, 1996; Paysan and Fritschy, 1996). This subunit switch does not reflect receptor expression in different cells but occurs in the same neuron (Fritschy et al., 1994). The timing of the switch is the same in rat and marmoset monkey (Hornung and Fritschy, 1996), although at birth the monkey brain is more mature than the rat brain. This suggests that GABA$_A$ receptors containing the α1-subunit are dispensable during embryonic development but are required for information processing after birth. These findings point to intricate developmental cues regulating receptor subtype expression.

To determine whether the factors that trigger the switch in gene expression are intrinsic to the GABA-receptive neurons, or whether they depend on extrinsic signals, receptor maturation in the rat cortical primary sensory areas was investigated (Paysan and Fritschy, 1996). Unilateral lesioning of the thalamus shortly after birth resulted in a dramatic alteration of the expression pattern of the α1- and α5-subunits in the cerebral cortex in seven-day-old animals. On the lesioned side, the expression of the α1-subunit in layer IV of primary visual cortex was strongly reduced as compared to the innervated control side of the cortex. By contrast, the expression of the α5-subunit, which is normally down-regulated in layer IV, remained prominent on the lesioned side. These results suggest that epigenetic factors derived from afferent thalamic neurons regulate the maturation of the α1- and α5-subunits in primary sensory areas of the rat neocortex. In the absence of these factors, an intrinsic program of receptor expression is revealed, which operates throughout the neocortex. Besides brain development, changes in $GABA_A$-receptor subunit composition appear to play a role also in adult brain. Tolerance to diazepam was correlated with alterations in $GABA_A$-receptor subunit expression. In the frontoparietal motor cortex, a decrease of the $\alpha 1$-subunit expression was paralleled by an increase in particular of the $\alpha 5$-subunit following chronic diazepam. No changes were observed after chronic imidazenil treatment which failed to induce tolerance (Impagnatiello et al., 1996)

7.2. Regulation of Receptor Number

Changes in the number of receptors have been reported under various conditions, based on radioligand binding studies. Alterations of the level of subunit mRNA in response to behavioral and pharmacological challenges, such as stress, sensory deprivation, or chronic alcohol, or BZ administration support this notion (Kang et al., 1991; Montpied et al., 1991; Primus and Gallager, 1992; Tietz et al., 1993; Hendry et al., 1994; Huntsman et al., 1994; Mhatre and Ticku, 1994; Wu et al., 1994). The visual system presents the best-studied example of the regulation of receptor number. Visual deprivation induced in adult monkeys by unilateral intraocular injection of tetrodotoxin resulted in a down-regulation of the $\alpha 1$-, $\beta 2$-, and $\gamma 2$-subunits in layer IV of primary visual cortex (area 17). This effect, which is evident at both the mRNA and the protein levels, is restricted to the ocular dominance columns corresponding to the deprived eye (Hendry et al., 1994; Huntsman et al., 1994). It appears thus that transcriptional control of $GABA_A$ receptor expression can be driven by neuronal activity. The clarification of the signal transduction pathway, which links GABA-ergic synaptic activity with the regulation of receptor subunit gene expression, will be a major challenge.

7.3. Receptor Phosphorylation

Phosphorylation of $GABA_A$ receptors is expected to be of importance for both short-term and long-term regulation of receptor function (Browning et al., 1990). However, the physiological significance of $GABA_A$ receptor phosphorylation remains controversial in view of the multitude of kinases, receptor subtypes, and cellular responses involved (Macdonald and Olsen, 1994; Macdonald, 1995). For instance, receptor regulation by PKA in spinal cord neurons (injection of PKA catalytic subunit) results in a reduction of GABA currents (Porter et al., 1990); activation of PKA in Purkinje cells (application of 8-bromo-cyclic AMP) enhances the GABA current. In recombinant receptors ($\alpha 1 \beta 1 \gamma 2$ in HEK cells), a reduction of receptor function by PKA (and PKC) being mediated by a serine residue (409) of the $\beta 1$-subunit was observed (Moss et al., 1992). However, when the same subunit combination was expressed in stably transfected L929 fibroblasts, the GABA$_A$ receptor currents were enhanced upon application of PKC (Lin et al., 1994). Recently, phosphorylation of the tyrosine residues 365 and 367 of the γ2L-subunit by tyrosine kinase has been shown to enhance GABA-induced currents (Moss et al., 1995).

Of particular interest is the proposal that the sensitivity of GABA$_A$ receptors to ethanol is linked to the phosphorylation status. In recombinant receptors, ethanol enhanced the function of GABA$_A$ receptors only when the long, but not short, variant of the γ2-subunit is present (γ2L in α1β1γ2 receptors) (Wafford et al., 1991), which contains an additional PKC phosphorylation site (Whiting et al., 1990). Mutant mice lacking the γ-isoform of PKC displayed reduced sensitivity to ethanol and the enhancing effect of ethanol on GABA$_A$ receptor function was abolished (Harris et al., 1995). Although the substrate of PKCγ-phosphorylation and its link to the behavioral actions of ethanol requires further analysis (Macdonald, 1995; Sigel, 1995), these studies provide a considerable stimulus for continued research into the function of GABA$_A$ receptor phosphorylation.

7.4. Receptor Regulation by Conformational Changes

Like other allosteric proteins (Galzi and Changeux, 1994), GABA$_A$ receptors display multiple conformational states, most clearly demonstrated by the analysis of channel kinetics, by the allosteric interaction between ligand binding sites, and by functional alterations induced by covalent receptor modifications (Sieghart, 1992; Macdonald and Olsen, 1994; Möhler et al., 1995a). Of major pharmacological significance are potential changes in receptor conformation as part of the reduced GABA$_A$ receptor sensitivity following chronic BZ treatment (Gallager and Primus, 1993). Changes in protein conformation have been analyzed recently for recombinant GABA$_A$ receptors, using the GABA shift assay as an indicator (Klein et al., 1994; D. W. Gallager, personal communication). Following chronic BZ agonist exposure, a decrease in allosteric coupling that replicated changes measured in rat cortical membranes following in vivo BZ exposure was demonstrated. The uncoupling was not accompanied by changes in the number or affinity of the receptors, but was correlated with agonist efficacy and was reversed by a brief exposure to the antagonist flumazenil. Thus, receptor desensitization by chronic BZ agonist exposure might include conformational changes. A differential susceptibility of GABA$_A$ receptor subtypes to conformational desensitization would be of major pharmacological relevance.

References

Amin, J. and Weiss, D. S. (1993) GABA$_A$ receptor needs two homologous domains of the β-subunit for activation by GABA but not by pentobarbital. *Nature* **366,** 565–567.

Angelman, H. (1965) 'Puppet' children. *Dev. Med. Child Neurol.* **7,** 681–683.

Auta, J., Giusti, P., Guidotti, A., and Costa, E. (1994) Imidazenil, a partial positive allosteric modulator of GABA$_A$ receptors, exhibits low tolerance and dependence liabilities in the rat. *J. Pharmacol. Exp. Ther.* **270,** 1262–1269.

Backus, K. H., Arigoni, M., Drescher, U., Scheurer, L., Malherbe, P., Möhler, H., and Benson, J. A. (1993) Stoichiometry of a recombinant GABA$_A$-receptor deduced from mutation-induced rectification. *Neuroreport* **5,** 285–288.

Barnard, E. A. (1995) The molecular biology of GABA$_A$ receptors and their structural determinants, in *GABA$_A$ Receptors and Anxiety. From Neurobiology to Treatment, Advances in Biochemical Psychoparmacology,* vol. 48 (Biggio, G., Sanna, E., Serra, M., and Costa, E., eds.), Raven, New York, pp. 1–16.

Bell, M. V., Bloomfield, J., McKinley, M., Patterson, M. N., Darlison, M. G., Barnard, E. A., and Davies, K. E. (1989) Physical linkage of a GABA$_A$ receptor subunit gene to the DXS374 locus in human Xq28. *Am. J. Hum. Genet.* **45,** 883–888.

Benke, D., Fritschy, J. M., Trzeciak, A., Bannwarth, W., and Möhler, H. (1994) Distribution, prevalence and drug-binding profile of GABA$_A$-receptors subtypes differing in β-subunit isoform. *J. Biol. Chem.* **269,** 27,100–27,107.

Benke, D., Mertens, S., Trzeciak, A., Gillessen, D., and Möhler, H. (1991) GABA$_A$ receptors display association of γ2-subunit with α1- and β2/3 subunits. *J. Biol. Chem.* **266,** 4478–4483.

Benke, D., Honer, M., Michel, C., and Mohler, H. (1996) GABA$_A$-receptor subtypes differentiated by their γ-subunit variants: prevalence, pharmacology and subunit architecture. *Neuropharmacol.* (in press).

Berninger, B., Marty, S., Zafra, F., Berzaghi, M. P., Thoenen, H., and Lindholm, D. (1995) GABAergic stimulation switches from enhancing to repressing BDNF expression in rat hippocampal neurons during maturation in vitro. *Development* **121,** 2327–2335.

Betz, H. (1990) Ligand-gated ion channels in the brain: the amino acid receptor superfamily. *Neuron* **5,** 383–392.

Bohlhalter, S., Weinmann, O., Möhler, H., and Fritschy, J. M. (1996) Laminar compartmentalization of GABA$_A$-receptor subtypes in the spinal cord. *J. Neurosci.* **16,** 283–297.

Browning, M. D., Bureau, M., Dudek, E. M., and Olsen, R. W. (1990) Protein kinase C and cAMP-dependent protein kinase phosphorylate the β subunit of the purified γ-aminobutyric acid A receptor. *Proc. Natl. Acad. Sci. USA* **87,** 1315–1318.

Buckle, V. J., Fujita, N., Ryder-Cook, A., Derry, J. M. J., Barnard, P. J., Lebo, R. V., Schofield, P. R., Seeburg, P. H., Bateson, A. N., Darlison, M. G., and Barnard, E. A. (1989) Chromosomal localization of GABA$_A$ receptor subunit genes: relationship to human genetic disease. *Neuron* **3,** 647–654.

Busto, U., Kaplan, H. L., Zawertailo, L., and Sellers, E. M. (1994) Pharmacologic effects and abuse liability of bretazenil, diazepam, and alprazolam in humans. *Clin. Pharmacol. Ther.* **55,** 451–463.

Clark, M., Massenburg, G. S., Weiss, S. R. B., and Post, R. M. (1994) Analysis of the hippocampal GABA$_A$ receptor system in kindled rats by autoradiographic and in situ hybridization techniques: contingent tolerance to carbamazepine. *Mol. Brain. Res.* **26,** 309–319.

Costa, E., Auta, J., Caruncho, H., Guidotti, A., Impagnatiello, F., Pesold, C., and Thompson, D. M. (1995) A search for a new anticonvulsant and anxiolytic benzodiazepine devoid of side effects and tolerance liability, in *GABA_A Receptors and Anxiety. From Neurobiology to Treatment, Advances in Biochemical Psychopharmacology*, vol. 48 (Biggio, G., Sanna, E., Serra, M., and Costa, E., eds.), Raven, New York, pp. 75–92.

Culiat, C. T., Stubbs, L. J., Montgomery, C. S., Russell, L. B., and Rinchik, E. M. (1994) Phenotypic consequences of deletion of the $\gamma3$, $\alpha5$, or $\beta3$ subunit of the type A γ-aminobutyric acid receptor in mice. *Proc. Natl. Acad. Sci. USA* **91**, 2815–2818.

Culiat, C. T., Stubbs, L., Nicholls, R. D., Montgomery, C. S., Russell, L. B., Johnson, D. K., and Rinchik, E. M. (1993) Concordance between isolated cleft palate in mice and alterations within a region including the gene encoding the $\beta3$ subunit of the type A γ-aminobutyric acid receptor. *Proc. Natl. Acad. Sci. USA* **90**, 5105–5109.

Culiat, C. T., Stubbs, L., Woychik, R. P., Russell, L. B., Johnson, D. K., and Riuchik, E. M. (1995) Deficiency of the $\beta3$-subunit of the type A γ-aminobutyric acid receptor causes cleft palate in mice. *Nature Genet.* **11**, 344–346.

Ducic, I., Puia, G., Vicini, S., and Costa, E. (1993) Triazolam is more efficacious than diazepam in a broad spectrum of recombinant receptors. *Eur. J. Pharmacol.* **244**, 29–35.

Duggan, M. J., Pollard, S., and Stephenson, F. A. (1991) Immunoaffinity purification of GABA_A receptor α-subunit iso-oligomers. Demonstration of receptor populations containing $\alpha1\alpha2$, $\alpha1\alpha3$, and $\alpha2\alpha3$ subunit pairs. *J. Biol. Chem.* **266**, 24,778–24,784.

Duggan, M. J., Pollard, S., and Stephenson, F. A. (1992) Quantitative immunoprecipitation studies with anti-γ-aminobutyric acid_A receptor $\gamma2$ 1–15 cys antibodies. *J. Neurochem.* **58**, 72–77.

Duka, T., Krause, W., Dorow, R., Rohloff, A., Hott, H., and Voet B. (1993) Abecarnil, a new β-carboline anxiolytic: preliminary clinical pharmacology, in *Anxiolytic β-Carbolines* (Stephens, D. N., ed.), Springer-Verlag, Berlin, pp. 132–148.

During, M. J., Ryder, K. M., and Spencer, D. D. (1995) Hippocampal GABA transporter function in temporal-lobe epilepsy. *Nature* **376**, 174–177.

During, M. J. and Spencer, D. D. (1993) Extracellular hippocampal glutamate and spontaneous seizure in the conscious human brain. *Lancet* **341**, 1607–1610.

Endö, S. and Olsen, R. W. (1993) Antibodies specific for α-subunit subtypes of GABA_A receptors reveal brain regional heterogeneity. *J. Neurochem.* **60**, 1388–1398.

Enz, R., Brandstatter, J. H., Hartveit, E., Wassle, H., and Bormann, J. (1995) Expression of GABA receptor $\rho1$ and $\rho2$ subunits in the retina and brain of the rat. *Eur. J. Neurosci.* **7**, 1495–1501.

Faull, R. L. M., Waldvogel, H. J., Nicholson, L. F. B., and Synek, B. J. L. (1993) The distribution of GABA_A-benzodiazepine receptors in the basal ganglia in Huntington's disease and in the quinolinic acid-lesioned rat. *Prog. Brain Res.* **99**, 105–123.

ffrench-Constant, R. H., Steichen, J. C., Rocheleau, T. A., Aronstein, K., and Roush, R. T. (1993) A single-amino acid substitution in a γ-aminobutyric acid subtype A receptor locus is associated with cyclodiene insecticide resistance in Drosophila populations. *Proc. Natl. Acad. Sci. USA* **90**, 1957–1961.

Fritschy, J. M. and Möhler, H. (1995) GABA_A-receptor heterogeneity in the adult rat brain: differential regional and cellular distribution of seven major subunits. *J. Comp. Neurol.* **359**, 154–194.

Fritschy, J. M., Benke, D., Mertens, S., Gao, B., and Möhler, H. (1993) Immunochemical distinction of GABA_A-receptor subtypes differing in drug binding profiles and cellular distribution. *Soc. Neurosci. Abstracts* **19**, 476.

Fritschy, J. M., Benke, D., Mertens, S., Oertel, W. H., Bachi, T., and Möhler, H. (1992) Five subtypes of type A γ-aminobutyric acid receptors identified in neurons by double and triple immunofluorescence staining with subunit-specific antibodies. *Proc. Natl. Acad. Sci. USA* **89,** 6726–6730.

Fritschy, J. M., Paysan, J., Enna, A., and Möhler, H. (1994) Switch in the expression of rat GABA$_A$-receptor subtypes during postnatal development: an immunohistochemical study. *J. Neurosci.* **14,** 5302–5324.

Gale, K. (1992) GABA and epilepsy: basic concepts from preclinical research. *Epilepsia* **33(Suppl. 5),** S3–S12.

Gallager, D. W. and Primus, R. J. (1993) Benzodiazepine tolerance and dependence: GABA$_A$ receptor complex locus of change. *Biochem. Soc. Symp.* **59,** 135–151.

Galzi, J. L. and Changeux, J. P. (1994) Neurotransmitter-gated ion channels as unconventional allosteric proteins. *Curr. Opin. Struct. Biol.* **4,** 554–565.

Gao, B. and Fritschy, J. M. (1994) Selective allocation of GABA$_A$-receptors containing the α1-subunit to neurochemically distinct subpopulations of hippocampal interneurons. *Eur. J. Neurosci.* **6,** 837–853.

Gao, B., Fritschy, J. M., Benke, D., and Möhler, H. (1993) Neuron-specific expression of GABA$_A$-receptor subtypes: differential associations of the α1- and α3-subunits with serotonergic and GABAergic neurons. *Neuroscience* **54,** 881–892.

Gao, B., Hornung, J. P., and Fritschy, J. M. (1995) Identification of distinct GABA$_A$-receptor subtypes in cholinergic and parvalbumin-positive neurons of the rat and marmoset medialseptum-diagonal band complex. *Neuroscience* **65,** 101–117.

Gunther, U., Benson, J., Benke, D., Fritschy, J. M., Reyes, G. H., Knoflach, F., Crestani, F., Aguzzi, A., Arigoni, M., Lang, Y., Bluthmann, H., Möhler, H., and Lüscher, B. (1995) Benzodiazepine-insensitive mice generated by targeted disruption of the γ2-subunit gene of γ-aminobutyric acid type A receptors. *Proc. Natl. Acad. Sci. USA* **92,** 7749–7753.

Haefely, W. (1994) Allosteric modulation of the GABA$_A$ receptor channel: a mechanism for interaction with a multitude of central nervous system functions, in *The Challenge of Neuropharmacology. A Tribute to the Memory of Willy Haefely* (Möhler, H. and Da Prada, M., eds.), Editiones Roche, Basel, pp. 15–40.

Haefely, W., Martin, J. R., and Schoch, P. (1990) Novel anxiolytics that act as partial agonists at benzodiazepine receptors. *Trends Pharmacol. Sci.* **11,** 452–456.

Harris, R. A., McQuilkin, S. J., Paylor, R., Abeliovich, A., Tonegawa, S., and Wehner, J. M. (1995) Mutant mice lacking the γ isoform of protein kinase C show decreased behavioral actions of ethanol and altered function of γ-aminobutyrate type A receptors. *Proc. Natl. Acad. Sci. USA* **92,** 3658–3662.

Hayden, M. R. (1981) *Huntington's Chorea.* Springer-Verlag, New York.

Hendry, S. H. C., Huntsman, M. M., Vinuela, A., Möhler, H., de Blas, A. L., and Jones, E. G. (1994) GABA$_A$ receptor subunit immunoreactivity in primate visual cortex: distribution in macaques and humans and regulation by visual input in adulthood. *J. Neurosci.* **14,** 2383–2401.

Herb, A., Wisden, W., Luddens, H., Puia, G., Vicini, S., and Seeburg, P. H. (1992) The third γ subunit of the γ-aminobutyric acid type A receptor family. *Proc. Natl. Acad. Sci. USA* **89,** 1433–1437.

Holthoff, V. A., Koeppe, R. A., Frey, K. A., Penney, J. B., Markel, D. S., Kuhl, D. E., and Young, A. B. (1993) Positron emission tomography measures of benzodiazepine receptors in Huntington's disease. *Ann. Neurol.* **34,** 76–81.

Hornung, J. P. and Fritschy, J. M. (1996) Developmental profile of GABA$_A$-receptors in the marmoset monkey: expression of distinct subtypes in pre- and postnatal brain. *J. Comp. Neurol.* **367,** 413–430.

Huntington's Disease Collaborative Research Group (1993) A novel gene containing a trinucleotide repeat that is expanded and unstable on Huntington's disease chromosomes. *Cell* **72,** 971–983.

Huntsman, M. M., Isackson, P. J., and Jones, E. G. (1994) Lamina-specific expression and activity-dependent regulation of seven GABA$_A$ receptor subunit mRNAs in monkey visual cortex. *J. Neurosci.* **14,** 2236–2259.

Im, H. K., Im, W. B., Judge, T. M., Gamill, R. B., Hamilton, B. J., Carter, D. B., and Pregenzer, J. F. (1993) Substituted pyrazinones, a new class of allosteric modulators for γ-aminobutyric acid A receptors. *Mol. Pharmacol.* **44,** 468–472.

Im, H. K., Im, W. B., Pregenzer, J. F., Carter, D. B., and Hamilton, B. J. (1995) U 89843 is a novel allosteric modulator of GABA$_A$-receptors. *J. Pharmacol. Exp. Ther.* **275,** 1390–1395.

Impagnatiello, F., Pesold, C., Longone, P., Caruncho, H., Fritschy, J. M., Costa, E., and Guidotti, A. (1996) Modifications of γ-aminobutyric acid$_A$ receptor subunit expression in rat neocortex during tolerance to diazepam. *Mol. Pharmacol.* **49,** 822–831.

Johnston, G. A. R. (1994) GABA$_C$ receptors. *Prog. Brain Res.* **100,** 61–65.

Kamphuis, W., De Rijk, T. C., and da Silva, F. H. L. (1994) GABA$_A$ receptor β1–3 subunit gene expression in the hippocampus of kindled rats. *Neurosci. Lett.* **174,** 5–8.

Kamphuis, W., De Rijk, T. C., and da Silva, F. H. L. (1995) Expression of GABA$_A$ receptor subunit mRNAs in hippocampal pyramidal and granular neurons in the kindling model of epileptogenesis: an in situ hybridization study. *Mol. Brain. Res.* **31,** 33–47.

Kang, I., Thompson, M. L., Heller, J., and Miller, L. G. (1991) Persistent elevation in GABA$_A$ receptor subunit mRNAs following social stress. *Brain Res. Bull.* **26,** 809–812.

Klein, R. L., Whiting, P. J., and Harris, R. A. (1994) Benzodiazepine treatment causes uncoupling of recombinant GABA$_A$ receptors expressed in stably transfected cells. *J. Neurochem.* **63,** 2349–2352.

Knoflach, F., Benke, D., Wang, Y., Scheurer, L., Luddens, H., Hamilton, B. J., Carter, D. B., Möhler, H., and Benson, J. A. (1996) Pharmacological modulation of the "diazepamin-sensitive" recombinant GABA$_A$ receptors α4β2γ2 and α6β2γ2. *Mol. Pharmacol.* (in press).

Knoflach, F., Drescher, U., Scheurer, L., Malherbe, P., and Möhler, H. (1993) Full and partial agonism displayed by benzodiazepine receptor ligands at different recombinant GABA$_A$ receptor subtypes. *J. Pharmacol. Exp. Ther.* **266,** 385–391.

Knoflach, F., Rhyner, T., Villa, M., Kellenberger, S., Drescher, U., Malherbe, P., Sigel, E., and Möhler, H. (1991) The γ3-subunit of the GABA$_A$-receptor confers sensitivity to benzodiazepine receptor ligands. *FEBS Lett.* **293,** 191–194.

Knoll, J. H., Sinnett, D., Wagstaff, J., Glatt, K., Wilcox, A. S., Whiting, P. M., Wingrove, P., Sikela, J. M., and Lalande, M. (1993) FISH ordering of reference markers and of the gene for the α5 subunit of the γ-aminobutyric acid receptor (GABAR5) within the Angelman and Prader-Willi syndrome chromosomal regions. *Hum. Mol. Gen.* **2,** 183–189.

Kokaia, M., Pratt, G. D., Elmer, E., Bengzon, J., Fritschy, J. M., Lindvall, O., and Möhler, H. (1994) Biphasic differential changes of GABA$_A$-receptor subunit mRNA levels in dentate gyrus granule cells following recurrent kindling induced seizures. *Mol. Brain. Res.* **23**, 323–332.

Kusama, T., Spivak, C. E., Whiting, P., Dawson, V. L., Schaffer, J. C., and Uhl, G. R. (1993) Pharmacology of GABA ρ1 and GABA α/β receptors expressed in Xenopus oocytes and COS cells. *Br. J. Pharmacol.* **109**, 200–206.

Lambert, J. J., Belelli, D., Hill Venning, C., and Peters, J. A. (1995) Neurosteroids and GABAA receptor function. *Trends Pharmacol. Sci.* **16**, 295–303.

Laurie, D. J., Seeburg, P. H., and Wisden, W (1992) The distribution of 13 GABA$_A$ receptor subunit mRNAs in the rat brain. II. Olfactory bulb and cerebellum. *J. Neurosci.* **12**, 1063–1076.

Lin, Y. F., Browning, M. D., Dudek, E. M., and Macdonald, R. L. (1994) Protein kinase C enhances recombinant bovine α1β1γ2L GABA$_A$ receptor whole-cell currents expressed in L929 fibroblasts. *Neuron* **13**, 1421–1431.

Luddens, H., Korpi, E. R., and Seeburg, P. H. (1995) GABA$_A$/benzodiazepine receptor heterogeneity: neurophysiological implications. *Neuropharmacology* **34**, 245–254.

Luddens, H., Pritchett, D. B., Kohler, M., Killisch, I., Keinanen, L., Monyer, H., Sprengel, R., and Seeburg, P. H. (1990) Cerebellar GABA$_A$-receptor selective for a behavioral alcohol antagonist. *Nature* **346**, 648–651.

Luddens, H., Seeburg, P. H., and Korpi, E. R. (1994) Impact of β and γ variants on ligand-binding properties of γ-aminobutyric acid type A receptors. *Mol. Pharmacol.* **45**, 810–814.

Lyon, M. F., King, T. R., Gondo, Y., Gardner, J. M., Nakatsu, Y., Eicher, E. M., and Brilliant, M. H. (1992) Genetic and molecular analysis of recessive alleles at the pink-eyed dilution (p) locus of the mouse. *Proc. Natl. Acad. Sci. USA* **89**, 6968–6972.

Macdonald, R. L. (1995) Ethanol, γ-aminobutyrate type A receptors, and protein kinase C phosphorylation. *Proc. Natl. Acad. Sci. USA* **92**, 3633–3635.

Macdonald, R. L. and Olsen, R. W. (1994) GABA$_A$ receptor channels. *Annu. Rev. Neurosci.* **17**, 569–602.

Marksitzer, R., Benke, D., Fritschy, J. M., and Möhler, H. (1993) GABA$_A$-receptors: drug binding profile and distribution of receptors containing the α2-subunit in situ. *J. Recept. Res.* **13**, 467–477.

McDonald, J. W., Garofalo, E. A., Hood, T., Sackellares, J. C., Gilman, S., McKeever, P. E., Troncoso, J. C., and Johnston, M. V. (1991) Altered excitatory and inhibitory amino acid receptor binding in hippocampus of patients with temporal lobe epilepsy. *Ann. Neurol.* **29**, 529–541.

McKernan, R. M., Quirk, K., Prince, R., Cox, P. A., Gillard, N. P., Ragan, C. I., and Whiting, P. (1991) GABA$_A$ receptor subtypes immunopurified from rat brain with α subunit-specific antibodies have unique pharmacological properties. *Neuron* **7**, 667–676.

McKernan, R. M. and Whiting, P. J. (1996) Which GABA$_A$-receptor subtypes really occur in the brain? *Trends Neurosci.* **19**, 139–143.

Meldrum, B. (1979) Convulsant drugs, anticonvulsants and GABA-mediated neuronal inhibition, in *GABA-Neurotransmitters* (Krogsgard-Larsen, P., Scheell-Kruger, J., and Kofod, H., eds.), Munksgaard, Copenhagen, pp. 390–405.

Meldrum, B. (1995) Taking up GABA again. *Nature* **376**, 122,123.

Mertens, S., Benke, D., and Möhler, H. (1993) GABA$_A$ receptor populations with novel subunit combinations and drug binding profiles identified in brain by α5- and δ-subunitspecific immunopurification. *J. Biol. Chem.* **268**, 5965–5973.

Mhatre, M. and Ticku, M. K. (1994) Chronic ethanol treatment upregulates the GABA_A receptor β subunit expression. *Mol. Brain. Res.* **23,** 246–252.

Möhler, H., Fritschy, J. M., Lüscher, B., Rudolph, U., Benson, J., and Benke, D. (1995a) The GABA_A-receptors: from subunits to diverse functions, in *Ion Channels*, vol. 4 (Narahashi, T., ed.), Plenum, New York, pp. 89–113.

Möhler, H., Knoflach, F., Paysan, J., Motejlek, K., Benke, D., Lüscher, B., and Fritschy, J. M. (1995b) Heterogeneity of GABA_A-receptors: cell-specific expression, pharmacology, and regulation. *Neurochem. Res.* **20,** 631–636.

Montpied, P., Morrow, A. L., Karanian, J. W., Ginns, E. I., Martin, B. M., and Paul, S. M. (1991) Prolonged ethanol inhalation decreases γ-aminobutyric acid_A receptor α subunit mRNAs in the rat cerebral cortex. *Mol. Pharmacol.* **39,** 157–163.

Moss, S. J., Gorrie, G. H., Amato, A., and Smart, T. G. (1995) Modulation of GABA_A receptors by tyrosine phosphorylation. *Nature* **377,** 344–348.

Moss, S. J., Smart, T. G., Blackstone, C. D., and Huganir, R. L. (1992) Functional modulation of GABA_A receptors by cAMP-dependent protein phosphorylation. *Science* **257,** 661–665.

Nakatsu, Y., Tyndale, R. F., DeLorey, T. M., Durham-Pierre, D., Gardner, J. M., McDanel, H. J., Nguyen, Q., Wagstaff, J., Lalande, M., Sikela, J. M., Olsen, R. W., Tobin, A. J., and Brilliant, M. H. (1993) A cluster of three GABA_A receptor subunit genes is deleted in a neurological mutant of the mouse p locus. *Nature* **364,** 448–450.

Nicholls, R. D., Gottlieb, W., Russell, L. B., Davda, M., Horsthemke, B., and Rinchik, E. M. (1993) Evaluation of potential models for imprinted and nonimprinted components of human chromosome 15q11-q13 syndromes by fine-structure homology mapping in the mouse. *Proc. Natl. Acad. Sci. USA* **90,** 2050–2054.

Nobrega, J. N., Kish, S. J., and Burnham, W. M. (1990) Regional brain [^{3}H]muscimol binding in kindled rat brain: a quantitative autoradiographic examination. *Epilepsy Res.* **6,** 102–109.

Olsen, R. W. and Sapp, D. W. (1995) Neuroactive steroid modulation of GABA_A receptors. *Adv. Biochem. Psychopharmacol.* **48,** 57–74.

Olsen, R. W., Bureau, M., Houser, C. R., Delgado-Escueta, A. V., Richards, J. G., and Möhler, H. (1990) GABA/Benzodiazepine receptors in human focal epilepsy, in *Neurotransmitters in Epilepsy, Advances in the Neurobiology of Epilepsy*, vol. 1 (Avanzini, G., Engel, J., Fariello, R. G., and Heinemann, U., eds.), Demos, New York, pp. 515–527.

Olsen, R. W., Bureau, M., Houser, C. R., Delgado-Escueta, A. V., Richards, J. G., and Möhler, H. (1992) GABA/benzodiazepine receptors in human focal epilepsy. *Epilepsy Res.* **Suppl. 8,** 383–391.

Olsen, R. W., Wamsley, J. K., McCabe, R. T., Lee, R. J., and Lomax, P. (1985) Benzodiazepine/γ-aminobutyric acid receptor deficit in the midbrain of the seizure-susceptible gerbils. *Proc. Natl. Acad. Sci. USA* **82,** 6701–6705.

Paysan, J. and Fritschy, J. M. (1996) GABA_A-receptor subtypes in developing brain: actors or spectators? *Perspect. Dev. Neurobiol.* (in press).

Pollard, S., Duggan, M. J., and Stephenson, F. A. (1991) Promiscuity of GABA_A-receptor β3 subunits as demonstrated by their presence in α1, α2 and α3 subunit-containing receptor subpopulations. *FEBS Lett.* **295,** 81–83.

Porter, N. M., Twyman, R. E., Uhler, M. D., and Macdonald, R. L. (1990) Cyclic AMP-dependent protein kinase decreases GABA_A receptor current in mouse spinal neurons. *Neuron* **5,** 789–796.

Pribilla, I., Neuhaus, R., Huba, R., Hillman, M., Turner, J. D., Stephens, D. N., and Schneider, H. H. (1993) Abercanil is a full agonist at some, and a partial agonist at other recombinant GABA$_A$ receptor subtypes, in Anxiolytic β-Carbolines (Stephens, D. N., ed.), Springer-Verlag, Berlin, pp. 50–61.

Primus, R. J. and Gallager, D. W. (1992) GABA$_A$ receptor subunit mRNA are differentially influenced by chronic FG 7142 and diazepam exposure. *Eur. J. Pharmacol.* **226,** 21–28.

Pritchett, D. B. and Seeburg, P. H. (1990) γ-Aminobutyric acid$_A$ receptor α5-subunit creates novel type II benzodiazepine receptor pharmacology. *J. Neurochem.* **54,** 1802–1804.

Pritchett, D. B., Sontheimer, H., Shivers, B. D., Ymer, S., Kettenmann, H., Schofield, P. R., and Seeburg, P. H. (1989) Importance of a novel GABA$_A$ receptor subunit for benzodiazepine pharmacology. *Nature* **338,** 582–585.

Puia, G., Dudic, I., Vicini, S., and Costa, F. (1992) Molecular mechanisms of the partial allosteric modulatory effects of bretazenil at γ-aminobutyric acid type A receptor. *Proc. Natl. Acad. Sci. USA* **89,** 3620–3624.

Reis, A., Kunze, J., Ladanyi, L., Enders, H., Klein-Vogler, U., and Niemann, G. (1993) Exclusion of the GABA$_A$-receptor β3 subunit gene as the Angelman's syndrome gene. *Lancet* **341,** 122–123.

Richards, G., Schoch, P., and Haefely, W. (1991) Benzodiazepine receptors: new vistas. *Semin. Neurosci.* **3,** 191–203.

Ruano, D., Araujo, F., Machado, A., de Blas, A. L., and Vitorica, J. (1994) Molecular characterization of type I GABA$_A$ receptor complex from rat cerebral cortex and hippocampus. *Mol. Brain. Res.* **25,** 225–233.

Saitoh, S., Kubota, T., Ohta, T., Jinno, Y., Niikawa, N., Sugimoto, T., Wagstaff, J., and Lalande, M. (1992) Familial Angelman Syndrome caused by imprinted submicroscopic deletion encompassing GABA$_A$ receptor b3-subunit gene. *Lancet* **339,** 366,367.

Savic, I., Roland, P., Sedvall, G., Persson, A., Pauli, S., and Widen, L. (1988) In vivo demonstration of reduced benzodiazepine receptor binding in human epileptic foci. *Lancet* **2,** 863–866.

Saxena, N. C. and Macdonald, R. L. (1994) Assembly of GABA$_A$ receptor subunits: role of the δ subunit. *J. Neurosci.* **14,** 7077–7086.

Scharf, M. B., Mayleben, D. W., Kaffeman, M., Krall, R., and Ochs, R. (1991) Dose response effects of zolpidem in normal geriatric subjects. *J. Clin. Psychiatry* **52,** 77–83.

Schoch, P., Moreau, J. L., Martin, J. R., and Haefely, W. E. (1993) Aspects of benzodiazepine receptor structure and function with relevance to drug tolerance and dependence. *Biochem. Soc. Symp.* **59,** 121–134.

Shimada, S., Cutting, G., and Uhl, G. R. (1992) γ-aminobutyric acid A or C receptor? γ-Aminobutyric acid ro1 receptor RNA induces bicuculline-, barbiturate-, and benzodiazepineinsensitive γ-aminobutyric acid responses in Xenopus oocytes. *Mol. Pharmacol.* **41,** 683–687.

Sieghart, W. (1992) GABA$_A$ receptors: ligand-gated Cl- ion channels modulated by multiple drug binding sites. *Trends Pharmacol. Sci.* **13,** 446–450.

Sieghart, W. (1995) Structure and pharmacology of γ-aminobutyric acid$_A$ receptor subtypes. *Pharmacol. Rev.* **47,** 181–234.

Sigel, E. (1995) Functional modulation of ligand-gated GABA$_A$ and NMDA receptor channels by phosphorylation. *J. Recept. Res.* **15,** 325–332.

Sinnett, D., Wagstaff, J., Glatt, K., Woolf, E., Kirkness, E. J., and Lalande, M. (1993) High-resolution mapping of the γ-aminobutyric acid receptor subunit β3 and α5 gene cluster on chromosome 15q11-q13, and localization of breakpoint in two Angelman syndrome patients. *Am. J. Hum. Genet.* **52,** 1216–1229.

Smith, G. B. and Olsen, R. W. (1995) Functional domains of GABA$_A$-receptors. *Trends Pharmacol. Sci.* **16,** 162–168.

Stephenson, F. A. (1995) The GABA$_A$ receptors. *Biochem. J.* **310,** 1–9.

Thompson, C. L., Bodewitz, G., Stephenson, F. A., and Turner, J. D. (1992) Mapping of GABA$_A$ receptor α5 and α6 subunit-like immunoreactivity in rat brain. *Neurosci. Lett.* **144,** 53–56.

Tietz, E. I., Huang, X., Weng, X., Rosenberg, H. C., and Chiu, T. H. (1993) Expression of α1, α5, and γ2 GABA$_A$ receptor subunit mRNAs measured in situ in rat hippocampus and cortex following chronic flurazepam administration. *J. Mol. Neurosci.* **4,** 277–292.

Titulaer, M. N. G., Kamphuis, W., Pool, C. W., van Heerikhuize, J. J., and da Silva, F. H. L. (1994) Kindling induces time-dependent and regional specific changes in the [^{3}H]muscimol binding in the rat hippocampus: a quantitative autoradiographic study. *Neuroscience* **59,** 817–826.

Titulaer, M. N. G., Kamphuis, W., and da Silva, F. H. L. (1995) Long-term and regional specific changes in ^{3}H-flunitrazepam binding in kindled rat hippocampus. *Neuroscience* **68,** 399–406.

Togel, M., Mossier, B., Fuchs, K., and Sieghart, W. (1994) γ-Aminobutyric acid$_A$ receptors displaying association of γ3-subunits with β2/3 and different α-subunits exhibit unique pharmacological properties. *J. Biol. Chem.* **269,** 12,993–12,998.

Varecka, L., Wu, C. H., Rotter, A., and Frostholm, A. (1994) GABA$_A$-benzodiazepine receptor α6 subunit mRNA in granule cells of the cerebellar cortex and cochlear nuclei: expression in developing and mutant mice. *J. Comp. Neurol.* **339,** 341–352.

Wada, T. and Fukuda, N. (1991) Pharmacologic profile of a new anxiolytic, DN-2327: effect of Ro-15 788 and interaction with diazepam in rodents. *Psychopharmacology* **103,** 314–322.

Wafford, K. A., Burnett, D. M., Leidenheimer, N. J., Burt, D. R., Wand, J. B., Kofuji, P., Dunwiddie, T. V., Harris, R. A., and Sikela, J. M. (1991) Ethanol sensitivity of the GABA$_A$ receptor expressed in *Xenopus* oocytes requires 8 amino acids contained in the γ2L subunit. *Neuron* **7,** 27–33.

Wafford, K. A., Whiting, P. J., and Kemp, J. A. (1993) Differences in affinity and efficacy of benzodiazepine receptor ligands at recombinant γ-aminobutyric acid receptor subtypes. *Mol. Pharmacol.* **43,** 240–244.

Wee, E. L. and Zimmerman, E. F. (1983) Involvement of GABA in palate morphogenesis and its relation to diazepam teratogenesis in two mouse strains. *Teratology* **28,** 15–22.

Whitehouse, P. J., Trifeletti, R. R., Jones, B. E., Folstein, S., Price, D. L., Snyder, S. H., and Kuhar, M. J. (1985) Neurotransmitter alterations in Huntington's disease: autoradiographic and homogenate studies with special reference to benzodiazepine receptor complexes. *Ann. Neurol.* **18,** 202–210.

Whiting, P., McKernan, R. M., and Iversen, L. L. (1990) Another mechanism for creating diversity in γ-aminobutyrate type A receptors: RNA splicing directs expression of two forms of γ2-subunit, one of which contains a protein kinase C phosphorylation site. *Proc. Natl. Acad. Sci. USA* **87,** 9966–9970.

Wieland, H. A., Luddens, H., and Seeburg, P. H. (1992) A single histidine in GABA$_A$

receptors is essential for benzodiazepine agonist binding. *J. Biol. Chem.* **267,** 1426–1429.

Wisden, W., Herb, A., Wieland, H., Keinanen, K., Luddens, H., and Seeburg, P. H. (1991) Cloning, pharmacological characteristics and expression pattern of the rat $GABA_A$ receptor $\alpha 4$ subunit. *FEBS Lett.* **289,** 227–230.

Wolf, H. K., Spanle, M., Muller, M. B., Elger, C. E., Schramm, J., and Wiestler, O. D. (1994) Hippocampal loss of the $GABA_A$ receptor $\alpha 1$ subunit in patients with chronic pharmacoresistant epilepsies. *Acta Neuropathol.* **88,** 313–319.

Wong, G. and Skolnik, P. (1992) Ro15-4513 binding to $GABA_A$ receptors: subunit composition determines ligand efficacy. *Pharmacol. Biochem. Behav.* **42,** 107–110.

Wu, Y. X., Rosenberg, H. C., Chiu, T. H., and Zhao, T. J. (1994) Subunit- and brain region-specific reduction of $GABA_A$ receptor subunit mRNAs during chronic treatment of rats with diazepam. *J. Mol. Neurosci.* **5,** 105–120.

Yasumatsu, H., Morimoto, Y., Yamamoto, Y., Takehara, S., Fukuda, T., Nakao, T., and Setoguchi, M. (1994) The pharmacological properties of Y-23684, a benzodiazepine receptor partial agonist. *Br. J. Pharmacol.* **111,** 1170–1178.

Ymer, S., Draguhn, A., Wisden, W., Werner, P., Keinanen, K., Schofield, P. R., Sprengel, R., Pritchett, D. B., and Seeburg, P. H. (1990) Structural and functional characterization of the $\gamma 1$ subunit of $GABA_A$/benzodiazepine receptors. *EMBO J.* **9,** 3261–3267.

CHAPTER 3

GABA$_A$ Receptor Agonists, Partial Agonists, and Antagonists

*Povl Krogsgaard-Larsen,
Bente Frølund, and Bjarke Ebert*

1. GABA in the Central Nervous System: Inhibition and Disinhibition

The neutral amino acid, γ-aminobutyric acid (GABA), is an inhibitory transmitter in the central nervous system (CNS). Furthermore, GABA is involved as a neurotransmitter and/or a paracrine effector in the regulation of a variety of physiological mechanisms in the periphery. Some of these latter functions may be under central GABA control; others are managed by local GABA neurons. A large percentage, perhaps the majority, of central neurons are under GABA control. The complex mechanisms underlying the GABA-mediated neurotransmission have been extensively studied, using a broad spectrum of electrophysiological, neurochemical, pharmacological, and in recent years, molecular biological techniques (Krnjevic, 1974; Curtis and Johnston, 1974; Olsen and Venter, 1986; Redburn and Schousboe, 1987; Bowery and Nistico, 1989; Bowery et al., 1990; Biggio and Costa, 1990; Schousboe et al., 1992a).

The overall activity of the brain is basically determined by two superior functions: excitation by the major excitatory amino acid transmitter, glutamic acid (Glu), which depolarizes neurons through a large number of receptor subtypes; and inhibition by GABA, which hyperpolarizes neurons, also through multiple receptors. However, depolarizing actions of GABA may occur, particularly during early postnatal development of the brain (Lodge, 1988; Wheal and Thompson, 1991; Krogsgaard-Larsen and Hansen, 1992; Walton et al., 1993).

The GABA Receptors Eds.: S. J. Enna and N. G. Bowery
Humana Press Inc., Totowa, NJ

It has been proposed that a third mechanism may play a fundamental role in the function of the brain, namely, disinhibition (Roberts, 1976, 1991). This indirect neuronal excitation implies synaptic contact between two inhibitory neurons. The operation of this indirect excitatory mechanism in the CNS has never been unequivocally proved or disproved, but many apparently paradoxical observations have been explained on the basis of disinhibition (Kardos et al., 1994).

2. GABA in the Peripheral Nervous System: Transmitter and Paracrine Effector

The role of GABA as a central transmitter is fully established, and there is rapidly growing evidence that GABA also has a broad spectrum of physiological functions in the peripheral nervous system (PNS) (Erdö, 1985; Erdö and Bowery, 1986; Bowery and Nistico, 1989; Bowery et al., 1990; Ong and Kerr, 1990). In a wide range of peripheral tissues, notably parts of the PNS, endocrine glands, smooth muscles, and the female reproductive systems, GABA receptors have been detected. In all tissues so far analyzed, $GABA_A$, and $GABA_B$ receptors (Fig. 1), have been identified.

There are many unsolved questions regarding the peripheral actions of GABA and its interactions with other physiological mechanisms using acetylcholine (ACh), norepinephrine, serotonin, and various peptides as transmitter or paracrine mediators (Ong and Kerr, 1990). It is possible that disinhibitory mechanisms between GABA neurons or between $GABA_A$ and $GABA_B$ receptors at the cellular level (Kardos et al., 1994), also contribute to the apparently very complex functions of GABA in the periphery.

The peripheral GABA receptors, or other GABA-ergic synaptic mechanisms, obviously have interest as drug targets. So far, GABA drug design projects have been focused on sites at central GABA-operated synapses. It should, however, be emphasized that even for GABA-ergic drugs, which easily penetrate the blood-brain barrier (BBB), most of the drug administered is found in the periphery, where it may cause adverse effects. On the other hand, most GABA analogs of pharmacological interest do not easily penetrate the BBB, making it possible to develop GABA-ergic drugs specifically targeted at peripheral GABA receptors.

As a result of the identification of GABA receptors different from $GABA_A$ or $GABA_B$, such as the $GABA_C$ type in retina (Fig. 1), it seems likely that other types of GABA receptors may be identified in peripheral tissues. There is, for example, circumstantial evidence of an involvement of nonclassical $GABA_A$ receptors in the regulation of the release of luteinizing hormone from rat pituitary cells (Virmani et al., 1990). Such atypical GABA receptors

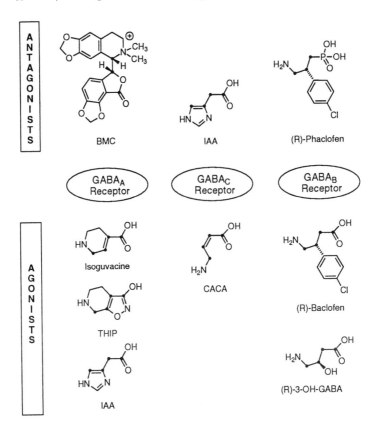

Fig. 1. Schematic illustration of the different classes of GABA receptors and the structures of some key agonists and antagonists.

in tissues showing specific physiological responsiveness to GABA may be particularly interesting targets for drug design.

The function of GABA, mediated by GABA$_A$ and GABA$_B$ receptors, in the enteric nervous system has been studied quite extensively (Kerr and Ong, 1986). Although it seems unlikely that GABA plays a major role in intestinal secretory activity, GABA$_A$ receptors and perhaps GABA$_B$ may play important roles in the control of gut motility. Peristalsis can be markedly reduced and ultimately stopped after administration of GABA$_A$ and GABA$_B$ antagonists, separately or in combination (Ong and Kerr, 1990). GABA receptors in the gut, as well as GABA receptors in the gallbladder, the lung, and the urinary bladder, may give rise to adverse effects in GABA drug therapies, or may be important new therapeutic targets in drug-induced or pathological dysfunctions of these organs (Erdö and Bowery, 1986).

The involvement of GABA in the regulation of blood pressure has been the object of numerous studies (Dannhardt et at., 1993). The relative importance of $GABA_A$ and $GABA_B$ receptors in these very complex mechanisms is still unclear, and the effects of GABA mimetics are, to some extent, species-dependent. In this area, the $GABA_A$ receptor-mediated dilatation of cerebral blood vessel is of particular interest and may have major therapeutic implications (Edvinsson et al., 1980). It is possible that this dilatation actually is mediated by ACh released via a $GABA_A$ receptor-regulated mechanism (Saito et al., 1985). The effect of the $GABA_A$ agonist 4,5,6,7-tetrahydroisoxazolo[5,4-c]pyridin-3-ol (THIP) on cortical blood flow in humans has been used for diagnostic purposes as a new test for hemispheric dominance (Roland and Friberg, 1988). THIP decreases, in a dose-dependent manner, blood flow in nonactivated brain areas. This submaximal depression can be counteracted physiologically by the patient (Roland and Friberg, 1988).

The involvement of GABA in the endocrine pancreatic functions is an area of growing therapeutic interest (Erdö, 1985; Solimena and De Camilli, 1993). Autoantibodies to glutamic acid decarboxylase (GAD) appear to play an important role in the initiation of insulin-dependent diabetes, underlining the importance of the GABA system in pancreatic function (Tirsch et al., 1993). GABA is present in the endocrine part of the pancreas at concentrations comparable to those encountered in the CNS, and co-localizes with insulin in the pancreatic β-cells. GABA seems to mediate part of the inhibitory action of glucose on glucagon secretion by activating $GABA_A$ receptors in α2 cells (Rorsman et al., 1989). $GABA_A$ receptors probably are playing a key role in the feedback regulation of glucagon release, which seems to be an important mechanism in the hypersecretion of glucagon, frequently associated with diabetes. These $GABA_A$ receptors, of as yet undisclosed subunit composition, are potential targets for therapeutic GABA intervention.

There is rapidly growing interest in the role of GABA as a transmitter in hearing mechanisms. This interest has been stimulated by the demonstration of a substantial, selective, and age-related loss of GABA in the central nucleus of the inferior colliculus (CIC) in rat (Caspary et al., 1990). There is immunocytochemical evidence for the existence of a GABA-ergic system in the guinea pig vestibule and for a role of GABA as a vestibular afferent transmitter (Ryan and Schwartz, 1986; Usami et al., 1989; Lopez et al., 1992). Impairment of inhibitory GABA-ergic transmission in the CIC may contribute to abnormal auditory perception and processing in neural presbycusis (Caspary et al., 1990). These observations may lead to the identification of novel targets for GABA-ergic therapeutic intervention in different age-related diseases and conditions involving defective hearing.

In the PNS, $GABA_A$ agonists and antagonists are potential therapeutic agents. The latter class of GABA-ergic drugs may be rather difficult to use therapeutically in CNS diseases because of seizure potential (*see* Section 4.2.), but $GABA_A$ antagonists, being unable to penetrate the BBB, may be of great therapeutic value in the periphery.

3. GABA Receptors

3.1. Multiplicity

The discovery of GABA in the early 1950s and the identification of the alkaloid, bicuculline, and its quaternized analog, bicuculline methochloride (BMC), as competitive GABA antagonists in CNS tissues, initiated the pharmacological characterization of GABA receptors (Curtis et al., 1970; Johnston et al., 1972; Roberts, 1986). The subsequent design of isoguvacine, THIP (Fig. 1), and piperidine-4-sulfonic acid (P4S) as a novel class of specific GABA agonists, further stimulated studies of the pharmacology of the GABA receptors (Krogsgaard-Larsen et al., 1977, 1981).

The GABA analog, baclofen, did however disturb the picture of a uniform class of GABA receptors. Baclofen, which was designed as a lipophilic analog of GABA capable of penetrating the BBB, is an antispastic agent, but its GABA agonistic effect could not be antagonized by BMC (Burke et al., 1971; Curtis et al., 1974). In the early 1980s, Bowery and co-workers demonstrated that baclofen, or rather *(R)*-(–)-baclofen was selectively recognized as an agonist by a distinct subpopulation of GABA receptors, which were named $GABA_B$ receptors (Bowery et al., 1980; Bowery, 1983). The classical GABA receptors were designated $GABA_A$ receptors. This receptor classification represents an important step in the development of the pharmacology of GABA.

During this period, the exploration of the GABA receptors was dramatically intensified by the observation that the binding site for the benzodiazepines (BZDs) was associated with the $GABA_A$ receptors (Möhler and Okada, 1977; Squires and Braestrup, 1977; Tallman et al., 1980; Haefely and Polc, 1986; Barnard and Costa, 1989; Biggio and Costa, 1990). After the cloning of a large number of $GABA_A$ receptor subunits, this area of the pharmacology of GABA continues to be in a state of rapid development (*see* Section 3.2.1. and Möhler, Chapter 2 of this volume).

Substitution of a phosphono group for the carboxyl group of baclofen gives a $GABA_B$ antagonist, phaclofen, and, in agreement with the competitive nature of this antagonism, the $GABA_B$ receptor affinity of phaclofen resides in the *(R)*-enantiomer (Fig. 1) (Kerr et al., 1987; Frydenvang et al., 1994). On the other hand, replacement of the aromatic group of baclofen by a hydroxy group to give 3-hydroxy-4-aminobutyric acid (3-OH-GABA), gives a $GABA_B$ agonist. It is the *(R)*-form of 3-OH-GABA that interacts with the $GABA_B$ receptors, and since the aromatic substituent of baclofen and the hydroxy group of 3-OH-GABA have opposite orientations, these groups probably bind to different substructures of the $GABA_B$ receptor site (Falch et al., 1986). This observation has been exploited in the $GABA_B$ antagonist field and has led to the development of new effective antagonists (Kristiansen et al., 1992; Froestl et al., 1995a,b; Froestl et al., Chapter 8 of this volume).

In connection with the design of conformationally restricted analogs of GABA, another disturber of the peace appeared on the GABA scene, namely, *cis*-4-aminopent-2-enoic acid (CACA) (Fig. 1) (Johnston, 1975a, 1986). This compound is a GABA-like neuronal depressant that is not sensitive to BMC and that binds to a class of GABA receptor sites that do not recognize isoguvacine or *(R)*-baclofen. These receptors have been named $GABA_C$ receptors or non-$GABA_A$, non-$GABA_B$ (NANB) receptors (Drew and Johnston, 1992; *see also* Chapter 11 of this volume). It is possible that this not well-understood class of GABA receptors is heterogeneous (Johnston, 1986). It has been proposed that a recently cloned GABA receptor subunit (ρ_1), showing some homology with the α and β subunits of $GABA_A$ receptors, may confer BMC-resistant properties of ionotropic GABA receptors structurally related to $GABA_A$ receptors (Cutting et al., 1991; Drew and Johnston, 1992). $GABA_A$-like receptors containing this subunit may be identical with or similar to the proposed $GABA_C$ receptors. A NANB receptor sensitive to CACA (Fig. 1) has been identified in the retina, and this ionotropic receptor probably contains the $\rho1$ subunit (Feigenspan et al., 1993; Woodward et al., 1993).

The physiology and pharmacology of NANB GABA receptors are still very incompletely elucidated, but these receptors, which seem to exist in the PNS, as well as in the CNS, may be novel targets for drug development (Drew and Johnston, 1992). Imidazole-4-acetic acid (IAA) has recently been shown to be an antagonist at the retinal GABA receptors, probably of the $GABA_C$ type (Fig. 1) (Qian and Dowling, 1993a,b; Qian and Dowling, 1994). At least some of the $GABA_C$ receptors may be homomeric $\rho1$ subunit-containing ligand-gated chloride channels (Fig. 2) (Djamgoz, 1995).

3.2. Structure, Function, and Modulation

The introduction of molecular biological techniques has revolutionized receptor research, and during the past few years the number of papers describing structure and function of G protein-coupled receptors and ligand-gated ion channels has exploded (Biggio and Costa, 1990; Olsen and Tobin, 1990; Verdoorn et al., 1990; Olsen et al., 1991; Barnard, 1992;

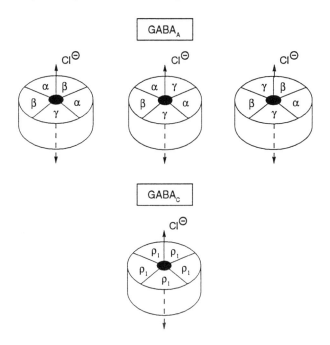

Fig. 2. Schematic illustration of some proposed subunit combinations of GABA$_A$ and GABA$_C$ receptors.

DeLorey and Olsen, 1992; Sieghart, 1992, 1995). A detailed review of this research area is beyond the scope of this chapter, and only a few aspects of particular relevance to the design and development of GABA$_A$ receptor ligands will be mentioned.

GABA$_A$ receptors are known, from cDNA cloning and expression studies, to contain a combination of homologous subunits, primarily from three classes, α, β, and γ; additional types, notably δ and ρ (*see* Section 3.1.), have been identified in certain types of neurons (Möhler et al., 1995; Sieghart, 1995; *see also* Chapter 2 of this volume). Each subunit is present in the brain in several independently expressed isoforms, and so far six α-subunits (α1–α6), four β-subunits (β1–β4), four γ-subunits (γ1–γ4), one δ-subunit, and two ρ subunits have been identified. The GABA$_A$ receptor is probably assembled as a pentameric structure (Fig. 2) from different subunit families, making it possible that a very large number of such heteromeric GABA$_A$ receptors exist in the mammalian CNS and PNS (Nayeem et al., 1994). The number of physiologically relevant GABA$_A$ receptors, their subunit stoichiometry, and their regional distributions are, however, far from being fully elucidated (Barnard, 1992; Möhler et al., 1995; Sieghart, 1995).

The gating properties of recombinant $GABA_A$ receptors vary markedly with subunit subtype combinations (Macdonald and Olsen, 1994). Subunits assemble with different efficiencies, and, when expressed in fibroblasts, for example $\alpha1\beta1$, but not $\alpha1\gamma2$ or $\beta1\gamma2$, subtypes assemble to produce BZD-insensitive $GABA_A$ receptor channels. In contrast to $\alpha1\beta1$ channels, which have only two open states, $\alpha1\beta1\gamma2$ $GABA_A$ channels (Fig. 2) have gating properties similar to those of neuronal $GABA_A$ receptors. The importance of the α subunit is emphasized by the observation that $\alpha6\beta1\gamma2$ channels show different properties (Sieghart, 1995).

Recombinant techniques have made it possible to determine the primary structure of receptor glycoproteins and to disclose a degree of heterogeneity of all classes of receptors, which was beyond imagination only a decade ago. Although the present models of ligand-gated ion channels, including $GABA_A$ and the *N*-methyl-D-aspartic acid (NMDA) subtype of Glu receptors, as well as G protein-coupled receptors, probably represent oversimplifications of the structure and structural diversity of these membrane-bound sites, they are useful as working models. A broad spectrum of problems regarding structure and function of receptors remains to be elucidated, and molecular biologists and pharmacologists are faced with a number of unanswered questions. Which type of cells express the individual receptor protein mRNAs? Do all subunit subtypes assemble into $GABA_A$ pentameric receptors? How many different heteromeric $GABA_A$ receptors actually become inserted into the cell membrane? Do all $GABA_A$ receptors assembled form functional and physiologically relevant $GABA_A$ and, perhaps, $GABA_C$ receptors (Macdonald and Olsen, 1994; Möhler et al., 1995; Sieghart, 1995)? These and many other problems regarding structure and function of receptors will probably be intensively studied during the next decade.

A major goal of such studies is to uncover the mechanisms underlying the extremely complex operational and regulatory mechanisms of the $GABA_A$ receptor complex. Such future studies undoubtedly will uncover the molecular mechanisms of key importance for receptor activation and desensitization. Elucidation of these aspects of $GABA_A$ receptors may make possible the rational design of nondesensitizing partial agonists and novel types of $GABA_A$ receptor-modulating drugs.

There is an urgent need for $GABA_A$ agonists, partial agonists, and antagonists with specific effects at physiologically relevant and pharmacologically important $GABA_A$ receptors of different subunit composition. The observations that THIP binds selectively to a β-subunit of such receptors, and that affinity and relative efficacy of partial $GABA_A$ agonists such as THIP and P4S, is dependent on the receptor subunit composition (Fig. 3), suggest that this is not an unrealistic objective (Bureau and Olsen, 1990; Ebert et al., 1994).

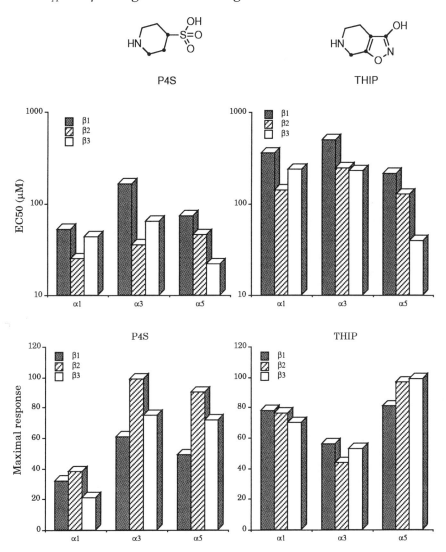

Fig. 3. Relationships between potencies or maximal responses of the GABA$_A$ agonists, piperidine-4-sulfonic acid (P4S) and 4,5,6,7-tetrahydroisoxazolo[5,4-*c*] pyridin-3-ol (THIP), and subunit combinations of recombinant GABA$_A$ receptors expressed in *Xenopus* oocytes. All of the subunit combinations tested contain a γ2 subunit (Ebert et al., 1994).

In the GABA$_A$ receptor field there are many examples of design of specific receptor ligands following systematic stereochemical and bioisosteric approaches. Identification and topographical analysis of the GABA$_A$ recognition site(s) using molecular modeling and X-ray crystallography may

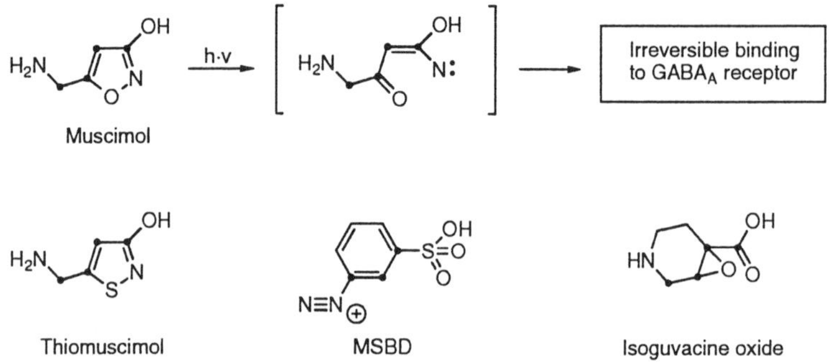

Fig. 4. Structures of the GABA$_A$ receptor photoaffinity labels, muscimol and thio-muscimol, the irreversible GABA$_A$ receptor ligand, m-benzenesulfonic acid diazo-nium ion (MSBD), and the reversible GABA$_A$ receptor agonist, isoguvacine oxide.

allow rational design of new specific drugs in the future. Identification and localization of the GABA$_A$ recognition site(s) may be facilitated by the availability of agents capable of binding irreversibly to different amino acid residues at these sites. m-Benzenesulfonic acid diazonium ion (MSBD) (Fig. 4) has been introduced as a compound capable of alkylating GABA$_A$ binding sites, whereas the potent and specific GABA$_A$ agonist, isoguvacine oxide, which contains a chemically reactive epoxy group, has been shown not to bind irreversibly to GABA$_A$ receptors in vitro or in vivo (Krogsgaard-Larsen et al., 1980; Bouchet et al., 1992). Muscimol has been used with varying degrees of success as a photoaffinity label of GABA$_A$ receptor sites. It has been proposed that photochemical cleavage of the N–O bond converts muscimol into chemically reactive species at the receptor sites (Fig. 4) (Cavalla and Neff, 1985). More recently, thiomuscimol (Fig. 4) has been shown to be an effective photolabel for the GABA$_A$ receptor (Frølund et al., 1995a; Nielsen et al., 1995). Thiomuscimol, which is a specific GABA$_A$ agonist approximately equipotent with muscimol, contains a 3-isothiazolol heterocyclic unit (Krogsgaard-Larsen et al., 1979). Since the pK_aI value (6.1) of the acidic group of thiomuscimol is higher than the pK_aI value (4.8) of muscimol, the fraction of thiomuscimol molecules containing an un-ionized acidic group is markedly higher than that of monoionized muscimol molecules (Fig. 5). Since it is the un-ionized forms of these heterocyclic units that appear to be sensitive to irradiation by UV light (*see* Fig. 4), and since thiomuscimol absorbs UV light of higher wavelength than muscimol, thiomuscimol was predicted and subsequently shown to be more effective than muscimol as a GABA$_A$ receptor photoaffinity ligand (Nielsen et al., 1995; Frølund et al., 1995a). Thiomuscimol has been tritiated, and Fig. 6

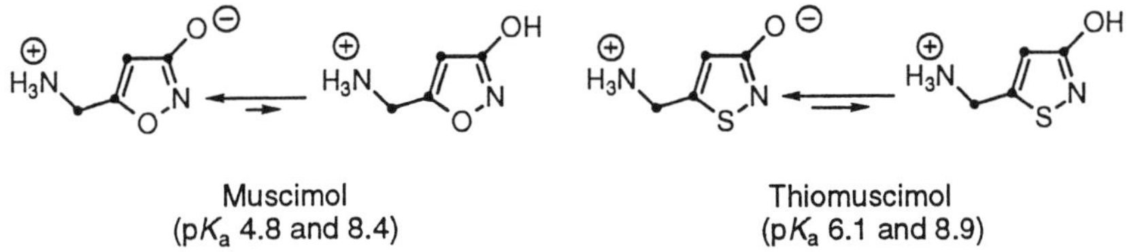

Muscimol
(pK_a 4.8 and 8.4)

Thiomuscimol
(pK_a 6.1 and 8.9)

Fig. 5. Structures, pK_a values, and equilibrium between mono- and diionized species of the photosensitive GABA$_A$ agonists, muscimol and thiomuscimol.

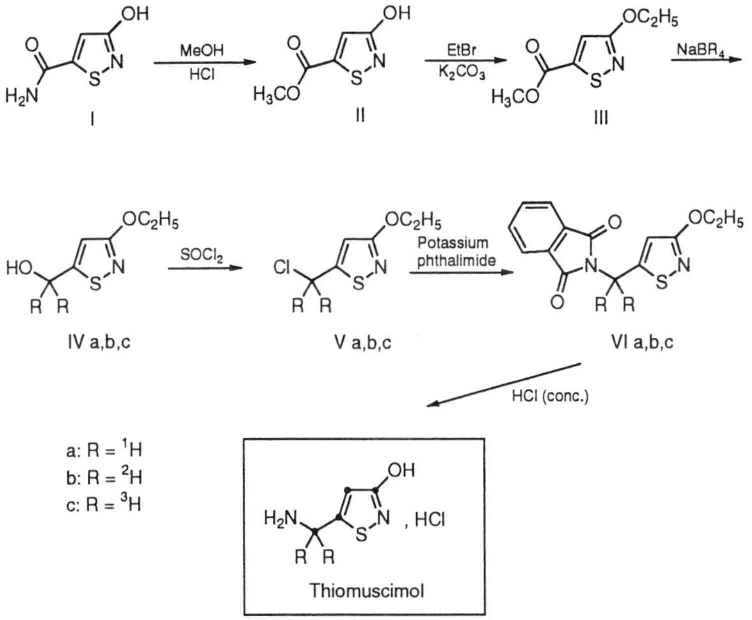

a: R = ^{1}H
b: R = ^{2}H
c: R = ^{3}H

Thiomuscimol

Fig. 6. Illustration of the last steps of the synthetic sequences for the syntheses of ^{1}H-hiomuscimol (thiomuscimol), ^{2}H-thiomuscimol, and ^{3}H-thiomuscimol.

outlines the synthesis of thiomuscimol (R = ^{1}H) and thiomuscimol labeled with deuterium (R = ^{2}H) or tritium (R = ^{3}H) in the aminomethyl side chain (Frølund et al., 1995a). Tritiated thiomuscimol may be a useful tool for the localization of the GABA$_A$ receptor recognition site.

Molecular biologists have disclosed a very high degree of heterogeneity of the GABA$_A$ receptors. The challenge for medicinal chemists is to further develop these observations into rational drug design projects and to develop receptor ligands that show specificity at the level of receptor subtypes.

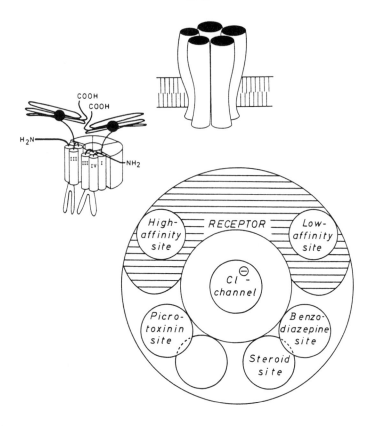

Fig. 7. Schematic illustrations of the proposed structure of GABA$_A$ receptors and the multiplicity of binding sites at GABA$_A$ receptor complex.

3.2.1. Benzodiazepines

The GABA$_A$ receptor complex (Fig. 7) is composed of a large number of binding sites for drugs, notably BZDs, steroids, barbiturates, and the compounds shown in Fig. 8; virtually all steps in the recognition and gating processes of the GABA$_A$ receptor have been shown to be subject to modulation by such drugs (Tallman et al., 1980; Haefely and Polc, 1986; Olsen and Venter, 1986; Barnard and Costa, 1989; Macdonald and Olsen, 1994; Möhler et al., 1995; Sieghart, 1995). The binding step(s) appear to be modified by BZDs, β-carbolines acting at the BZD site, and possibly by steroids, including endogenous and synthetic steroids (*see* Section 3.2.2.). The gating process is apparently regulated by steroids and barbiturates, and the open state of the channel can be occluded by penicillin. The sensitivity of the desensitization mechanism(s) and state(s) to such drugs has, so far, not been studied

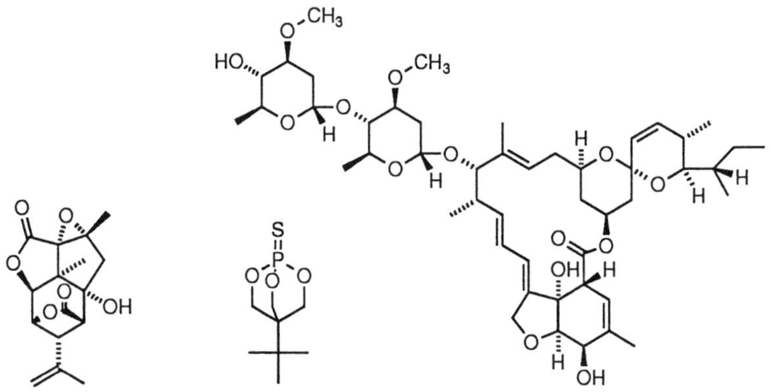

Fig. 8. Structures of the noncompetitive GABA$_A$ receptor antagonists, TBPS and picrotoxinin, and the GABA$_A$ receptor modulatory agent, avermectin B$_{1a}$.

in detail. This degree of complexity of the GABA$_A$ receptor function is comparable to that of the NMDA subtype of Glu receptor channels (Lodge, 1988; Wheal and Thompson, 1995; Krogsgaard-Larsen and Hansen, 1992).

The relationship between GABA$_A$ receptor subunit composition and molecular pharmacology of the GABA$_A$ receptor modulating BZDs has been extensively studied and, on the basis of mutation studies, it has been possible to identify a single amino acid residue of key importance for the binding of BZD ligands (Wieland et al., 1992; Gammill and Carter, 1993). It may be possible to identify and localize distinct subtypes of GABA$_A$ receptors associated with different physiological and pathophysiological functions. The aim of such studies in the BZD field is to design compounds with appropriately balanced agonist/antagonist or inverse agonist/antagonist properties capable of interacting selectively with GABA$_A$ receptors of particular relevance to anxiety, epilepsy, and sleep disorders (Gammill and Carter, 1993).

The pharmacological profile of ligands binding to the BZD sites spans the entire continuum from full and partial agonists, through antagonists, to partial and full inverse agonists. The BZD agonists act by increasing the channel function in response to GABA or a GABA$_A$ agonist; the inverse agonists exert the opposite effect by decreasing the channel function (Hunkeler et al., 1981). Antagonists do not influence GABA-induced chloride flux, but antagonize the action of agonists or inverse agonists (Hunkeler et al., 1981). The spectrum of different efficacies produces a wide variety of behavioral pharmacological effects (Günther et al., 1995). The full BZD

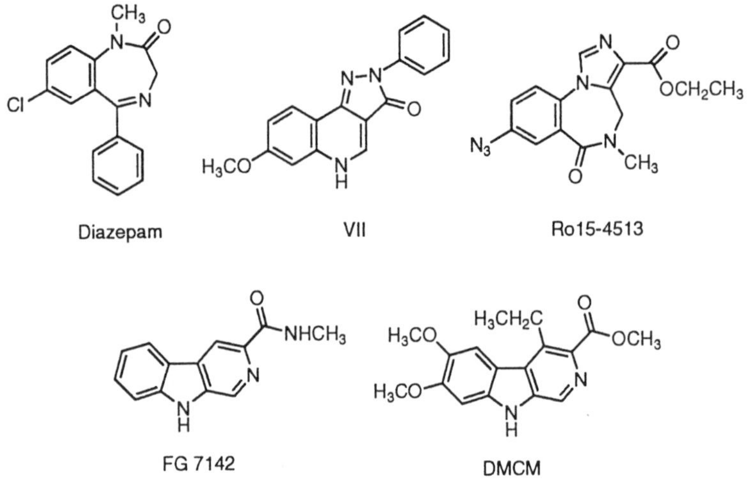

Fig. 9. Structures of some compounds interacting with different types of BZD receptor sites.

agonists show anxiolytic, anticonvulsant, sedative, and muscle relaxant effects; the inverse agonists produce anxiety and convulsions. Of particular therapeutic interest are the reports of partial agonists at the BZD site displaying potent anxiolytic and anticonvulsive effects with markedly less sedation and muscle relaxation (Guidotti, 1992; Serra et al., 1992). The BZD sites do not only recognize and react to BZDs having different efficacies, but they also accept ligands of very different structures, e.g., β-carbolines, imidazo-benzodiazepines, pyrazoloquinolinones, and triazolopyridazines (Fig. 9) (Gammill and Carter, 1993).

It is generally accepted that heterogeneity exists in BZD binding sites. This has been demonstrated by differences in binding properties of several BZD ligands from different chemical classes. Ro15-4513, a partial inverse agonist, was found to bind to sites in the cerebellum where BZDs (e.g., diazepam, flunitrazepam), some β-carbolines (e.g., 3-carbomethoxy-β-carbo-line), and triazolopyridazines (e.g., CL 218872) which are high-affinity ligands at other diazepam-sensitive BZD binding sites, show only low-affinity (Sieghart et al., 1987; Malminiemi and Korpi, 1989). The $\alpha6$ subunit, which is only expressed in cerebellar granule cells, appears to be responsible for this diazepam-insensitive receptor isoform (Luddens et al., 1990; Wieland et al., 1992).

A number of structural classes, including β-carbolines (e.g., FG 7142 and DMCM) and pyrazoloquinolinones (e.g., VII), depicted in Fig. 9, bind to

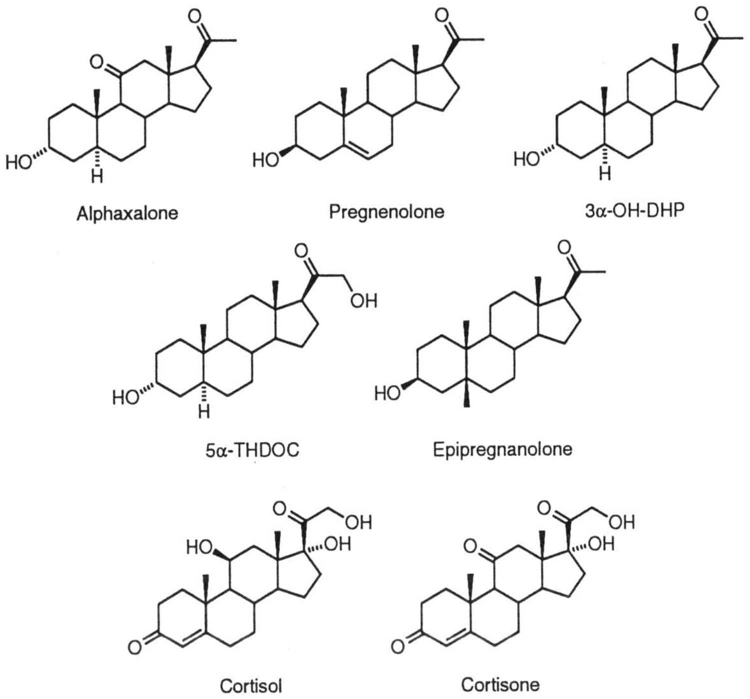

Fig. 10. Structures of some neurosteroids and neuroactive steroids.

the diazepam-insensitive sites with high to low affinity and low selectivity, compared to diazepam-sensitive BZD binding sites. This makes the characterization of the physiological and pharmacological role of the diazepam insensitive binding site difficult (Korpi et al., 1992; Zhang et al., 1995).

3.2.2. Neurosteroids and Neuroactive Steroids

There is strong and rapidly growing interest in the steroid binding site of the GABA$_A$ receptor complex as a target for pharmacological and therapeutic intervention (McNeil et al., 1992). The physiological role of this receptor site is still not fully understood, and steroids interacting with this site should be classified as neurosteroids and neuroactive steroids (Sieghart, 1995). The former class of steroids is synthesized in the brain; neuroactive steroids show pharmacological effects in the CNS, but are not necessarily synthesized in CNS tissue. Pregnenolone and its metabolites, such as 3α-hydroxy-5α-pregnan-20-one (3α-OH-DHP), are synthesized from cholesterol in brain tissue and these compounds belong to the class of neurosteroids (Fig. 10) (Baulieu, 1991). 3α,21-Dihydroxy-5α-pregnan-

20-one (5α-THDOC) and 3β-hydroxy-5β-pregnan-20-one (epipregnano-lone) are neuroactive steroids, and the results of analyses of the antagonism by epipregnanolone of the effects of neuroactive steroids are consistent with the existence of more than one class of steroid binding sites at the $GABA_A$ receptor complex (Fig. 7) (Prince and Simmonds, 1993).

Alphaxalone (Fig. 10) is a potent steroid anesthetic agent, that has been shown electrophysiologically to enhance the activation of $GABA_A$ receptors by GABA (Harrison and Simmonds, 1984). As a result of this observation of fundamental importance, a large number of industrial and academic drug research groups initiated projects to identify or develop drugs acting specifi-cally at the steroid site of the $GABA_A$ receptor complex (McNeil et al., 1992). These research activities were stimulated by the observation that cortisol is a potent bidirectional modulator of $GABA_A$ receptors, being an enhancer at low concentrations, but an inhibitor at higher concentrations (Ong et al., 1987). This corticosteroid and cortisone (Fig. 10), which is a noncompetitive antagonist at the steroid site of the $GABA_A$ receptor and the most potent agent acting at this site, may have a physiological modulatory function (Ong et al., 1990; Möhler et al., 1995; Sieghart, 1995).

3.3. Interaction Between $GABA_A$ and $GABA_B$ Receptors

Neurons intrinsic to cerebellum utilize either Glu or GABA as the neu-rotransmitter (Palay and Chan-Palay, 1982). The glutamatergic excitatory innervation of the Purkinje neurons by granule cell parallel fibers is fine-tuned by GABA-ergic interneurons. GABA exerts a modulatory action in-hibiting glutamatergic activity, a process involving activation of both $GABA_A$ and $GABA_B$ receptors. The molecular mechanisms for this fine-tuning of the excitatory glutamatergic activity are not fully clarified, but are likely to involve an interaction between $GABA_A$ and $GABA_B$ receptors, leading to disinhibitory phenomena at the level of single neurons, i.e., the granule cells (Kardos et al., 1994).

Cerebellar granule neurons have been shown to have specific binding sites for baclofen, and using cultured cells it has recently been demonstrated that the number of binding sites can be increased by exposure of the neurons to THIP during the culture period (Kardos et al., 1994; Huston et al., 1990; Travagli et al., 1991; DeErasquin, 1992). This appears to be analogous to the ability of THIP to induce low-affinity $GABA_A$ receptors on these neurons. The $GABA_B$ receptors on the granule cells are functionally involved in regu-lation of transmitter release, since (R)-baclofen has been shown to inhibit K^+-stimulated Glu release from these neurons (Belhage et al., 1990; Huston et al., 1990, 1993; Travagli et al., 1991; Kardos et al., 1994). The inhibitory actions of $GABA_A$ and $GABA_B$ receptors on evoked Glu release in cerebellar granule neurons were recently characterized. It was shown that the inhibitory actions of baclofen and isoguvacine were not additive, which strongly indicates that the two receptors are functionally coupled to each other (Kardos et al., 1994). An inhibitory action of GABA$_B$ receptors on GABA$_A$ receptors, as also previously suggested, will result in a disinhibitory action of the GABA$_B$ receptors at the cellular level, which could possibly explain numerous reports on excitatory actions of GABA or baclofen in multicellular systems, or in the intact brain (Mitchell, 1980; Levi and Gallo, 1981; Nielsen et al., 1989; Cherubini et al., 1991; Hahner et al., 1991). Such a disinhibitory interaction between GABA$_A$ and GABA$_B$ receptors at the cellular level may be functionally indistinguishable from the originally described disinhibitory organization of neuronal networks (Roberts, 1976, 1991).

Cerebellar granule neurons are rich in GABA$_A$ receptors, which based on analysis of GABA binding can be divided into high- and low-affinity receptors with affinity constants of 5–10 and 500 nM, respectively (Meier et al., 1984). Using a monotypic cerebellar culture system, it has been shown that expression of the low-affinity receptors is dependent upon whether or not the neurons are exposed to GABA or THIP during early development (Meier et al., 1984). Since cerebellar granule neurons in culture can be grown under conditions in which either high-affinity GABA receptors are expressed alone, or the two distinct receptors are expressed together, it is possible to obtain information about the functional properties of these receptors.

As mentioned, the granule neurons in cerebellum are excitatory in nature, using Glu as the neurotransmitter; transmitter release can be inhibited by GABA, depending upon the expression of the two types of GABA$_A$ receptors, as well as the depolarizing signal (Stone, 1979). In cells expressing only high-affinity GABA receptors, GABA inhibits transmitter release evoked by a moderately depolarizing signal (30 mM KCl), but not that evoked by a strong depolarizing pulse (55 mM KCl). On the contrary, in neurons expressing both high- and low-affinity GABA receptors, GABA is able to inhibit transmitter release regardless of the depolarizing condition. This action of GABA can be mimicked by THIP and muscimol (Fig. 11) and blocked by bicuculline, in keeping with the notion that the low-affinity GABA binding sites are GABA$_A$ receptors. The action of GABA mediated by the low-affinity GABA receptor has been shown to be insensitive to the chloride channel blocker, picrotoxinin (Fig. 8), indicating these receptors may be mechanistically different from the high-affinity receptors, which are clearly coupled to a chloride channel and blocked by picrotoxinin (Belhage et al., 1991).

The inhibition of evoked Glu release mediated by high-affinity GABA$_A$ receptors clearly is dependent upon the GABA$_A$ receptor gated chloride channels, since this action of GABA can be blocked by picrotoxinin (Belhage et

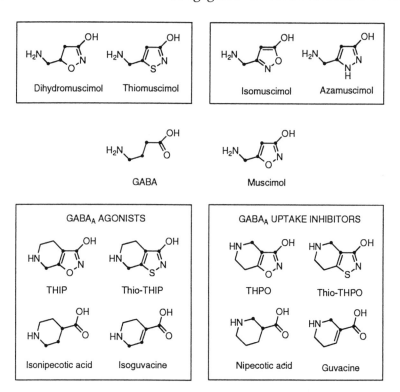

Fig. 11. Structures of some GABA$_A$ agonists and GABA uptake inhibitors.

al., 1991). It is not clear how the inhibitory action of GABA mediated by the inducible low-affinity receptors may be mediated. Since this action of GABA cannot be inhibited by picrotoxinin, it is unlikely that the classical mechanism involving the chloride channel plays a major role (Belhage et al., 1991). It was, however, shown that the induction of the low-affinity GABA$_A$ receptors is closely associated with a similar increase in the number of voltage gated calcium channels (Hansen et al., 1992). More importantly, it was observed that in nerve processes, but not in cell bodies, there was a tight spatial coupling between GABA$_A$ receptors and calcium channels in neurons expressing the low-affinity GABA$_A$ receptors but not in cells expressing high-affinity receptors alone (Hansen et al., 1992). This led to the suggestion that the inhibitory action of GABA mediated by the low-affinity receptors could involve a regulation of the activity of voltage gated calcium channels (Belhage et al., 1991; Schousboe, et al., 1992b). GABA$_B$ receptors in cerebellar granule neurons regulate intracellular level via a G protein-dependent mechanism (Sivilotti and Nistri, 1991; Kardos et al., 1994). If a coupling between $GABA_A$ and $GABA_B$ receptors in these neurons is of functional importance, this could explain how $GABA_A$ receptors may modulate transmitter release in a manner involving calcium channels.

4. $GABA_A$ Agonists

The inhibitory nature of the central GABA neurotransmission prompted the design and development of different structural types of GABA agonists. Conformational restriction of various parts of the molecule of GABA and bioisosteric replacements of the functional groups of this amino acid have led to a broad spectrum of specific $GABA_A$ agonists. Some of these molecules have played a key role in the development of the pharmacology of the $GABA_A$ receptor family (Krogsgaard-Larsen et al., 1994).

The histamine metabolite, IAA, is a relatively potent $GABA_A$ agonist and $GABA_C$ antagonist (Fig. 1), which may play a role as a central and/or peripheral endogenous GABA receptor ligand.

Muscimol, a constituent of the mushroom *Amanita muscaria*, has been extensively used as a lead for the design of different classes of GABA analogs (Fig. 11). The 3-hydroxyisoxazole carboxyl group bioisostere of muscimol can be replaced by a 3-hydroxyisothiazole or 3-hydroxyisoxazoline group to give thiomuscimol and dihydromuscimol, respectively, without significant loss of $GABA_A$ receptor agonism (Krogsgaard-Larsen et al., 1979). *(S)*Dihydromuscimol is the most potent $GABA_A$ agonist described thus far (Krogsgaard-Larsen et al., 1986). The structurally related muscimol analogs, isomuscimol and azamuscimol (Fig. 11), on the other hand, are virtually inactive, emphasizing the strict structural constraints imposed on agonist molecules by $GABA_A$ receptors (Krogsgaard-Larsen et al., 1979).

Conversion of muscimol into THIP and the isomeric compound 4,5,6,7-tetrahydroisoxazole[4,5-*c*]pyridin-3-ol (THPO) effectively separated $GABA_A$ receptor and GABA uptake affinity, because THIP is a specific $GABA_A$ agonist and THPO is a GABA uptake inhibitor (Figs. 11 and 12) (Krogsgaard-Larsen and Johnston, 1975; Krogsgaard-Larsen et al., 1977).

Using THIP as a lead, a series of specific monoheterocyclic $GABA_A$ agonists, including isoguvacine and isonipecotic acid, were developed (Krogsgaard-Larsen et al., 1985, 1988) (Fig. 11). Thio-THIP is weaker than THIP as a $GABA_A$ agonist, but recent studies have disclosed a unique pharmacological profile of this compound. Although Thio-THIP shows distinct $GABA_A$ agonist effects on cat spinal neurons (Fig. 13), recent studies using human brain recombinant $GABA_A$ receptors have disclosed that, at such receptors, Thio-THIP expresses very low efficacy partial agonism (Fig. 14) (Krogsgaard-Larsen et al., 1983; Ebert et al., 1996).

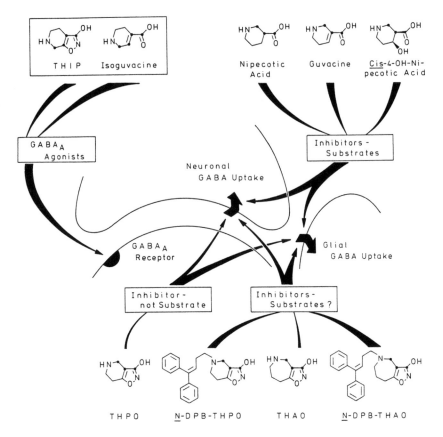

Fig. 12. Structures and sites of action of some GABA$_A$ agonists and GABA uptake substrates and/or inhibitors. The GABA uptake inhibitors containing the 4,4-diphenyl-3-butenyl (DPB) *N*-substituent are capable of penetrating the BBB.

As a result of the structural similarity of THIP and Thio-THIP (Figs. 11 and 14), the markedly different pharmacology of these compounds is noteworthy and emphasizes the very strict structural requirements of GABA$_A$ receptors. The pK_a values of THIP (4.4; 8.5) and Thio-THIP (6.1; 8.5) are different, and a significant fraction of the molecules of the latter compound must contain a nonionized 3-hydroxyisothiazole group at physiological pH (Krogsgaard-Larsen et al., 1983). Furthermore, the different degree of charge delocalization of the zwitterionic forms of THIP and Thio-THIP and other structural parameters of these two compounds, as well as the bioisosteric 3-hydroxyisoxazole and 3-hydroxyisothiazole groups, may have to be considered to explain their different potencies and efficacies at GABA$_A$ receptors.

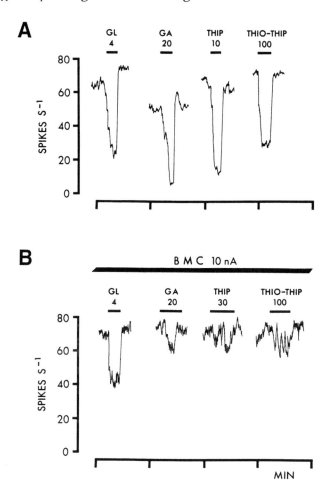

Fig. 13. Effects of microelectrophoretically administered glycine (GL), GABA (GA), THIP, and Thio-THIP on the firing of a cat spinal neuron in the absence **(A)** or presence **(B)** of the GABA$_A$ antagonist BMC. (Reprinted with permission from Krogsgaard-Larsen et al., 1983.)

A series of cyclic amino acids derived from THPO, including nipecotic acid and guvacine (Fig. 11), was developed as GABA uptake inhibitors (Krogsgaard- Larsen and Johnston, 1975; Johnston et al., 1975b). Nipecotic acid and guvacine potently inhibit neuronal, as well as glial, GABA uptake, but THPO interacts selectively with the latter uptake system (Fig. 12) (Schousboe et al., 1979, 1981; Krogsgaard-Larsen et al., 1987). Thio-THPO is slightly weaker than THPO as an inhibitor of GABA uptake (Krogsgaard-Larsen et al., 1983).

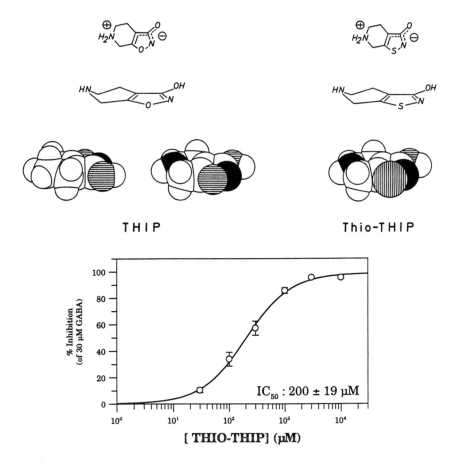

Fig. 14. Structures of THIP and Thio-THIP, illustrated in different versions, and the dose dependent inhibition by Thio-THIP of GABA-induced responses at recombinant (α3β2γ2) human GABA$_A$ receptors expressed in *Xenopus* oocytes.

4.1. Stereostructure-Activity Relationships for GABA$_A$ Agonists

The degree of stereoselectivity of chiral GABA analogs of known absolute stereochemistry (Fig. 15) depends on the structure of the compounds and is a function of the conformational flexibility of the molecules (Krogsgaard-Larsen et al., 1985, 1988; Krogsgaard-Larsen, 1988). Thus, the *(S)*- and *(R)*-forms of the flexible GABA analog 4-aminopentanoic acid (4-Me-GABA) are equally effective at GABA$_A$ receptor sites, and both enantiomers interact with neuronal, as well as glial, GABA uptake systems in vitro (Schousboe et

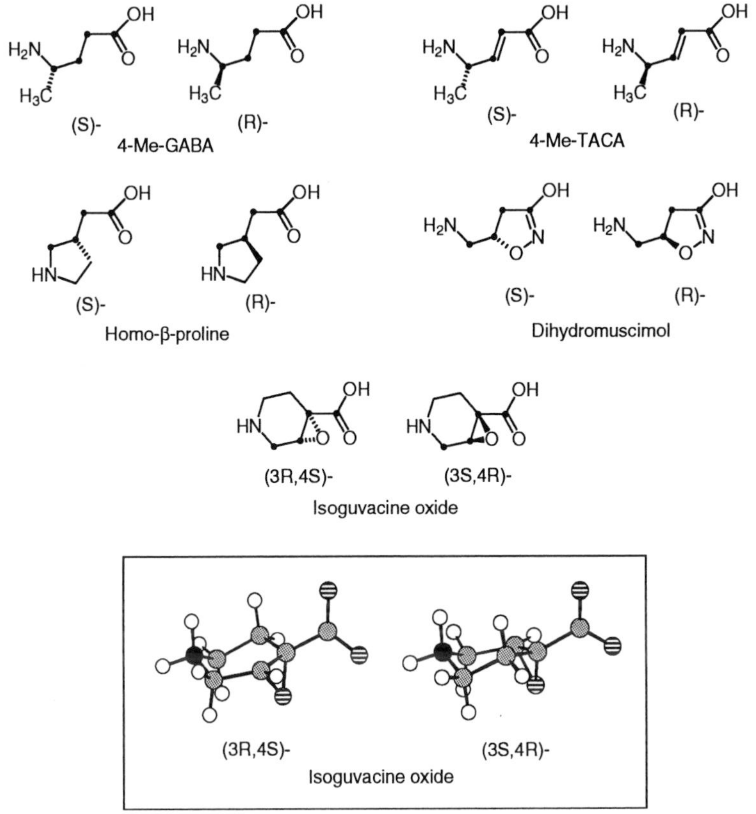

Fig. 15. Structures of the enantiomers of some chiral GABA analogs.

al., 1979). Introduction of a double bond into these molecules to give the *(S)*- and *(R)*-forms of *trans*-4-aminopent-2-enoic acid (4-Me-TACA) has quite dramatic consequences. *(S)*-4-Me-TACA interacts specifically with $GABA_A$ receptors in vivo and in vitro; *(R)*-4-Me-TACA interacts with the GABA uptake systems and does not affect $GABA_A$ receptor binding (Schousboe et al., 1979; Krogsgaard-Larsen et al., 1988).

Homo-β-proline is a cyclic but still rather flexible analog of GABA (Fig. 15). *(R)*-Homo-β-proline is about an order of magnitude more potent than *(S)*-homo-β-proline as an inhibitor of $GABA_A$ receptor binding, but the latter enantiomer selectively binds to $GABA_B$ receptor sites, and both enantiomers bind with equal affinity to the synaptosomal GABA uptake system (Nielsen et al., 1990). Dihydromuscimol is a more rigid analog of GABA, *(S)*-dihydromuscimol is a selective and extremely potent $GABA_A$ agonist, but

(R)-dihydromuscimol is a weak GABA$_A$ agonist and an inhibitor of GABA uptake (Krogsgaard-Larsen et al., 1986).

Isoguvacine oxide, which contains a chemically reactive epoxy group (Fig. 15), was designed as a GABA$_A$ agonist capable of interacting irreversibly with the GABA$_A$ receptor (Krogsgaard-Larsen et al., 1980). Although isoguvacine oxide is a potent and high-affinity GABA$_A$ agonist, it shows no sign of irreversible receptor interaction. Isoguvacine oxide has recently been resolved, and, surprisingly, the (3R,4S)- and the (3S,4R)-enantiomers were shown to be equally active as GABA$_A$ agonists (Frølund et al., 1995b). The equipotency of the enantiomers of this GABA$_A$ agonist, containing a rather bulky epoxy group (Fig. 15), indicates that a relatively spacious cavity is present at the GABA$_A$ recognition site, and that this proposed cavity does not contain an appropriately positioned nucleophilic group capable of reacting with the epoxy group of isoguvacine oxide (*see also* Section 3.2.).

4.2. Behavioral and Clinical Effects of GABA$_A$ Agonists

4.2.1. GABA in Analgesia and Anxiety

The involvement of central GABA$_A$ receptors in pain mechanisms and analgesia has been thoroughly studied, and the results have been discussed and reviewed (Krogsgaard-Larsen et al., 1984, 1985, 1988; DeFeudis, 1989; Sawynok, 1989). The demonstration of potent antinociceptive effects of the specific and metabolically stable GABA$_A$ agonist THIP in different animal models, and the potent analgesic effects of THIP in human, greatly stimulated studies in this area of pain research. THIP-induced analgesic effects were shown to be insensitive to the opiate antagonist naloxone, indicating these effects are not mediated by the opiate receptors (Kendall et al., 1982). THIP analgesia could not be reversed by bicuculline, which may reflect the involvement of a distinct class of GABA$_A$ receptors or, perhaps, a NANB-type of GABA receptor. On the other hand, THIP-induced analgesia could be reduced by atropine and potentiated by cholinergics, such as physostigmine, reflecting as yet unclarified functional interactions between GABA and ACh neurons and, possibly, the central opiate systems, rather than a direct action of THIP on muscarinic ACh receptors (Zorn and Enna, 1987).

THIP and morphine are approximately equipotent as analgesics, although their relative potencies are dependent on the animal species, and experimental models used. Acute injection of THIP potentiates morphine-induced analgesia, and chronic administration of THIP produces a certain degree of functional tolerance to its analgesic effects. In contrast to morphine, THIP does not cause respiratory depression. Clinical studies on postoperative patients, and patients with chronic pain of malignant origin, have revealed potent analgesic effects of THIP, in the latter group of patients at total doses of 5–30 mg (im).

In these cancer patients, and also in patients with chronic anxiety, the desired effects of THIP were accompanied by sedation, nausea, and in a few cases, euphoria (Hoehn-Saric, 1983). The side effects of THIP have been described as mild and similar in quality to those of other GABA-mimetics (Hoehn-Saric, 1983).

It is assumed that the postsynaptic $GABA_A$ receptor complex is mediating the anxiolytic effects of the BZDs, and, consequently, it is of interest to determine whether $GABA_A$ agonists have anxiolytic effects. Muscimol has proved effective in conflict tests, although with a pharmacological profile different from that of diazepam, and, in humans, muscimol in low doses was found to sedate and calm schizophrenic patients (Tamminga et al., 1979). In a number of patients with chronic anxiety, the effects of THIP were assessed on several measures of anxiety (Hoehn-Saric, 1983). Although these effects were accompanied by undesirable side effects, the combination of analgesic and anxiolytic effects of THIP would seem to have therapeutic prospects.

The neuronal and synaptic mechanisms underlying THIP- and, in general, GABA-induced analgesia are still not completely understood. The insensitivity of THIP-induced analgesia to naloxone has been consistently demonstrated. Sensitivity of THIP analgesia to a serotonin agonist seems to indicate an interaction between central GABA and serotonin systems. GABA-induced analgesia does not seem to be mediated primarily by spinal $GABA_A$ receptors, but rather by GABA mechanisms in the forebrain, and it appears also to involve neurons in the midbrain. The naloxone-insensitivity and apparent lack of dependence liability of $GABA_A$ agonist-mediated analgesia suggest that GABA-ergic drugs may play a role in the treatment of pain. Furthermore, it has been suggested that pharmacological manipulation of GABA mechanisms may have some relevance for future treatment of opiate addiction.

Other observations emphasize the complexity of the role of GABA in pain mechanisms. THIP has been shown to inhibit its own analgesic action at higher doses, producing a bell-shaped dose-response curve (Zorn and Enna, 1987). In addition, subconvulsant doses of bicuculline were shown to increase the latency of licking in the hot plate test in mice, an effect which was not modified by naloxone or atropine, but was antagonized by the $GABA_B$ antagonist CGP 35348 (Malcangio et al., 1992). These latter observations suggest that more than one type of $GABA_A$ receptor, perhaps including autoreceptors, are involved in pain mechanisms and, furthermore, that interactions between $GABA_A$ and $GABA_B$ receptors may be involved (*see* Section 3.3.).

The full GABA$_A$ agonist muscimol, the very efficacious partial GABA$_A$ agonist THIP (Fig. 3), and the GABA$_A$ antagonist bicuculline show potent antinociceptive effects. It is possible that the side effects of THIP in patients are associated with its high efficacy at GABA$_A$ receptors. If so, partial GABA$_A$ agonists may be of particular interest as analgesics (*see* Section 6.).

4.2.2. GABA in Neurological Disorders

There is an overwhelming amount of indirect evidence, derived from experimental models of epilepsy, supporting the view that pharmacological stimulation of the GABA neurotransmission may yield therapeutic benefit in the treatment of the condition (Morselli et al., 1981; Fariello et al., 1984; Nistico et al., 1986). The anticonvulsant effects of THIP and muscimol have been compared in a variety of animal models. THIP typically is 2–5 times weaker than muscimol in suppressing seizure activities. In mice and gerbils with genetically determined epilepsy, systemically administered THIP has proven very effective in suppressing seizure activity, and THIP is capable of reducing audiogenic seizures in DBA/2 mice. However, THIP failed to protect baboons with photosensitive epilepsy against photically induced myoclonic responses.

THIP has been subjected to a single-blind controlled trial in patients with epilepsy, in which THIP was added to the concomitant antiepileptic treatment. Under these conditions, no significant effects of THIP were detected, although a trend was observed for lower seizure frequency with submaximal doses of THIP (Petersen et al., 1983).

As a result of the surprising effects of THIP in photosensitive baboons, and the lack of clinical antiepileptic effects of this GABA$_A$ agonist, its effects on human brain glucose metabolism has been studied using positron emission tomography (PET) scanning techniques (Peyron et al., 1994a,b). In light of the sedative effects of THIP observed in animals and patients, the sleepiness and decrease of alpha rhythms observed in the patients and normal volunteers involved in these PET studies were expected (Krogsgaard-Larsen et al., 1984). Brain glucose hypometabolism was anticipated in these volunteers and epileptic patients receiving clinically relevant doses of THIP (0.2 mg/ kg). Paradoxically, brain glucose metabolism increased globally, showing an average increase in grey matter of 17% (Peyron et al., 1994b).

Dysfunctions of central GABA neurotransmitter system(s) have also been associated with other neurological disorders, such as Huntington's chorea and tardive dyskinesia (DiChiara and Gessa, 1981; Thaker et al., 1983, 1989). In Huntington's chorea there is a marked loss of GABA neurons and possible changes in GABA$_A$ receptors binding (Van Ness et al., 1982; *see also* Chapter 2 of this volume). Nevertheless, replacement therapies using the specific GABA$_A$ agonists muscimol or THIP did not significantly ameliorate the symptoms of choreic patients (Foster et al., 1983). THIP only marginally improved the symptoms of patients suffering from tardive dyskinesia (Korsgaard et al., 1982).

There are several possible explanations for these largely negative effects of THIP in the treatment of neurological disorders. Disinhibitory neuronal mechanisms, converting inhibitory effects into functional excitation (*see* Section 1.), may play a key role in the brain areas affected in these disorders. GABA$_A$ autoreceptors regulating GABA release may be more sensitive to the GABA$_A$ agonists studied than the hyperpolarizing postsynaptic GABA$_A$ receptors. The GABA$_A$ agonists studied may cause receptor desensitization. Moreover, the ρ-like receptors found in retina, where THIP shows very weak antagonist effects, may play a role in certain parts of the human brain (*see* Section 3.1.) (Mathers, 1987; Löscher, 1989; Feigenspan et al., 1993; Woodward et al., 1993).

These possibilities suggest it may be worthwhile to design new types of therapeutic GABA$_A$ receptor ligands. Antagonists at postsynaptic GABA$_A$ receptors, notably those involved in disinhibitory mechanisms, may in principle have therapeutic interest, but selective antagonists at GABA$_A$ autoreceptors seem to have major interest. There is, however, an obvious need for partial GABA$_A$ agonists showing different levels of efficacy (*see* Section 6.) and, in addition, showing selectivity for GABA$_A$ receptors in brain areas of particular relevance for individual neurological or psychiatric disorders.

4.2.3. GABA in Alzheimer's Disease

There is a well-documented loss of central ACh nerve terminals in certain brain areas of patients suffering from Alzheimer's disease (Wurtman et al., 1990). Consequently, most efforts for a therapeutic treatment of this neurodegenerative disease have been focused on the processes and mechanisms at cholinergic synapses.

Central cholinergic neurons appear to be under inhibitory GABA-ergic control; consequently, the function of such neurons may be indirectly stimulated by blockade of GABA$_A$ receptors involved in this regulation (Supavilai and Karobath, 1985; Friedman and Redburn, 1990). These GABA$_A$ receptors may be located pre- or postsynaptically on ACh neurons. Therapies based on agents with antagonist actions at GABA$_A$ receptors, or at one of the modulatory sites of the GABA$_A$ receptor complex could, at least theoretically, be useful in treating Alzheimer's disease. GABA$_A$ receptor partial agonists might stimulate ACh release, and thus improve learning and memory in Alzheimer patients without producing seizures.

The results of studies on different $GABA_A$ receptor ligands in animal models relevant to learning and memory support such GABA-ergic therapeutic approaches in Alzheimer's disease. Although administration of $GABA_A$ agonists impairs learning and memory in animals via modulation of cholinergic pathways, memory enhancement was observed after injection of the $GABA_A$ antagonist BMC (Brioni et al., 1989, 1990). Similarly, agonists and inverse agonists at the BZD site of the $GABA_A$ receptor complex impair and enhance, respectively, performance in learning and memory tasks (Venault et al., 1986). Administration of THIP to Alzheimer patients failed to significantly improve cognitive performance (Bruno et al., 1984).

The lack of positive and, in particular, negative effects of THIP in Alzheimer patients is very interesting and may reflect that THIP, as mentioned earlier, is a rather efficacious partial $GABA_A$ agonist. These observations seem to support the view that low-efficacy partial $GABA_A$ agonists may be of clinical interest in Alzheimer's disease (*see* Section 6.).

4.2.4. GABA in Schizophrenia

Evidence supporting the hypothesis of GABA receptor-mediated hyperactivity as an important component of schizophrenic symptoms is, as in the case of the Glu hypothesis, indirect. Increased GABA-ergic activity either via direct stimulation with $GABA_A$ agonists, such as muscimol or THIP, or indirect stimulation via inhibition of enzymes essential for the metabolism of GABA produce psychotomimetic effects (Theobald et al., 1968; Tamminga et al., 1978; Meldrum, 1982; Brodie and McKee, 1990; Ring and Reynolds, 1990; Robinson et al., 1990; Sander and Hart, 1990). Likewise, BZD agonists may produce schizophrenia-like symptoms in some patients, (Hall and Zisool, 1981; Bixler et al., 1987). Partial inverse agonists at the BZD site of the $GABA_A$ receptor complex reduce schizophrenic symptoms, which supports the view that hyperactivity of GABA-ergic pathways may be responsible for symptoms associated with this disorder (Haefely, 1984; Merz et al., 1988; Squires and Saederup, 1991). Receptor binding studies have revealed an increase in muscimol and flunitrazepam binding in brains from schizophrenic patients (Hanada et al., 1987; Benes et al., 1992; Kiuchi et al., 1989). However, flunitrazepam binding also has been reported to be significantly reduced in the brains of schizophrenics (Squires et al., 1993).

A possible role of hyperactive $GABA_A$ receptors in schizophrenic symptoms suggests that blockade of $GABA_A$ receptor-mediated synaptic transmission may be a relevant approach to the treatment of schizophrenia. A GABA-ergic strategy in the treatment of schizophrenia is analogous to a GABA-ergic strategy for the treatment of Alzheimer's disease (*see* Section 4.2.3.).

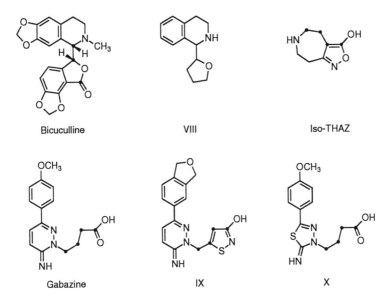

Fig. 16. Structures of some GABA$_A$ antagonists.

5. GABA$_A$ Antagonists

Specific receptor antagonists are essential tools for studies of the physiological and pharmacological importance of receptors. The classical GABA$_A$ antagonists bicuculline (Fig. 16) and BMC (Fig. 1) have played a key role in such studies on GABA$_A$ receptors.

In recent years, new structural classes of GABA$_A$ antagonists have been developed, and this line of GABA drug research has been stimulated by the growing interest in such compounds as potential therapeutic agents. The bicyclic 5-isoxazolol compound, Iso-THAZ (Fig. 16), derived from THIP, is a moderately potent GABA$_A$ antagonist but a series of arylaminopyridazine analogs of GABA, notably Gabazine, show very potent and selective GABA$_A$ antagonist effects (Arnt and Krogsgaard-Larsen, 1979; Chambon et al., 1985; Wermuth and Biziere, 1986; Wermuth et al., 1987; Rognan et al., 1992). These compounds bind tightly to GABA$_A$ receptor sites, and tritiated Gabazine is now used as a standard receptor ligand. Although Gabazine and related compounds containing a GABA-structural element show convulsant effects after systemic administration, these zwitterionic compounds do not easily penetrate the BBB (Melikian et al., 1992). Compound IX, in which the GABA-structural element has been replaced by a thiomuscimol unit (*see* Fig. 11), is the most potent GABA$_A$ antagonist in the arylaminopyridazine series (Melikian et al., 1992). This increased potency has been explained by the more pronounced lipophilic character of compound IX, compared with the corresponding analogs of GABA (Melikian et al., 1992). Bioisosteric substitution of a 2-amino-1,3,4-thiadiazole unit for the 3-aminopyridazine part of Gabazine gives compound X (Fig. 16), which also shows GABA$_A$ antagonistic properties, though markedly weaker than those of Gabazine (Allan et al., 1990).

GABA$_A$ autoreceptors, which regulate GABA release via a negative feedback mechanism, are novel targets for GABA-ergic drug design. Although such autoreceptors basically are GABA$_A$ receptors, they have pharmacological characteristics markedly different from those of postsynaptic GABA$_A$ receptors (Minchin et al., 1992a). Selective GABA$_A$ autoreceptor antagonists may function as positive modulators of GABA neurotransmission processes. Compound VIII, which is a peeled analog of bicuculline (Fig. 16), and a number of other related compounds, are two orders of magnitude more potent as GABA$_A$ autoreceptor antagonists than as antagonists at postsynaptic GABA$_A$ receptors (Minchin et al., 1992a,b). This particular class of GABA receptor antagonists may have therapeutic potential.

6. Partial GABA$_A$ Agonists

Full GABA$_A$ agonists or antagonists may be rather difficult to introduce as drugs of practical clinical applicability for treating disorders of the CNS (*see* Section 4.2.). The former class may induce rapid desensitization and the GABA$_A$ antagonists are potential anxiogenics, proconvulsants, or convulsants.

In clinical conditions where GABA$_A$ agonist therapies may be beneficial, the level of efficacy is probably dependent on the particular disease. The very potent analgesic effects of THIP (*see* Section 4.2.1.) indicate that the relatively high level of efficacy of this partial GABA$_A$ agonist (Fig. 3) is close to optimal for pain treatment, although it may be postulated that a slightly less efficacious GABA$_A$ agonist may display fewer side effects (Krogsgaard-Larsen et al., 1988; Maksay, 1994).

Analogously, very low-efficacy GABA$_A$ agonists may have clinical usefulness in certain diseases. Such compounds, showing sufficient GABA$_A$ receptor agonism to avoid seizures, may theoretically be useful therapeutic agents in Alzheimer's disease or, quite paradoxically, in epileptic disorders (*see* Section 4.2.2.).

The heterocyclic GABA bioisosteres IAA (Fig. 1) and P4S (Fig. 3) show the characteristics of partial GABA$_A$ agonists (Braestrup et al., 1979; Maksay, 1994). The nonfused THIP analog, 5-(4-piperidyl)isoxazol-3-ol (4-PIOL) (Fig. 17), is a moderately potent agonist at GABA$_A$ receptors in the cat spinal

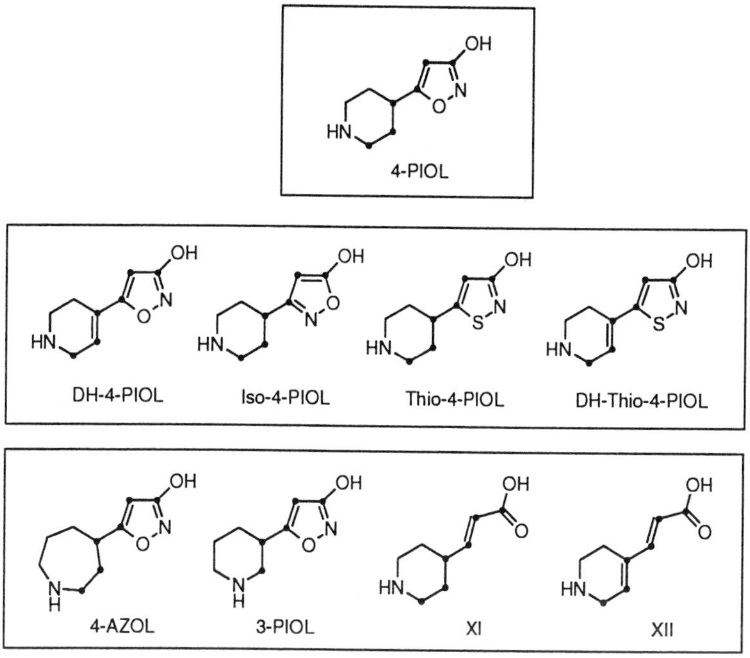

Fig. 17. Structures of the low-efficacy partial GABA$_A$ agonist, 4-PIOL, and some active (middle box) and inactive (bottom) analogs.

cord (Byberg et al., 1987, 1993). However, 4-PIOL did not show significant stimulatory effects on BZD binding; it antagonized dose-dependent muscimol-induced stimulation of BZD binding in a manner similar to that of the GABA$_A$ antagonist BMC (Falch et al., 1990).

Whole-cell patch-clamp recordings from cultured hippocampal or cerebral cortical neurons (Figs. 18 and 19) have been used to further characterize the action of 4-PIOL (Kristiansen et al., 1991; Frølund et al., 1995c). The action of 4-PIOL was compared with that of the full GABA$_A$ agonist isoguvacine (Figs. 18 and 19) and the GABA$_A$ antagonist BMC (Kristiansen et al., 1991; Frølund et al., 1995c). The response to 4-PIOL was competitively antagonized by BMC. 4-PIOL was about 200 times less potent as an agonist than isoguvacine. The maximum response to 4-PIOL was only a small fraction of that to submaximal concentrations of isoguvacine, and 4-PIOL antagonized the response to isoguvacine (Frølund et al., 1995c). On the basis of these studies it is concluded that 4-PIOL is a low-efficacy partial GABA$_A$ agonist showing a predominant GABA$_A$ antagonist profile, being about 30 times weaker than BMC as a GABA$_A$ antagonist. Repeated administration of

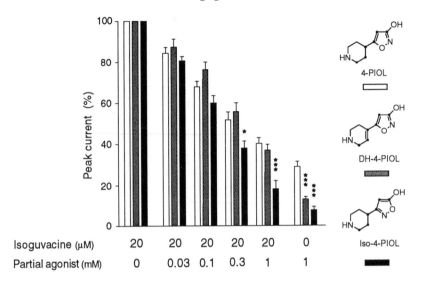

Fig. 18. The dose-dependent reduction by the partial $GABA_A$ agonists, 4-PIOL, DH-4-PIOL, and Iso-4-PIOL, of the effects of the full $GABA_A$ agonist, isoguvacine, on cultured cortical neurons using whole-cell patch-clamp techniques (Frølund et al., 1995c).

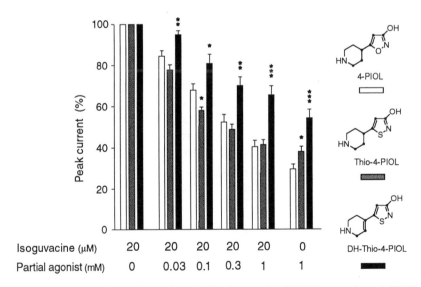

Fig. 19. The dose-dependent reduction by the partial $GABA_A$ agonists, 4-PIOL, Thio-4-PIOL, and DH-Thio-4-PIOL, of the effects of the full $GABA_A$ agonist, isoguvacine, on cultured cortical neurons using whole-cell patch-clamp techniques (Frølund et al., 1995c).

4-PIOL did not cause significant desensitization of $GABA_A$ receptors (Kristiansen et al., 1991). Unfortunately, 4-PIOL does not show pharmacological effects after systemic administration (Falch et al., 1990). In contrast to THIP, which penetrates the BBB very easily, the protolytic properties of 4-PIOL do not allow this compound to pass the BBB (Krogsgaard-Larsen et al., 1984; Falch et al., 1990) .

In an attempt to overcome this pharmacokinetic obstacle, and to shed further light on the relationship between structure and $GABA_A$ agonist efficacy of this class of heterocyclic GABA-ergic compounds, a number of 4-PIOL analogs have been synthesized and tested. Some of these analogs, notably 4-AZOL, 3-PIOL, and the monocyclic analogs XI and XII (Fig. 17) were completely inactive, emphasizing the very strict structural requirements for binding to, and activation of, $GABA_A$ receptors (*see also* Section 4.) (Krogsgaard-Larsen et al., 1985, 1988; Byberg et al., 1987, 1993; Frølund et al., 1992, 1995c).

On the other hand, the 4-PIOL analogs, DH-4-PIOL, Iso-4-PIOL, Thio-4-PIOL, and DH-Thio-4-PIOL (Fig. 17), showed qualitatively similar effects on cultured cortical neurons (Frølund et al., 1995c). Interestingly, however, the relative efficacies of these compounds as partial $GABA_A$ agonists ranged from levels markedly below that of 4-PIOL (Fig. 18) to significantly higher (Fig. 19). It should be stressed that neither potency nor efficacy of the compounds under study can be determined precisely under the present experimental conditions. On the assumption that each compound acts as a true partial agonist capable of completely displacing isoguvacine from the $GABA_A$ receptors, its maximal agonist effect must lie between the agonist levels produced by a high concentration (1 mM) of the compound in the absence or presence of isoguvacine (20 mM).

The 3-isothiazolol analog of 4-PIOL, Thio-4-PIOL, which binds more tightly to $GABA_A$ receptor sites than 4-PIOL itself, was equally effective with 4-PIOL; the unsaturated analog of Thio-4-PIOL, DH-Thio-4-PIOL, was significantly more efficacious (Fig. 19) (Frølund et al., 1995c). In light of these relative efficacies of Thio-4-PIOL and DH-Thio-4-PIOL, it was surprising to find the reverse relative efficacies of 4-PIOL and the corresponding unsaturated analog, DH-4-PIOL, which is somewhat less efficacious than 4-PIOL (Fig. 18). Like DH-4-PIOL, the 5-isoxazolol analog of 4-PIOL, Iso-4-PIOL, has a lower affinity for $GABA_A$ receptor sites than 4-PIOL. Furthermore, Iso-4-PIOL shows a relative efficacy comparable to, or lower than, DH-4-PIOL (Fig. 18) (Frølund et al., 1995c).

The results of receptor binding studies indicate these new compounds (Fig. 17) interact with $GABA_A$ receptor sites. In order to demonstrate that the partial agonist effects of DH-4-PIOL, Iso-4-PIOL, Thio-4-PIOL, and

DH-Thio-4-PIOL are also mediated by $GABA_A$ receptors, the reversal potential of all compounds, including the well-established $GABA_A$ receptor ligands isoguvacine and 4-PIOL, were determined (Krogsgaard-Larsen et al., 1977; Kristiansen, 1991). With the possible exception of Iso-4-PIOL, these compounds showed very similar reversal potential values indicating their effects on cultured cerebral cortex neurons involve the same ionic mechanism (Frølund et al., 1995c). In contrast to 4-PIOL, Thio-4-PIOL may be capable of penetrating the BBB, suggesting it may be useful for animal behavioral studies (Falch et al., 1990; Frølund, 1995c).

7. Future Developments

Molecular biologists have disclosed a very high degree of heterogeneity of the $GABA_A$ receptors. A necessary condition for elucidation of the physiological relevance, pharmacological importance, and potential as therapeutic targets of subtypes of this receptor is the availability of subtype-selective or -specific ligands. The design of such $GABA_A$ receptor ligands, following systematic stereochemical and bioisosteric approaches, represents a major challenge for medicinal and computational chemists.

Using affinity labeling techniques, site-directed mutagenesis, and domain-specific antibodies, the functional domains of $GABA_A$ receptors are being mapped (Smith and Olsen, 1995). One of the prerequisites for the design of $GABA_A$ receptor ligands on a strictly rational basis is very detailed information about the topography of the recognition site(s) derived from X-ray crystallographic structure determination of crystals of $GABA_A$ receptors or complexes of $GABA_A$ receptors and specific ligands. Neither $GABA_A$ receptors nor any other transmitter-gated ion channel proteins have, so far, been amenable to such studies. However, using conventional or novel crystallization techniques, studies along these lines are likely to be possible in a not too distant future.

For different reasons, neither full $GABA_A$ agonists nor antagonists may be useful therapeutic agents for the treatment of psychiatric and neurological diseases (*see* Section 4.2.). The high-efficacy partial $GABA_A$ agonist THIP shows very potent analgesic effects in humans, but it seems likely that low-efficacy partial $GABA_A$ agonists, such as Thio-4-PIOL or related 4-PIOL analogs may be more appropriate for treating CNS disorders (*see* Sections 4.2. and 6.).

$GABA_A$ receptor modulatory agents, notably different types of BZDs, neurosteroids or neuroactive steroids, will have growing therapeutic interest and utility in the future (*see* Sections 3.2.1. and 3.2.2.) (Gammill and Carter, 1993; Lambert et al., 1995). It seems likely that novel types of modulatory sites at the GABA$_A$ receptor complex may be disclosed and shown to be interesting targets for therapeutic intervention.

Acknowledgments

This work was supported by grants from the Lundbeck Foundation, the Danish Technical Research Council, and the Danish State Biotechnology Program (1991–1995). The secretarial assistance of Anne Nordly is gratefully acknowledged.

References

Allan, R. D., Apostopoulos, C., and Richardson, J. A. (1990) 2-Amino-1,3,4-thiadiazole derivatives of GABA as GABA$_A$ antagonists. *Aust. J. Chem.* **43,** 1767–1772.

Arnt, J. and Krogsgaard-Larsen, P. (1979) GABA agonists and potential antagonists related to muscimol. *Brain Res.* **177,** 395–400.

Barnard, E. A. (1992) Receptor classes and the transmitter-gated ion channels. *Trends Biochem. Sci.* **17,** 368–374.

Barnard, E. A. and Costa, E., eds. (1989) *Allosteric Modulation of Amino Acid Receptors: Therapeutic Implications*, Raven, New York.

Baulieu, E. E. (1991) Neurosteroids: a new function in the brain. *Biol. Cell.* **71,** 3–10.

Belhage, B., Damgaard, I., Saederup, E., Squires, R. F., and Schousboe, A. (1991) High- and low-affinity GABA-receptors in cultured cerebellar granule cells regulate transmitter release by different mechanisms. *Neurochem. Int.* **19,** 475–482.

Belhage, B., Hansen, G. H., Meier, E., and Schousboe, A. (1990) Effects of inhibitors of protein synthesis and intracellular transport on the GABA agonist induced functional differentiation of cultured cerebellar granule cells. *J. Neurochem.* **55,** 1107–1113.

Benes, F. M., Vincent, S. L., Alsterberg, G., Bird, E. D., and SanGiovanni, J. P. (1992) Increased GABA$_A$ receptor binding in superficial layers of cingulate cortex in schizophrenics. *J. Neurosci.* **12,** 924–929.

Biggio, G. and Costa, E., eds. (1990) *GABA and Benzodiazepine Receptor Subtypes*, Raven, New York.

Bixler, E. O., Kales, A., Brubaker, B. H., and Kales, J. D. (1987) Adverse reactions to benzodiazepine hypnotics: spontaneous reporting system. *Pharmacology* **35,** 286–300.

Bouchet, M.-J., Jacques, P., Ilien, B., Goeldner, M., and Hirth, C. (1992) m-Sulfonate benzene diazonium chloride: a powerful affinity label for the γ-aminobutyric acid binding site from rat brain. *J. Neurochem.* **59,** 1405–1413.

Bowery, N. G. (1983) Classification of GABA receptors, in *The GABA Receptors* (Enna, S. J., ed.), Humana, Clifton, NJ, pp. 177–213.

Bowery, N. G., Bittiger, H., and Olpe, H.-R., eds. (1990) *GABA$_B$ Receptors in Mammalian Function*, John Wiley, Chichester.

Bowery, N. G., Hill, D. R., Hudson, A. L., Doble, A., Middlemiss, D. N., Shaw, J., and Turnbull, M. (1980) (–) Baclofen decreases neurotransmitter release in the mammalian CNS by an action at a novel GABA receptor. *Nature* **283,** 92–94.

Bowery, N. G. and Nistico, G., eds. (1989) *GABA: Basic Research and Clinical Applications*, Pythagora, Rome.

Braestrup, C., Nielsen, M., Krogsgaard-Larsen, P., and Falch, E. (1979) Partial agonists for brain GABA/benzodiazepine receptor complex. *Nature* **280,** 331–333.

Brioni, J. D., Decker, M. W., Gamboa, L. P., Izquierdo, I., and McGaugh, J. L. (1990) Muscimol injections in the medial septum impair spatial learning. *Brain Res.* **522,** 227–234.

Brioni, J. D., Nagahara, A. H., and McGaugh, J. L. (1989) Involvement of the amygdala GABAergic system in the modulation of memory storage. *Brain Res.* **487,** 105–112.

Brodie, M. J. and McKee, P. J. W. (1990) Vigabatrin and psychosis. *Lancet* **335,** 1279.

Bruno, G., Foster, N. L., Fedio, P., Mohr, E., Cox, C., Gillespie, M. M., and Chase, T. N. (1984) THIP therapy of Alzheimer's disease. *Neurology* **34 (Suppl.),** 225.

Bureau, M. and Olsen, R. W. (1990) Multiple distinct subunits of the γ-aminobutyric acid-A receptor protein show different ligand-binding affinities. *Mol. Pharmacol.* **37,** 497–502.

Burke, D., Andrews, C. J., and Knowles, L. (1971) The action of a GABA derivative in human spasticity. *J. Neurol.* **14,** 199–208.

Byberg, J. R., Hjeds, H., Krogsgaard-Larsen, P., and Jørgensen, F. S. (1993) Conformational analysis and molecular modelling of a partial $GABA_A$ agonist and a glycine antagonist related to the $GABA_A$ agonist, THIP. *Drug Des. Discovery* **10,** 213–229.

Byberg, J. R., Labouta, I. M., Falch, E., Hjeds, H., Krogsgaard-Larsen, P., Curtis, D. R., and Gynther, B. D. (1987) Synthesis and biological activity of a GABA-A agonist which has no effect on benzodiazepine binding and structurally related glycine antagonists. *Drug Des. Delivery* **1,** 261–274.

Caspary, D. M., Raza, A., Lawhorn Armour, B. A., Pippin, J., and Arneric, S. P. (1990) Immunocytochemical and neurochemical evidence for age-related loss of GABA in the inferior colliculus: implications for neural presbycusis. *J. Neurosci.* **10,** 2363–2372.

Cavalla, D. and Neff, N. H. (1985) Photoaffinity labeling of the $GABA_A$ receptor with [^{3}H]muscimol. *J. Neurochem.* **44,** 916–921.

Chambon, J.-P., Feltz, P., Heaulme, M., Restle, S., Schlichter, R., Biziere, K., and Wermuth, C. G. (1985) An arylaminopyridazine derivative of γ-aminobutyric acid (GABA) is a selective and competitive antagonist of the receptor sites. *Proc. Natl. Acad. Sci. USA* **82,** 1832–1836.

Cherubini, E., Gaiarsa, J. L., and Ben-Ari, Y. (1991) GABA: an excitatory transmitter in early postnatal life. *Trends Neurosci.* **14,** 515–519.

Curtis, D. R., Duggan, A. W., Felix, D., and Johnston, G. A. R. (1970) GABA, bicuculline and central inhibition. *Nature* **226,** 1222–1224.

Curtis, D. R., Game, C. J. A., Johnston, G. A. R., and McCulloch, R. M. (1974) Central effects of β-(p-chlorophenyl)-γ-aminobutyric acid. *Brain Res.* **70,** 493–499.

Curtis, D. R. and Johnston, G. A. R. (1974) Amino acid transmitters in the mammalian central nervous system. *Ergebn. Physiol.* **69,** 97–188.

Cutting, G. R., Lu, L., O'Hara, B. F., Kasch, L. M., Montrose-Rafizaheh, C., Donovan, D. M., Shimada, S., Antonorakis, S. E., Guggino, W. B., Uhl, G. R., and Kazazian, H. H. (1991) Cloning of the γ-aminobutyric acid (GABA) r_1 cDNA: a GABA receptor subunit highly expressed in retina. *Proc. Natl. Acad. Sci. USA* **88,** 2673–2677.

Dannhardt, G., Dominiak, P., and Laufer, S. (1993) Hypertensive effects and structure-activity relationships of 5-ω-aminoalkyl isoxazoles. *Drug Res.* **43,** 441–444.

DeErasquin, G., Grooker, G., Costa, E., and Woscik, W. J. (1992) Stimulation of high affinity γ-aminobutyric acid$_B$ receptors potentiates the depolarization induced increase of intraneuronal ionised calcium content in cerebellar granule neurons. *Mol. Pharmacol.* **42**, 407–414.

DeFeudis, F. V. (1989) GABA agonists and analgesia. *Drug News Perspect.* **2**, 172,173.

DeLorey, T. M. and Olsen, R. W. (1992) γ-Aminobutyric acid_A receptor structure and function. *J. Biol. Chem.* **267**, 16,747–16,750.

DiChiara, G. and Gessa, G. L., eds. (1981) *GABA and the Basal Ganglia*, Raven, New York.

Djamgoz, M. B. A. (1995) Diversity of GABA receptors in the vertebrate outer retina. *Trends Neurosci.* **18**, 118–120.

Drew, C. A. and Johnston, G. A. R. (1992) Bicuculline- and baclofen-insensitive γ-aminobutyric acid binding to rat cerebellar membranes. *J. Neurochem.* **58**, 1087–1092.

Ebert, B., Brehm, L., Wafford, K. A., Kristiansen, U., Kemp, J. A., and Krogsgaard-Larsen, P. (1996) Structure and molecular pharmacology of thio-THIP. *Eur. J. Med. Chem.*, submitted.

Ebert, B., Wafford, K. A., Whiting, P. J., Krogsgaard-Larsen, P., and Kemp, J. A. (1994) Molecular pharmacology of γ-aminobutyric acid type A receptor agonists and partial agonists in oocytes injected with different α, β and γ receptor subunit combinations. *Mol. Pharmacol.* **46**, 957–963.

Edvinsson, L., Larsson, B., and Skarby, T. (1980) Effect of the GABA receptor agonist muscimol on regional cerebral blood flow in the rat. *Brain Res.* **185**, 445–448.

Erdo, S. L. (1985) Peripheral GABAergic mechanisms. *Trends Pharmacol. Sci.* **6**, 205–208.

Erdo, S. L. and Bowery, N. G., eds. (1986) *GABAergic Mechanisms in Mammalian Periphery*, Raven, New York.

Falch, E., Hedegaard, A., Nielsen, L., Jensen, B. R., Hjeds, H., and Krogsgaard-Larsen, P. (1986) Comparative stereostructure-activity studies on GABA_A and GABA_B receptor sites and GABA uptake using rat brain membrane preparations. *J. Neurochem.* **47**, 898–903.

Falch, E., Larsson, O. M., Schousboe, A., and Krogsgaard-Larsen, P. (1990) GABA-A agonists and GABA uptake inhibitors: structure-activity relationships. *Drug Dev. Res.* **21**, 169–188.

Fariello, R. G., Morselli, P. L., Lloyd, K. G., Quesney, L. F., and Engel, J., eds. (1984) *Neurotransmitters, Seizures, and Epilepsy II*, Raven, New York.

Feigenspan, A., Wassle, H., and Bormann, J. (1993) Pharmacology of GABA receptor Cl⁻ channels in rat retinal bipolar cells. *Nature* **361**, 159–162.

Foster, N. L., Chase, T. N., Denaro, A., Hare, T. A., and Tamminga, C. A. (1983) THIP treatment and Huntington's chorea. *Neurology* **33**, 637–639.

Friedman, D. E. and Redburn, D. A. (1990) Evidence for functionally distinct subclasses of γ-aminobutyric acid receptors in rabbit retina. *J. Neurochem.* **55**, 1189–1199.

Froestl, W., Mickel, S. J., Hall, R. G., von Sprecher, G., Strub, D., Baumann, P. A., Brugger, F., Gentsch, C., Jaekel, J., Olpe, H.-R., Rihs, G., Vassout, A., Waldmeier, P. C., and Bittiger, H. (1995a) Phosphinic acid analogues, of GABA. 1. New potent and selective GABA_B agonists. *J. Med. Chem.* **38**, 3297–3312.

Froestl, W., Mickel, S. J., von Sprecher, G., Diel, P. J., Hall, R. G., Maier, L., Strub, D., Melillo, V., Baumann, P. A., Bernasconi, R., Gentsch, C., Hauser, K., Jaekel, J., Karlsson, G., Klebs, K., Maître, L., Marescaux, C., Pozza, M. F., Schmutz, M., Steinmann, M. W., van Riezen, H., Vassout, A., Mondadori, C., Olpe, H.-R., Waldmeier, P. C., and Bittiger, H. (1995b) Phosphinic acid analogues of GABA. 2. Selective, orally active GABA_B antagonists. *J. Med. Chem.* **38**, 3313–3331.

Frølund, B., Ebert, B., Lawrence, L. W., Hurt, S. D., and Krogsgaard-Larsen, P. (1995a) Synthesis and receptor binding of 5-amino[^{3}H]$_2$methyl-3-isothiazolol ([^{3}H]thiomuscimol), a specific GABA$_A$ agonist photoaffinity label. *J. Labelled Compd. Radiopharm.* **36,** 877–889.

Frølund, B., Jeppesen, L., Krogsgaard-Larsen, P., and Hansen, J. J. (1995b) GABA$_A$ agonists: resolution and pharmacology of (+)- and (–)-isoguvacine oxide. *Chirality* **7,** 434–438.

Frølund, B., Kristiansen, U., Brehm, L., Hansen, A. B., Krogsgaard-Larsen, P., and Falch, E. (1995c) Partial GABA$_A$ receptor agonists. Synthesis and in vitro pharmacology of a series of nonannulated analogs of 4,5,6,7-tetrahydroisoxazolo[5,4-*c*]pyridin-3-ol. *J. Med. Chem.* **38,** 3287–3296.

Frølund, B. F., Kristiansen, U., Nathan, T., Falch, E., Lambert, J. D. C., and Krogsgaard-Larsen, P. (1992) 4-PIOL, a low-efficacy partial GABA$_A$ agonist, in *Drug Research Related to Neuroactive Amino Acids, Alfred Benzon Symposium 32* (Schousboe, A., Diemer, N. H., and Kofod, H., eds.), Munksgaard, Copenhagen, pp. 449–460.

Frydenvang, K., Krogsgaard-Larsen, P., Hansen, J. J., Mitrovic, A., Tran, H., Drew, C. A., and Johnston, G. A. R. (1994) GABA$_B$ antagonists: resolution, absolute stereochemistry and pharmacology of (*R*)- and (*S*)-phaclofen. *Chirality* **6,** 583–589.

Gammill, R. B. and Carter, D. B. (1993) Neuronal BZD receptors: new ligands, clones and pharmacology. *Annu. Rep. Med. Chem.* **28,** 19–27.

Guidotti, A. (1992) Imidazenil: a new partial positive allosteric modulator of the GABA$_A$ receptor. *Neurosci. Facts* **3,** 71–72.

Günther, U., Benson, J., Benke, D., Fritschy, J.-M., Reyes, G., Knoflach, F., Crestani, F., Aguzzi, A., Arigoni, M., Lang, Y., Bluethmann, H., Möhler, H., and Luscher, B. (1995) Benzodiazepine-insensitive mice generated by targeted disruption of the γ_2 subunit gene of γ-aminobutyric acid type A receptors. *Proc. Natl. Acad. Sci. USA* **92,** 7749–7753.

Haefely, W. (1984) Pharmacological profile of two benzodiazepine partial agonists: Ro 16-6028 and Ro 17-1812. *Clin. Neuropharmacol.* **7 (Suppl. 1),** 670–671.

Haefely, W. and Polc, P. (1986) Physiology of GABA enhancement by benzodiazepines and barbiturates, in *Benzodiazepine/GABA Receptors and Chloride Channels: Structural and Functional Properties* (Olsen, R. W., Venter, J. C., eds.), Alan R. Liss, New York, pp. 97–133.

Hahner, L., McQuilkin, S., and Harris, R. A. (1991) Cerebellar GABA$_B$ receptors modulate function of GABA$_A$ receptors. *FASEB J.* **5,** 2466–2472.

Hall, R. C. and Zisool, S. (1981) Paradoxical reactions to benzodiazepines. *Br. J. Clin. Pharmacol.* **11,** 99S–104S.

Hanada, S., Mita, S., Nishino, N., and Tanaka, C. (1987) [^{3}H]Muscimol binding sites increased in autopsied brains of chronic schizophrenics. *Life Sci.* **40,** 259–266.

Hansen, G. H., Belhage, B., and Schousboe, A. (1992) First direct electron microscopic visualization of a tight spatial coupling between GABA$_A$-receptors and voltage sensitive calcium channels. *Neurosci. Lett.* **137,** 14–18.

Harrison, N. L. and Simmonds, M. A. (1984) Modulation of the GABA receptor complex by a steroid anaesthetic. *Brain Res.* **323,** 287–292.

Hoehn-Saric, R. (1983) Effects of THIP on chronic anxiety. *Psychopharmacology* **80,** 338–341.

Hunkeler, W., Möhler, H., Pieri, L., Polc, P., Bonetti, E. P., Cumin, R., Schaffner, R., and Haefely, W. (1981) Selective antagonists of benzodiazepines. *Nature* **290,** 514–516.

Huston, E., Gullen, G., Sweeney, M. I., Pearson, H., Fazeli, M. S., and Dolphin, A. C. (1993) Pertussis toxin treatment increases glutamate release and dihydropyridine binding sites in cultured rat cerebellar granule neurons. *Neuroscience* **52**, 787–798.

Huston, E., Scott, R. H., and Dolphin, A. C. (1990) A comparison of the effect of calcium channel ligands and $GABA_B$ agonists and antagonists in transmitter release and somatic calcium currents in cultured neurons. *Neuroscience* **38**, 721–729.

Johnston, G. A. R. (1986) Multiplicity of GABA receptors, in *Benzodiazepine/GABA Receptors and Chloride Channels: Structural and Functional Properties* (Olsen, R. W. and Venter, J. C., eds.), Alan R. Liss, New York, pp. 57–71.

Johnston, G. A. R., Beart, P. M., Curtis, D. R., Game, C. J. A., McCulloch, R. M., and MacLachlan, R. M. (1972) Bicuculline methochloride as a GABA antagonist. *Nature (New Biol.)* **240**, 219,220.

Johnston, G. A. R., Curtis, D. R., Beart, P. M., Game, C. J. A., McCulloch, R. M., and Twitchin, B. (1975a) Cis- and Trans-4-aminocrotonic acid as GABA analogues of restricted conformation. *J. Neurochem.* **24**, 157–160.

Johnston, G. A. R., Krogsgaard-Larsen, P., and Stephanson, A. (1975b) Betel nut constituents as inhibitors of γ-aminobutyric acid uptake. *Nature* **258**, 627–628.

Kardos, J., Elster, L., Damgaard, I., Krogsgaard-Larsen, P., and Schousboe, A. (1994) Role of $GABA_B$ receptors in intracellular Ca^{2+} homeostasis and possible interaction between $GABA_A$ and $GABA_B$ receptors in regulation of transmitter release in cerebellar granule neurons. *J. Neurosci. Res.* **39**, 646–655.

Kendall, D. A., Browner, M., and Enna, S. J. (1982) Comparison of the antinociceptive effect of GABA agonists: evidence for a cholinergic involvement. *J. Pharmacol. Exp. Ther.* **220**, 482–487.

Kerr, D. I. B. and Ong, J. (1986) $GABA_B$-receptors in peripheral function, in *GABAergic Mechanisms in Mammalian Periphery* (Erdo, S. L. and Bowery, N. G., eds.), Raven, New York, pp. 239–259.

Kerr, D. I. B., Ong, J., Prager, R. H., Gynther, B. D., and Curtis, D. R. (1987) Phaclofen: a peripheral and central baclofen antagonist. *Brain Res.* **405**, 150–154.

Kiuchi, Y., Kobayashi, T., Takeuchi, J., Shimuzu, H., Ogata, H., and Toru, M. (1989) Benzodiazepine receptors increase in post-mortem brain of chronic schizophrenics. *Eur. Arch. Psychiat. Neurol. Sci.* **239**, 71–78.

Korpi, E. R., Uusi-Oukari, M., and Wegelius, K. (1992) Substrate specificity of diazepam-insensitive cerebellar [³H]Ro 15–4513 binding sites. *Eur. J. Pharmacol.* **213**, 323–329.

Korsgaard, S., Casey, D. E., Gerlach, J., Hetmar, O., Kaldan, B., and Mikkelsen, L. B. (1982) The effect of tetrahydroisoxazolopyridinol (THIP) in tardive dyskinesia. *Arch. Gen. Psychiatry* **39**, 1017–1021.

Kristiansen, U., Hedegaard, A., Herdeis, C., Lund, T. M., Nielsen, B., Hansen, J. J., Falch, E., Hjeds, H., and Krogsgaard-Larsen, P. (1992) Hydroxylated analogues of 5-aminovaleric acid as 4-aminobutyric acid$_B$ receptor antagonists: stereostructure-activity relationships. *J. Neurochem.* **58**, 1150–1159.

Kristiansen, U., Lambert, J. D. C., Falch, E., and Krogsgaard-Larsen, P. (1991) Electrophysiological studies of the $GABA_A$ receptor ligand, 4-PIOL, on cultured hippocampal neurones. *Br. J. Pharmacol.* **104**, 85–90.

Krnjevic, K. (1974) Chemical nature of synaptic transmission in vertebrates. *Physiol. Rev.* **54**, 418–540.

Krogsgaard-Larsen, P. (1988) GABA synaptic mechanisms: stereochemical and conformational requirements. *Med. Res. Rev.* **8**, 27–56.

Krogsgaard-Larsen, P., Falch, E., and Christensen, A. V. (1984) Chemistry and pharmacology of the GABA agonists THIP (Gaboxadol) and isoguvacine. *Drugs Fut.* **9,** 597–618.

Krogsgaard-Larsen, P., Falch, E., and Hjeds, H. (1985) Heterocyclic analogues of GABA: chemistry, molecular pharmacology and therapeutic aspects. *Prog. Med. Chem.* **22,** 67–120.

Krogsgaard-Larsen, P., Falch, E., Larsson, O. M., and Schousboe, A. (1987) GABA uptake inhibitors: relevance to antiepileptic drug research. *Epilepsy Res.* **1,** 77–93.

Krogsgaard-Larsen, P., Frølund, B., Jørgensen, F. S., and Schousboe, A. (1994) $GABA_A$ receptor agonists, partial agonists, and antagonists. Design and therapeutic prospects. *J. Med. Chem.* **37,** 2489–2505.

Krogsgaard-Larsen, P. and Hansen, J. J., eds. (1992) *Excitatory Amino Acid Receptors: Design of Agonists and Antagonists,* Ellis Horwood, Chichester, UK.

Krogsgaard-Larsen, P., Hjeds, H., Curtis, D. R., Lodge, D., and Johnston, G. A. R. (1979) Dihydromuscimol, thiomuscimol and related heterocyclic compounds as GABA analogues. *J. Neurochem.* **32,** 1717–1724.

Krogsgaard-Larsen, P., Hjeds, H., Falch, E., Jørgensen, F. S., and Nielsen, L. (1988) Recent advances in GABA agonists, antagonists and uptake inhibitors: structure- activity relationships and therapeutic potential. *Adv. Drug Res.* **17,** 381–456.

Krogsgaard-Larsen, P., Jacobsen, P., Brehm, L., Larsen, J.-J., and Schaumburg, K. (1980) GABA agonists and uptake inhibitors designed as agents with irreversible actions. *Eur. J. Med. Chem.* **15,** 529–535.

Krogsgaard-Larsen, P. and Johnston, G. A. R. (1975) Inhibition of GABA uptake in rat brain slices by nipecotic acid, various isoxazoles and related compounds. *J. Neurochem.* **25,** 797–802.

Krogsgaard-Larsen, P., Johnston, G. A. R., Lodge, D., and Curtis, D. R. (1977) A new class of GABA agonist. *Nature* **268,** 53–55.

Krogsgaard-Larsen, P., Mikkelsen, H., Jacobsen, P., Falch, E., Curtis, D. R., Peet, M. J., and Leah, J. D. (1983) 4,5,6,7-Tetrahydroisothiazolo[5,4-c]pyridin-3-ol and related analogues of THIP. Synthesis and biological activity. *J. Med. Chem.* **26,** 895–900.

Krogsgaard-Larsen, P., Nielsen, L., Falch, E., and Curtis, D. R. (1986) GABA agonists. Resolution, absolute stereochemistry, and enantioselectivity of (*S*)-(+)- and (*R*)-(–) dihydromuscimol. *J. Med. Chem.* **28,** 1612–1617.

Krogsgaard-Larsen, P., Snowman, A., Lummis, S. C., and Olsen, R. W. (1981) Characterization of the binding of the GABA agonist [³H]piperidine-4-sulfonic acid to bovine brain synaptic membranes. *J. Neurochem.* **37,** 401–409.

Lambert, J. J., Belelli, D., Hill-Venning, C., and Peters, J. A. (1995) Neurosteroids and $GABA_A$ receptor function. *Trends Pharmacol. Sci.* **16,** 295–303.

Levi, G. and Gallo, V. (1981) Glutamate as a putative transmitter in the cerebellum: stimulation by GABA of glutamic acid release from specific pools. *J. Neurochem.* **37,** 22–31.

Lodge, D., ed. (1988) *Excitatory Amino Acids in Health and Disease,* John Wiley, Chichester, UK.

Lopez, I., Wu, J. Y., and Meza, G. (1992) Immunocytochemical evidence for an afferent GABAergic neurotransmission in the guinea pig vestibular system. *Brain Res.* **589,** 341–348.

Loscher, W. (1989) GABA and the epilepsies. Experimental and clinical conditions, in *GABA: Basic Research and Clinical Applications* (Bowery, N. G. and Nistico, G., eds.), Pythagora, Rome, pp. 260–300.

Lüddens, H., Pritchett, D. B., Kohler, M., Killisch, I., Keinänen, K., Moneyer, H., Sprengel, R., and Seeburg, P. H. (1990) Cerebellar GABA$_A$ receptor selective for a behavioural alcohol antagonist. *Nature* **346**, 648–651.

Macdonald, R. L. and Olsen, R. W. (1994) GABA$_A$ receptor channels. *Annu. Rev. Neurosci.* **17**, 569–602.

Maksay, G. (1994) Thermodynamics of γ-aminobutyric acid type A receptor binding differentiate agonists from antagonists. *Mol. Pharmacol.* **46**, 386–390.

Malcangio, M., Malmberg-Aiello, P., Giotti, A., Ghelardini, C., and Bartolini, A. (1992) Desensitization of GABA$_B$ receptors and antagonism by CGP 35348 prevent bicuculline- and picrotoxin-induced antinociception. *Neuropharmacology* **31**, 783–791.

Malminiemi, O. and Korpi, E. S. (1989) Diazepam-insensitive [^{3}H]Ro 15-4513 binding in intact cultured cerebellar granule cells. *Eur. J. Pharmacol.* **169**, 53–60.

Mathers, D. A. (1987) The GABA$_A$ receptor: new insights from single-channel recording. *Synapse* **1**, 96–101.

McNeil, R. G., Gee, K. W., Bolger, M. B., Lan, N. C., Wieland, S., Belelli, D., Purdy, R. H., and Paul, S. M. (1992) Neuroactive steroids that act at GABA$_A$ receptors. *Drug News Perspect.* **5**, 145–152.

Meier, E., Drejer, J., and Schousboe, A. (1984) GABA induces functionally active low-affinity GABA receptors on cultured cerebellar granule cells. *J. Neurochem.* **43**, 1737–1744.

Meldrum, B. (1982) GABA and acute psychoses. *Psychol. Med.* **12**, 1–5.

Melikian, A., Schlewer, G., Chambon, J.-P., and Wermuth, C. G. (1992) Condensation of muscimol or thiomuscimol with aminopyridazines yields GABA-A antagonists. *J. Med. Chem.* **35**, 4092–4097.

Merz, W. A., Alterwain, P., Ballmer, U., Bechelli, L., Capponi, R., Munoz, J. G., Marquez, C., Nestoros, J., Almanzor, L. R., Udabe, R. U., and Versiani, M. (1988) Treatment of paranoid schizophrenia with the partial benzodiazepine agonist, Ro 16-6028. *Psychopharmacol.* **95-96 (Suppl.)**, 237.

Minchin, M. C. W., Ennis, C., Lattimer, N., White, J. F., White, A. C., and Lloyd, K. G. (1992a) The GABA$_A$-like autoreceptor is a pharmacologically novel GABA receptor, in *GABAergic Synaptic Transmission* (Biggio, G., Concas, A., and Costa, E., eds.), Raven, New York, pp. 199–203.

Minchin, M. C. W., White, A. C., and White, J. F. (1992b) Novel GABA autoreceptor antagonists. *Current Drugs* **2**, 1878–1880.

Mitchell, R. (1980) A novel GABA receptor modulates stimulus induced glutamate release from cortico-striatal terminals. *Eur. J. Pharmacol.* **67**, 119–122.

Möhler, H., Knoflach, F., Paysan, J., Motejlek., K., Benke, D., Luscher, B., and Fritschy, J. M. (1995) Heterogeneity of GABA$_A$-receptors: cell-specific expression, pharmacology, and regulation. *Neurochem. Res.* **20**, 631–636.

Möhler, H. and Okada, T. (1977) Benzodiazepine receptors: demonstration in the central nervous system. *Science* **198**, 849–851.

Morselli, P. L., Loscher, W., Lloyd, K. G., Meldrum, B., and Reynolds, E. H., eds. (1981) *Neurotransmitters, Seizures, and Epilepsy*, Raven, New York.

Nayeem, N., Green, T. P., Martin, I. L., and Barnard, E. A. (1994) Quaternary structure of the native GABA$_A$ receptor determined by electron microscopic image analysis. *J. Neurochem.* **62**, 815–818.

Nielsen, E. Ø., Aarslew-Jensen, M., Diemer, N. H., Krogsgaard-Larsen, P., and Schousboe, A. (1989) Baclofen-induced, calcium-dependent stimulation of *in vivo* release of

D-[³H]aspartate from rat hippocampus monitored by intracerebral microdialysis. *Neurochem. Res.* **14**, 321–326.

Nielsen, L., Brehm, L., and Krogsgaard-Larsen, P. (1990) GABA agonists and uptake inhibitors. Synthesis, absolute stereochemistry, and enantioselectivity of (R)-(–)- and (S)-(+)-homo-β-proline. *J. Med. Chem.* **33**, 71–77.

Nielsen, M., Witt, M.-R., Ebert, B., and Krogsgaard-Larsen, P. (1995) Thiomuscimol, a new photoaffinity label for the GABA$_A$ receptor. *Eur. J. Pharmacol. Mol. Pharmacol. Sect.* **289**, 109–112.

Nistico, G., Morselli, P. L., Lloyd, K. G., Fariello, R. G., and Engel, J., eds. (1986) *Neurotransmitters, Siezures, and Epilepsy III*, Raven, New York.

Olsen, R. W., Bureau, M. H., Edno, S., and Smith, G. (1991) The GABA$_A$ receptor family in the mammalian brain. *Neurochem. Res.* **16**, 317–325.

Olsen, R. W. and Tobin, A. J. (1990) Molecular biology of GABA$_A$ receptors. *FASEB J.* **4**, 1469–1480.

Olsen, R. W. and Venter, J. C., eds. (1986) *Benzodiazepine/GABA Receptors and Chloride Channels: Structural and Functional Properties*, Alan R. Liss, New York.

Ong, J. and Kerr, D. I. B. (1990) GABA-receptors in peripheral tissues. *Life Sci.* **46**, 1489–1501.

Ong, J., Kerr, D. I. B., Capper, H. R., and Johnston, G. A. R. (1990) Cortisone, a potent GABA$_A$ antagonist in the guinea-pig isolated ileum. *J. Pharm. Pharmacol.* **42**, 662–664.

Ong, J., Kerr, D. I. B., and Johnston, G. A. R. (1987) Cortisol: a potent biphasic modulator at GABA$_A$-receptor-complexes in the guinea-pig isolated ileum. *Neurosci. Lett.* **82**, 101–106.

Palay, S. and Chan-Palay, V. (1982) The cerebellum-new vistas. *Exp. Brain. Res. Suppl.* **6**, 1–620.

Petersen, H. R., Jensen, I., and Dam, M. (1983) THIP: a single-blind controlled trial in patients with epilepsy. *Acta Neurol. Scand.* **67**, 114–117.

Peyron, R., Cinotti, L., Le Bars, D., Garcia-Larrea, L., Galy, G., Landais, P., Millet, P., Lavenne, F., Froment, J. C., Krogsgaard-Larsen, F., and Mauguiere, F. (1994b) Effects of GABA$_A$ receptor activation on brain glucose metabolism in normal subjects and temporal lobe epilepsy (TLE) patients. A positron emission tomography (PET) study. II. The focal hypometabolism is reactive to GABA$_A$ agonist administration in TLE. *Epilepsy Res.* **19**, 55–62.

Peyron, R., Le Bars, D., Cinotti, L., Garcia-Larrea, L., Galy, G., Landais, P., Millet, P., Lavenne, F., Froment, J. C., Krogsgaard-Larsen, P., and Mauguiere, F. (1994a) Effects of GABA$_A$ receptor activation on brain glucose metabolism in normal subjects and temporal lope epilepsy (TLE) patients. A positron emission tomography (PET) study. I. Brain glucose metabolism is increased after GABA$_A$ receptors activation. *Epilepsy Res.* **19**, 45–54.

Prince, R. J. and Simmonds, M. A. (1993) Differential antagonism by epipregnanolone of alphaxalone and pregnanolone potentiation of [³H]flunitrazepam binding suggests more than one class of binding site for steroids at GABA$_A$ receptors. *Neuropharmacology* **32**, 59–63.

Qian, H. and Dowling, J. E. (1993a) Novel GABA responses from rod-driven retinal horizontal cells. *Nature* **361**, 162–164.

Qian, H. and Dowling, J. E. (1993b) GABA responses on retinal bipolar cells. *Biol. Bull.* **185**, 312.

Qian, H. and Dowling, J. E. (1994) Pharmacology of novel GABA receptors found on rod horizontal cells of the white perch retina. *J. Neurosci.* **14,** 4299–4307.

Redburn, D. A. and Schousboe, A., eds. (1987) *Neurotrophic Activity of GABA During Development*, Alan R. Liss, New York.

Ring, H. A. and Reynolds, E. H. (1990) Vigabatrin and behaviour disturbance. *Lancet* **335,** 970.

Roberts, E. (1976) Disinhibition as an organizing principle in the nervous system—the role of the GABA system. Application to neurologic and psychiatric disorders, in *GABA in Nervous System Function* (Roberts, E., Chase, T. N., and Tower, D. B., eds.), Raven, New York, pp. 515–539.

Roberts, E. (1986) GABA: the road to neurotransmitter status, in *Benzodiazepine/GABA Receptors and Chloride Channels: Structural and Functional Properties* (Olsen, R. W., and Venter, J. C., eds.), Alan R. Liss, New York, pp. 1–39.

Roberts, E. (1991) Living systems are tonically inhibited, autonomous optimizers, and disinhibition coupled to a variability generation is their major organizing principle: inhibitory command-control at levels of membrane, genome, metabolism, brain, and society. *Neurochem. Res.* **16,** 409–421.

Robinson, M. K., Richens, A., and Oxley, R. (1990) Vigabatrin and behaviour disturbances. *Lancet* **336,** 504.

Rognan, D., Boulanger, T., Hoffmann, R., Vercauteren, D. P., Andre, J.-M., Durant, F., and Wermuth, C. G. (1992) Structure and molecular modeling of GABA_A receptor antagonists. *J. Med. Chem.* **35,** 1969–1977.

Roland, P. E. and Friberg, L. (1988) The effect of the GABA_A agonist THIP on regional cortical blood flow in humans. A new test of hemispheric dominans. *J. Cereb. Blood Flow Metab.* **8,** 314–323.

Rorsman, P., Berggren, P.-O., Bokvist, K., Ericson, H., Möhler, H., Ostenson, C.-G., and Smith, P. A. (1989) Glucose-inhibition of glucagon secretion involves activation of GABA_A-receptor chloride channels. *Nature* **341,** 233–236.

Ryan, A. F. and Schwartz, I. R. (1986) Nipecotic acid: preferential accumulation in the cochlea by GABA uptake systems and selective retrograde transport to brainstem. *Brain Res.* **399,** 399–403.

Saito, A., Wu, J. Y., and Lee, T. J. (1985) Evidence for the presence of cholinergic nerves in cerebral arteries: an immunohistochemical demonstration of choline acetyltransferase. *J. Cereb. Blood Flow Metab.* **5,** 327–334.

Sander, J. W. and Hart, Y. M. (1990) Vigabatrin and behaviour disturbances. *Lancet* **335,** 57.

Sawynok, J. (1989) GABAergic agents as analgesics, in *GABA: Basic Research and Clinical Applications* (Bowery, N. G. and Nistico, G., eds.), Pythagora, Rome, pp. 383–399.

Schousboe, A., Diemer, N. H., and Kofod, H., eds. (1992a) *Drug Research Related to Neuroactive Amino Acids*, Munksgaard, Copenhagen.

Schousboe, A., Hansen, G. H., and Belhage, B. (1992b) Regulation of neurotransmitter release by GABA_A receptors in glutamatergic neurons, in *New Leads and Targets in Drug Research* (Krogsgaard-Larsen, P., Christensen, S. B., and Kofod, H., eds.), Munksgaard, Copenhagen, pp. 176–186.

Schousboe, A., Larsson, O. M., Hertz, L., and Krogsgaard-Larsen, P. (1981) Heterocyclic GABA analogues as new selective inhibitors of astroglial GABA transport. *Drug Dev. Res.* **1,** 115–127.

Schousboe, A., Thorbek, P., Hertz, L., and Krogsgaard-Larsen, P. (1979) Effects of GABA analogues of restricted conformation on GABA transport in astrocytes and brain cortex slices and on GABA receptor binding. *J. Neurochem.* **33**, 181–189.

Serra, M., Foddi, M. C., Ghiani, C. A., Melis, M. A., Motzo, C., Concas, A., Sanna, E., and Biggio, G. (1992) Pharmacology of γ-aminobutyric acid$_A$ receptor complex after the *in vivo* administration of the anxioselective and anticonvulsant β-carboline derivative abecarnil. *Pharmacol. Exp. Ther.* **263**, 1360–1368.

Sieghart, W. (1992) GABA$_A$ receptors: ligand-gated Cl– ion channels modulated by multiple drug-binding sites. *Trends Pharmacol. Sci.* **13**, 446–450.

Sieghart, W. (1995) Structure and pharmacology of γ-aminobutyric acid$_A$ receptor subtypes. *Pharmacol. Rev.* **47**, 181–234.

Sieghart, W., Eichinger, A., Richards, J. G., and Möhler, H. (1987) Photoaffinity labeling of benzodiazepine receptor proteins with the partial inverse agonist [³H]Ro 15-4513: a biochemical and autoradiographic study. *J. Neurochem.* **48**, 46–52.

Sivilotti, L. and Nistri, A. (1991) GABA inhibits neuronal activity by activating GABA$_B$ receptors coupled to K$^+$ channels. *Prog. Neurobiol.* **36**, 35–92.

Smith, G. B. and Olsen, R. W. (1995) Functional domains of GABA$_A$ receptors. *Trends Pharmacol. Sci.* **16**, 162–168.

Solimena, M. and De Camilli, P. (1993) Spotlight on a neuronal enzyme. *Nature* **366**, 15–17.

Squires, R. F. and Braestrup, C. (1977) Benzodiazepine receptors in rat brain. *Nature* **266**, 732–734.

Squires, R. F., Lajtha, A., Saederup, E., and Palkovits, M. (1993) Reduced [³H]flunitrazepam binding in cingulate cortex and hippocampus of post mortem schizophrenic brains: is selective loss of glutamatergic neurons associated with major psychoses. *Neurochem. Res.* **18**, 219–223.

Squires, R. F. and Saederup, E. (1991) A review of evidence for GABAergic predominance/glutamertergic deficit as a common etiological factor in both schizophrenia and affective psychoses: more support for a continuum hypothesis of "functional" psychosis . *Neurochem. Res.* **16**, 1099–1111.

Stone, T. W. (1979) Glutamate as the neurotransmitter of cerebellar granule cells in the rat: electrophysiological evidence. *Br. J. Pharmacol.* **66**, 291–296.

Supavilai, P. and Karobath, M. (1985) Modulation of acetylcholine release from rat striatal slices by the GABA/benzodiazepine receptor complex. *Life Sci.* **36**, 417–426.

Tallman, J. F., Paul, S. M., Skolnick, P., and Gallager, D. W. (1980) Receptors for the age of anxiety: pharmacology of the benzodiazepines. *Science* **207**, 274–281.

Tamminga, C. A., Crayton, J. W., and Chase, T. N. (1978) Muscimol: GABA agonist therapy in schizophrenia. *Am. J. Psychiat.* **135**, 746–747.

Tamminga, C. A., Crayton, J. W., and Chase, T. N. (1979) Improvement of tardive dyskinesia after muscimol therapy. *Arch. Gen. Psychiat.* **36**, 595–598.

Thaker, G. K., Hare, T. A., and Tamminga, C. A. (1983) GABA system: clinical research and treatment of tardive dyskinesia. *Mod. Probl. Pharmacopsychiat.* **21**, 155–167.

Thaker, G. K., Nguyen, J. A., and Tamminga, C. A. (1989) Increased saccadic distractability in tardive dyskinesia: functional evidence for subcortical GABA dysfunction. *Biol. Psychiatry* **25**, 49–59.

Theobald, W., Buch, O., Kunz, H. A., Krupp, P., Stenger, E. G., and Heimann, H. (1968) Pharmakologische und experimentalpsychologische untersuchungen mit 2 inhaltsstoffen des fliegenpilzes (amanita muscaria). *Arzneim. Forsch.* **18**, 311–315.

Tirsch, R., Yang, X.-D., Singer, S. M., Liblau, R. S., Fugger, L., and McDevitt, H. O. (1993) Immune response to glutamic acid decarboxylase correlates with insulitis in non-obese diabetic mice. *Nature* **366,** 72–75.

Travagli, R. A., Ulivi, M., and Wojcik, W. J (1991) γ-Aminobutyric acid-B receptors inhibit glutamate release from cerebellar granule cells: consequences of inhibiting cyclic AMP formation and calcium influx. *J. Pharm. Exp. Ther.* **258,** 903–909.

Usami, S., Hozawa, J., Tazawa, M., Igarashi, M., Thompson, G. C., Wu, J. Y., and Wenthold, R. J. (1989) Immunocytochemical study of the GABA system in chicken vestibular endorgans and the vestibular ganglion. *Brain Res.* **503,** 214–218.

Van Ness, P. C., Watkins, A. E., Bergman, M. O., Tourtelotte, W. W., and Olsen, R. W. (1982) γ-Aminobutyric acid receptors in normal human brain and Huntington's disease. *Neurology* **32,** 63–68.

Venault, P., Chapouthier, G., Prado de Carvalho, L., Simiand, J., Morre, M., Dodd, R. H., and Rossier, J. (1986) Benzodiazepine impairs and β-carboline enhances performance in learning and memory tasks. *Nature* **321,** 864–866.

Verdoorn, T. A., Draguhn, A., Ymer, S., Seeburg, P. H., and Sakmann, B. (1990) Functional properties of recombinant rat GABA$_A$ receptors depend upon subunit composition. *Neuron* **4,** 919–928.

Virmani, M. A., Stojilkovic, S. S., and Catt, K. J. (1990) Stimulation of luteinizing hormone release by γ-aminobutyric acid (GABA) agonists: mediation by GABA$_A$-type receptors and activation of chloride and voltage-sensitive calcium channels. *Endocrinology* **126,** 2499–2505.

Walton, M. K., Schaffner, A. E., and Barker, J. L. (1993) Sodium channels, GABA$_A$ receptors, and glutamate receptors develop sequentially on embryonic rat spinal cord cells. *J. Neurosci.* **13,** 2068–2084.

Wermuth, C. G. and Biziére, K. (1986) Pyridazinyl-GABA derivatives: a new class of synthetic GABA$_A$ antagonists. *Trends Pharmacol. Sci.* **7,** 421–424.

Wermuth, C. G., Bourguignon, J.-J., Schlewer, G., Gies, J.-P., Schoenfelder, A., Melikian, A., Bouchet, M.-J., Chantreux, D., Molimard, J.-C., Heaulme, M., Chambon, J.-P., and Biziére, K. (1987) Synthesis and structure-activity relationships of a series of aminopyridazine derivatives of γ-aminobutyric acid acting as selective GABA-A antagonists. *J. Med. Chem.* **30,** 239–249.

Wheal, H. and Thomson, A., eds. (1995) *Excitatory Amino Acids and Synaptic Transmission, 2nd ed.*, Academic, London.

Wieland, H. A., Luddens, H., and Seeburg, P. H. (1992) A single histidine in GABA$_A$ receptors is essential for benzodiazepine agonist binding. *J. Biol. Chem.* **267,** 1426–1429.

Woodward, R. M., Polenzani, L., and Miledi, R. (1993) Characterization of bicuculline/baclofen-insensitive (r-like) γ-aminobutyric acid receptors expressed in *Xenopus* oocytes. II. Pharmacology of γ-aminobutyric acid$_A$ and γ-aminobutyric acid$_B$ receptor agonists and antagonists. *Mol. Pharmacol.* **43,** 609–625.

Wurtman, R. J., Corkin, S., Growdon, J. H., and Ritter-Walker, E., eds. (1990) *Advances in Neurology,* vol. 51. *Alzheimer's Disease,* Raven, New York.

Zhang, P., Zhang, W., Liu, R., Harris, B., Skolnick, P., and Cook, J. M. (1995) Synthesis of novel imidazobenzodiazepines as probes of the pharmacophore for "diazepam-insensitive" GABA$_A$ receptors. *J. Med. Chem.* **38,** 1679–1688.

Zorn, S. H. and Enna, S. J. (1987) The GABA agonist THIP attenuates antinociception in the mouse by modifying central cholinergic transmission. *Neuropharmacology* **26,** 433–437.

CHAPTER 4

Pharmacology of Mammalian GABA$_A$ Receptors

Neil Upton and Thomas Blackburn

1. Introduction

γ-Aminobutyric acid (GABA) is the most prevalent neurotransmitter in the mammalian brain and exerts its main actions through GABA$_A$ receptors (GABA$_A$Rs). GABA$_A$Rs have proven to serve as the primary target for many important neuroactive drugs, including benzodiazepines (BZs), barbiturates, steroids, general anesthetics, and possibly ethanol (Macdonald and Olsen, 1994). Recent elegant studies of the molecular nature of GABA$_A$Rs have revealed the existence of multiple subtypes of these receptors, the composition of which is determined by the formation of pentameric structures from members of at least three distinct subunit families (α1–6, β1–3, γ1–3) (Lüddens et al., 1995). Furthermore, by using sophisticated in vitro techniques, the regulation of functional properties by GABA itself, as well as other modulators of GABA$_A$Rs, has now been shown to differ dramatically with the type of subunit variants in the pentameric complex (Lüddens et al., 1995; Sieghart, 1995).

This diversity of GABA$_A$Rs is presumed to be the means of providing several functionally distinct inhibitory pathways within the central nervous system (CNS). It has also led to speculation that it may be possible to target various GABA$_A$R subtypes in order to develop drugs of improved clinical profile over agents such as the BZs. This strategy does not negate the validity of an earlier theory proposing that agents with reduced intrinsic activity (relative to full agonist BZs) at BZ receptors would exhibit similarly enhanced therapeutic profiles (Haefely et al., 1990). Indeed, as would be predicted, both functional activity and GABA$_A$R subtype selectivity are the key determinants of the pharmacological actions of modulators at these sites (see Section 10.).

The GABA Receptors Eds.: S. J. Enna and N. G. Bowery
Humana Press Inc., Totowa, NJ

It has become increasingly evident that the many classes of agents that interact with central GABA$_A$Rs exhibit widely diverse pharmacological profiles. In this chapter, we will highlight the pharmacological properties of selected modulators of these receptors and discuss whether their varied actions can be used to provide an insight into the likely roles for the various subtypes of GABA$_A$Rs at the behavioral level.

2. Pharmacological Characteristics, Structure, and Distribution of GABA$_A$Rs

GABA transmits the majority of all inhibitory fast signaling in the mammalian brain via an action at GABA$_A$Rs. These receptors are multi-subunit Cl$^-$ ionophores possessing binding sites for many classes of drugs and their unique properties are exemplified by the different pharmacological profiles of the various allosteric modulators now known to act at GABA$_A$Rs. Thus, both in vitro and in vivo studies indicate that anxiolytic, anticonvulsant, muscle relaxant, and sedative-hypnotic BZs and some depressant barbiturates enhance the action of GABA at GABA$_A$Rs; conversely, anxiogenic or convulsant β-carbolines reduce GABA$_A$-ergic function. In addition, several anesthetics, neurotoxins, neuroactive steroids, and ethanol produce at least part of their pharmacological effects by interacting with GABA$_A$Rs. The rich pharmacology exhibited by the many agents that modulate GABA$_A$Rs also strongly indicates that these sites are intimately involved in neuronal systems mediating anxiety, seizures, cognition, motor coordination, arousal, and possibly reward. In retrospect, it is not surprising, given the diversity of these neurophysiological roles, that GABA$_A$Rs have evolved as a heterogenous population within the brain.

GABA$_A$Rs are members of a large superfamily of ligand-gated ion channels. Evaluation of receptor size and visualization by electron microscopy concluded that, like the nicotinic acetylcholine receptor, they are heteropentameric glycoproteins (Fig. 1) of approx 275 kDa (Olsen and Tobin, 1990). To date, at least 13 (α1–6, β1–3, γ1–3, δ) distinct mammalian subunits of GABA$_A$Rs have been identified and shown to have differing distributions between brain regions, and even between the cell types within those regions (Wisden et al., 1992). It is now recognized that an α subunit, a β subunit, and a γ subunit are required to form a fully functional GABA$_A$R (Pritchett et al., 1989b). Selection of at least one of each of these three types of subunits from the above 13 allows for the possible existence of more than 10,000 pentameric subunit combinations (McKernan and Whiting, 1996). This calculation does not take into account several subunits that exist as splice variants (Lüddens et al., 1995; Sieghart, 1995). However, based on studies

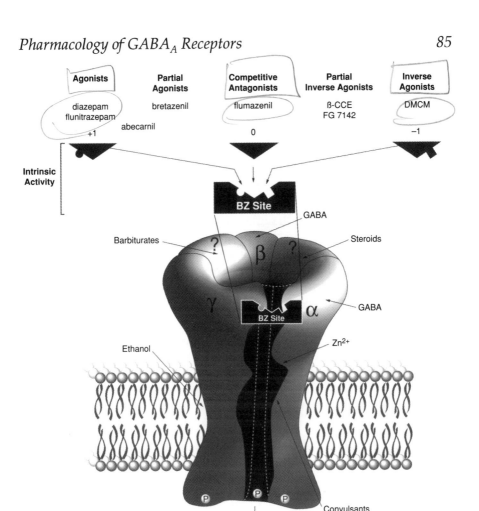

Fig. 1. Schematic representation of the proposed pentameric structure of GABA_ARs, depicted as containing the α, β, and γ subunits required to form fully functional receptors. Binding sites for GABA and receptor modulators are assigned to their respective subunits, where such evidence exists. Also illustrated is the spectrum of agonism through antagonism to inverse agonism displayed by agents that interact with the BZ binding sites associated with GABA_ARs.

using antibody, radioligand binding, and immunopurifying techniques, it has been suggested that less than ten major subtypes of GABA_ARs actually exist in adult mammalian brain (McKernan and Whiting, 1996) (although no functional subunit combination can be ignored, since even a rare receptor may have important functions for a limited neuronal population). The composition of these subtypes, together with their distribution and pharmacological characteristics, are summarized in Table 1 (*see* McKernan and Whiting, 1996; and Chapter 2, this volume, for further information). The localization and constitution of GABA$_A$Rs varies dramatically during postnatal development, with the observed rapid increase in the proportion of α1-subunit-containing receptors (corresponding to BZ1 sites; *see* Section 5.) being particularly striking (Brooks-Kayal and Pritchett, 1993; Fritschy et al., 1994; Paysan et al., 1994). These changes may be related to the functional maturation of inhibitory pathways in discrete brain regions (Payson et al., 1994; Schousboe and Redburn, 1995) but as yet, no clear physiological roles have been identified for the individual GABA$_A$R subtypes.

One of the most intriguing findings in the pharmacology of GABA$_A$Rs is the existence of the many modulatory sites on these receptors. This raises the possibility that, in addition to GABA, other endogenous ligands for GABA$_A$Rs may be present in brain. There have been numerous candidates for such roles; among the most likely are the polypeptides, diazepam binding inhibitor (DBI: which acts as a partial inverse agonist at GABA$_A$Rs) and its processing products (for review, *see* Costa and Guidotti, 1991), and a family of neuroactive steroids (*see* Section 7.). There appears to be a further link between these two classes of modulators because DBI regulates the synthesis of neuroactive steroids in the brain through an action at peripheral-type BZ receptors (Costa and Guidotti, 1991).

3. The GABA Binding Site of GABA$_A$Rs

Activation of GABA$_A$Rs by GABA results in an increase in neuronal membrane conductance for Cl$^-$ because of prolonged openings of the ion channel (Macdonald and Twyman, 1992). In turn, this causes a localized hyperpolarization of the neuronal membrane (as Cl$^-$ moves into the cell along its concentration gradient), which counteracts the effects of depolarizing stimuli (Bormann, 1988; Study and Barker, 1981). The inhibitory action of GABA can be competitively antagonized by bicuculline or mimicked by full agonists, such as muscimol. Partial agonists at GABA binding sites (e.g., piperidine 4-sulphonic acid) have also been described (*see* Sieghart, 1995).

[^{3}H]GABA or [^{3}H]muscimol binding studies in mammalian brain tissue reveal both high- and low-affinity states for GABA with K_D values in the low and high nanomolar range, respectively (Olsen et al., 1981). The low-affinity recognition site seems to be an antagonist-preferring site since it can be specifically labeled by bicuculline (Olsen and Snowman, 1983). However, it is now generally considered that GABA exerts its physiological effects by acting at an additional very low affinity binding site. Thus, micromolar con-

Table 1
Structure, Distribution, and Pharmacological Characteristics
of the Major GABA$_A$R Subtypes in Rat Brain

Subtype	Relative abundance in rat brain, %	Location	Pharmacological characteristics
α1β2γ2	43	Most brain areas. Localized to interneurons in hippocampus and cortex, and cerebral Purkinje cells	BZ1 Subtype
α2β2/3γ2	18	Spinal cord motorneurons and hippocampal pyramidal cells	BZ2 Subtype
α3βγ2/3	17	Cholinergic and monoaminergic neurons	BZ2 Subtype
α2βγ1	8	Bergmann glia, nuclei of the limbic systems	
α5β3γ2/3	4	Predominantly on hippocampal pyramidal cells	BZ2 Subtype (zolpidem insensitive)
α6βγ2	2	Cerebellar granule cells	Diazepam insensitive
α6βδ	2	Cerebellar granule cells	
α4βδ	3	Thalamus and hippocampal dentate gyrus	
Other minor subtypes	3	Throughout brain	

Adapted from McKernan and Whiting, 1996.

centrations of GABA are needed to open Cl⁻ channels in ion flux (Kardos and Cash, 1990) and electrophysiological experiments (Segal and Barker, 1984) and to modulate other binding sites on the GABA$_A$R complex (Karobath et al., 1979; Olsen, 1982; Squires et al., 1983).

The apparent separate existence of high-, low-, or very low-affinity binding sites for GABA can be explained in terms of different affinity states of the same receptor or, alternatively, if it is assumed that there are several distinct GABA binding sites on a single GABA$_A$R (Sieghart, 1995). In recombinant GABA$_A$Rs, homooligomeric channels consisting of α, β, γ, or δ subunits exhibit multiple conductance states in response to GABA, suggesting that the neurotransmitter binding site may be constitutively present on each of these subunits, or can form on assembly of homo- or hetrooligomeric channels. Theoretically, this allows for up to five GABA binding sites on each

GABA$_A$R (a similar argument can be made for barbiturate and neuroactive steroid binding sites) (Sieghart, 1995). Other studies indicate that a minimal composition of α and β subunits is required for fully effective GABA-dependent gating and that the agonist binding site may reside on the interface between these different subunits (*see* Smith and Olsen, 1995).

In agreement with the notion that GABA$_A$Rs contain a multiplicity of allosteric binding sites, GABA can modulate the binding of a variety of different compounds and vice versa. For example, the affinities of agonists, antagonists, or inverse agonists at BZ receptors are enhanced, unchanged, or reduced, respectively, by the presence of GABA. The extent of this so-called GABA shift (Möhler and Richards, 1981; Braestrup et al., 1982) also provides an indication of the level of intrinsic activity at BZ receptors, with partial agonists such as bretazenil and abecarnil, undergoing a smaller shift than the full agonist diazepam (e.g., Stephens et al., 1992).

4. The Convulsant Binding Site of GABA$_A$Rs

The cage convulsants *t*-butylbicyclophosphorothionate (TBPS) and picrotoxin share the same unique binding site on GABA$_A$Rs, where they act to inhibit the amplitude of neuronal GABA-activated Cl$^-$ currents (Bowery et al., 1976; Squires et al., 1983). As such, they are regarded as noncompetitive antagonists of GABA$_A$Rs, since they do not compete directly with GABA for its recognition site. There is some controversy about whether these agents bind to a modulatory site on GABA$_A$Rs or directly to the channel pore (Lüddens et al., 1995). Recent electrophysiological studies in recombinant GABA$_A$Rs indicate that TBPS and picrotoxin interact with both resting and GABA-bound receptors. Although displaying 10-fold greater affinity for the latter, these agents appeared to behave as allosteric modulators rather than as open channel blockers (Dillon et al., 1995). The binding site itself appears to be present on α, β, and γ subunits alike (Sieghart, 1995).

In addition to GABA, most other substances known to interact with GABA$_A$Rs allosterically modulate the convulsant binding site labeled by [^{35}S]TBPS. Thus, agents that facilitate the opening of Cl$^-$ channels, such as barbiturates and steroids, potently inhibit [^{35}S]TBPS binding; it is affected in the opposite manner by drugs that reduce GABA$_A$-ergic transmission (Squires et al., 1983; Supavilai and Korath, 1984; Gee et al., 1986; Concas et al., 1988). Importantly, BZs inhibit the binding of [^{35}S]TBPS only when micromolar GABA is included in the assay (Gee, 1988; Im and Blakeman, 1991), an observation in keeping with the finding that the neurotransmitter is an absolute requirement for this class of compounds to open Cl$^-$ channels (*see* Section 5.1.). These data suggest that the degree of [^{35}S]TBPS binding in the presence of GABA closely reflects the functional state of $GABA_ARs$ and may therefore be useful for characterization of allosteric interactions between various sites on these receptors (Im and Blakeman, 1991).

5. The BZ Binding Sites of $GABA_ARs$

There is little doubt that the BZs are one of the most important classes of drugs used in clinical psychopharmacology. For over 30 years they have been in widespread use as anxiolytics, anticonvulsants, and sedative hypnotics and have been shown to be remarkably well-tolerated, safe, and effective, although they are not without their problems (Woods et al., 1987, 1992; Hollister et al., 1993). Following the proposal that BZs act primarily by facilitating $GABA_A$-ergic neurotransmission (Costa et al., 1975; Haefely et al., 1975), a major advance in the understanding of the mode of action of these drugs came when it was demonstrated that they bind to high-affinity sites in the brain (Möhler and Okada, 1977; Braestrup, 1977; Squires and Braestrup, 1977). These sites, now referred to as BZ receptors, form an integral part of the $GABA_AR$ complex, at which BZ receptor agonists act to positively modulate the activity of GABA by allosterically influencing the conformation of the neurotransmitter recognition site.

The availability of a radioligand binding assay for BZ receptors (Squires and Braestrup, 1977) provided a powerful tool in the search for endogenous modulators of these sites and for BZ receptor ligands with improved pharmacological profiles (e.g., lacking unwanted effects, such as ataxia and cognitive impairment) compared to classical BZs. However, an unexpected consequence of these efforts was the discovery of compounds (e.g., FG 7142 and DMCM; methyl,6,7-dimethoxy-4-ethyl-β-carboline-3-carboxylate) which illustrated that BZ receptors could exert a bidirectional modulation of the $GABA_AR$ complex (Fig. 1). Such agents (which have been termed inverse agonists) reduced the actions of GABA and were anxiogenic and proconvulsant in vivo (Hunkeler et al., 1981). The effects of both classical agonists and inverse agonists were blocked by BZ receptor antagonists (i.e., compounds with no or negligible intrinsic activity, such as flumazenil), indicating that they acted through the same receptor (Hunkeler et al., 1981).

As the availability of new chemical classes of BZ receptor ligands increased, it also became apparent that the population of BZ receptors within the brain was not homogenous. On the basis of biochemical and pharmacological differences, it was initially suggested that BZ receptors could be designated as two distinct subtypes; so-called Type I (now called BZ1, or ω1) and Type II (BZ2, or ω2) receptors (Klepner et al., 1979; Lippa et al., 1979; Squires et al., 1979). BZ1 receptors constitute the major population of binding sites in most rodent brain structures and are particularly predominant in cerebellum. In contrast, BZ2 receptors are enriched in only a few brain areas, such as hippocampus, striatum, and spinal cord (Benavides et al., 1993).

Several compounds, most notably CL 218,872, zolpidem, and alpidem, show some selectivity for BZ1 receptors (Squires et al., 1979; Arbilla et al., 1985; Langer and Arbilla, 1988a,b) although no BZ2 selective agents have yet been identified.

A third type of BZ receptor has been described (variously referred to as the peripheral-type BZ, or mitochondrial diazepam binding inhibitor receptor), which is most abundant in peripheral tissues (Anholt et al., 1985), but also has a central localization, mainly in glial cells (Dubois et al., 1988). This binding site is structurally and functionally unrelated to central BZ receptors and is not associated with $GABA_ARs$ (Parola et al., 1993).

The advent of recent rapid developments in our knowledge of the molecular nature of $GABA_ARs$ has highlighted that, although the BZ1/BZ2 classification now appears to be something of an oversimplification, it does have a sound structural basis. From studies with recombinant $GABA_ARs$, it has become fairly well-established that the heterogeneity of BZ binding sites mainly arises from the existence of different α subunits; the presence of a $\gamma2$ subunit is required to convey a functional BZ site to the receptor (Pritchett et al., 1989a,b; Angelotti and Macdonald, 1993). The pharmacological and electrophysiological properties of BZ1 receptors can be mimicked only by recombinant receptors of the $\alpha1\beta x\gamma2$ type; BZ2 receptors assemble from $\alpha2$, $\alpha3$, or $\alpha5$ subunit variants together with the $\beta x\gamma2$ combination (Pritchett et al., 1989b; Pritchett and Seebury, 1990). BZ2 receptors can be further differentiated according to their intermediate ($\alpha2$ and $\alpha3\beta x\gamma2$) or very low affinities ($\alpha5\beta x\gamma2$) for zolpidem. $GABA_ARs$ containing $\alpha4$ or $\alpha6$ isotypes are insensitive to classical BZs (Sieghart, 1995).

The diverse pharmacological profiles of compounds with differing intrinsic activities at BZ receptors and/or relative selectivity for $GABA_A$/BZ receptor subtypes are described below.

5.1. Classical Full Agonist BZs

The modern era of the BZs as the most frequently prescribed psychotropic agents (Leonard, 1993) began in the early 1960s, with the introduction of chlordiazepoxide into clinical practice. Since that time, a whole host of BZs have been identified (e.g., diazepam, flunitrazepam, triazolam, alprazolam, clonazepam) and it is thought that as many as 50 of this class of compounds are now in use worldwide (Potokar and Nutt, 1994), principally for the treatment of anxiety, insomnia, and epilepsy. They are also used as myorelaxants for some specific circumstances, such as premedication in anesthesia. This profile of activity has now become established as that of a classical full agonist BZ (Gardner, 1989).

BZ agonists, such as diazepam, enhance the actions of GABA at the $GABA_A R$ complex both by facilitating its binding to the receptor and by increasing receptor-ion channel coupling (Study and Barker, 1981; Edgar and Schwarz, 1992); they do not, however, open channels in the absence of GABA (Study and Barker, 1981; Polc, 1988). This potentiation of GABA is mediated by an action at a specific BZ receptor that is an integral modulatory unit of the $GABA_A R$ complex (Haefely, 1989). As a result of the excellent correlation between the clinical potency of BZs and their affinity for the [^{3}H]flunitrazepam (BZ) binding site, it is believed that these sites are the pharmacological receptors by which the BZs exert their clinically important actions (Haefely et al., 1985). Evidence that the selective BZ receptor antagonist flumazenil blocks the central pharmacological effects of BZs (*see* Section 5.4.) supports this conclusion.

Photoaffinity labeling studies indicate that the BZ binding site is located on the α subunit, or perhaps at the α/γ subunit interface of the $GABA_A R$ (Fuchs et al., 1988; Stephenson et al., 1990). Classical BZs bind with similar high affinity to recombinant receptors containing α1, α2, α3, or α5 subunits, but have low affinity for receptors constituted with α4 or α6 isotypes (*see* Sieghart, 1995). This lack of α subunit selectivity (which is also evident in brain tissue, where BZs do not discriminate between BZ1 and BZ2 receptor subtypes; Braestrup and Nelsen, 1983) may account for the multiplicity of pharmacological effects of BZ receptor agonists. The presence of a γ (optimally γ2) subunit allows BZs to allosterically modulate $GABA_A Rs$ (Pritchett et al., 1989b). Genetically engineered mice lacking the γ2 subunit are insensitive to the behavioral effects of diazepam, and provide elegant confirmation of the importance of the γ2 subtype to the pharmacological properties of BZs (Günther et al., 1995).

The effects of BZ agonists on animal behavior have proven to be highly predictive of the observed pharmacological profile in man. This class of compounds produces what is considered to reflect marked anxiolytic activity in a wide variety of rodent (and to a lesser extent, primate) tests, which can be broadly categorized according to the type of anxiety-provoking stimulus that they utilize: conflict or conditioning (e.g., Geller-Seifter conflict and conditioned emotional response); novel situations (social interaction and elevated plus maze); and anxiogenic chemicals (e.g., FG 7142) (Thiebot and Soubrie, 1983; File and Pellow, 1987; Giusti and Arban, 1993). In addition, classical BZs attenuate several physiological, biochemical, and pathological correlates of stress, including a decrease in activation of the hypothalamic-pituitary-adrenocortical system, and in most situations reduce aggression (Thiebot and Soubrie, 1983; File and Pellow, 1987).

Another important property of BZ agonists is their ability to produce broad spectrum anticonvulsant activity in animal models. They inhibit seizures in genetically susceptible rodents and baboons and convulsions induced by various chemicals (e.g., pentylenetetrazol, bicuculline, and picrotoxin), electroshock, and repeated electrical stimulation of discrete brain areas (File and Pellow, 1987; Löscher and Schmidt, 1988). In rodents, it is generally possible to produce anxiolytic and anticonvulsant activity at doses of BZ agonists that are devoid of the well-known muscle relaxant and sedative properties of these agents (Gardner, 1989), although there can be an overlap, depending on the test systems used. This observation is consistent with the finding that the anxiolytic/anticonvulsant activities of diazepam and triazolam are elicited at a lower functional BZ receptor occupancy than their muscle relaxant/sedative actions (Facklam et al., 1992a). Other effects of BZs observed in animals include cognitive impairment (File and Pellow, 1987) and potentiation of the depressant action of ethanol.

Upon repeated administration, tolerance (loss of efficacy) has been demonstrated to most of the behavioral effects of BZs in animals, but the rate at which this phenomenon occurs is different for the various behavioral actions (e.g., in some studies, 3–5 d for sedative/anticonvulsant properties and 10–15 d for anxiolytic effects; File, 1985). Another consequence of long-term dosing with BZ agonists is the induction of a dependence state in which abrupt discontinuation of drug treatment, or administration of a BZ receptor antagonist, results in withdrawal symptoms that are usually of a nature that is opposite to the primary drug effects (File and Pellow, 1987; Schoh et al., 1993). The precise cellular and molecular mechanisms underlying tolerance to, and dependence on, BZs are not fully understood. However, down-regulation of BZ receptors (measured using in vivo binding techniques) (Miller et al., 1988, 1989) and a loss of allosteric coupling efficiency between BZ and GABA recognition sites (Gallager et al., 1984; Allan et al., 1992) have been demonstrated with reasonable consistency after prolonged treatment with BZ agonists. As yet, there is no clear link between such changes and differences in either mRNA levels or polypeptide expression of individual subunits of the $GABA_AR$ (Wu et al., 1995). The net effect of whatever receptor events do occur appears to be a shift in the set-point of the $GABA_AR$ complex, so that it becomes less sensitive to full agonists and more sensitive to inverse agonists (Nutt et al., 1992).

The most widespread clinical application of BZ agonists is in the treatment of pathological anxiety and panic disorder, where they have proven efficacy (Rickels and Schweizer, 1987; Charney and Woods, 1989) but can be associated with inappropriate sedation and muscle relaxation (Lader, 1994). The latter two properties are utilized therapeutically in their own right to alleviate insomnia and muscle tension, respectively. Cognitive impairment (File and Pellow, 1987) and a potentially lethal interaction with ethanol are other known disadvantages of this class of agents. Unfortunately, the rapid development of tolerance has severely limited the therapeutic use of BZs in epilepsy disorders, despite their excellent acute antiepileptic activity against a wide range of seizure types (Löscher and Schmidt, 1988). However, the greatest concern regarding BZ agonists is the growing recognition that they have a fairly high propensity to induce dependence (e.g., Marks, 1983). In humans, withdrawal from BZs can consist of psychological and somatic symptoms of anxiety, seizures, and, in extreme cases, death (Petursson and Lader, 1981; Owen and Tyrer, 1983; Woods, et al., 1992). Of little comfort is the conclusion reached by Lader and File (1987) that the same withdrawal syndrome occurs on termination of high or low doses of BZs, and regardless of whether they have been taken long- or short-term. Relatively few patients who receive BZs for medical indications begin to abuse their medication, but there are some individuals (often already involved in illicit use of other drugs) who specifically seek these compounds for their ability to produce a high. Among the abusers, there is a preference for BZs with a rapid onset, such as diazepam and alprazolam (O'Brien, 1996).

5.2. BZ Receptor Partial Agonists

One of the most popular approaches adopted in the search for anxiolytic agents that lack the untoward effects of BZs has been the design of partial agonists at BZ receptors. By definition, partial agonists have lower intrinsic efficacies than classical BZ full agonists. Because of this lower efficacy at the receptor, partial agonists require higher fractional receptor occupancies than full agonists in order to potentiate GABA-ergic function to the same extent. This will be true for all pharmacological measures, but it will be most apparent for those responses that are affected only at high receptor occupancies. For example, in rodents, anxiolytic effects usually require a lower fractional receptor occupancy than sedative effects (Facklam et al., 1992a); therefore, it may be possible to distinguish between partial and full receptor agonists using measures of sedation, but it should be more difficult to do so using measures of anxiolytic activity. (As a corollary, in those test systems in which partial agonists do not display sufficient efficacy to achieve the pharmacological end-point, they should antagonize the actions of full agonists). This concept underlies the theoretical basis for developing partial agonists for therapeutic purposes because they are more likely to display behavioral selectivity (Haefely et al., 1990).

A large number of chemically diverse BZ receptor partial agonists have been reported in the literature, and animal studies suggest they have less propensity to cause adverse events than classical BZs, while still retaining anxiolytic properties. Clinical experience with partial agonists is still rather limited, but early results appear promising. Efficacy comparisons with BZs are eagerly awaited, as are studies in epilepsy sufferers.

Bretazenil and abecarnil are highlighted as providing examples of the types of pharmacological profiles that characterize partial agonists with differing degrees of intrinsic activity at the BZ receptor. In addition, these agents have been evaluated clinically.

5.2.1. Bretazenil

Bretazenil has high (low nanomolar) affinity for BZ receptors (Giusti et al., 1993) and exhibits a characteristic partial agonist profile in a broad spectrum of in vitro and in vivo tests. For example, under experimental conditions where diazepam potentiates GABA-stimulated chloride flux into membrane vesicles of rat cortex by approximately 40%, bretazenil produces a maximal enhancement of only 20% (Facklam et al., 1992b). Similarly, the compound is significantly less effective than full BZ agonists in facilitating chloride currents in all the recombinant $GABA_A Rs$ so far tested, including $\alpha 1$, $\alpha 2$, $\alpha 3$, and $\alpha 5$ ($\beta x \gamma x$) combinations (Puia et al., 1992; Giusti et al., 1993; Knoflach et al., 1993). These latter studies, and others performed using native tissue (Richards et al., 1991), also suggest that bretazenil does not interact preferentially with any particular subtype of BZ receptors.

In animal models, bretazenil produced potent anticonflict effects (Haefely et al., 1990; Facklam et al., 1992a; Giusti et al., 1993; Jones et al., 1994) and inhibited seizures induced by a variety of chemical stimuli (Haefely et al., 1990; Facklam et al., 1992a; Giusti et al., 1993; Serra et al., 1994). In many cases, the compound had a smaller maximal effect than full agonists. Several studies have clearly demonstrated that, in comparison to diazepam and alprazolam, higher fractional BZ receptor occupancy is required for bretazenil to exert equivalent levels of anxiolytic or anticonvulsant activity (Facklam et al., 1992a; Giusti et al., 1993; Jones et al., 1994). In further distinction to BZ agonists, bretazenil failed to significantly alter motor activity, elicit ataxia, or potentiate ethanol or barbiturate sleep time, even at doses that occupied 100% of BZ receptors (Facklam et al., 1992a; Giusti et al., 1993). Moreover, bretazenil potently antagonized the motor impairing properties of diazepam (Facklam et al., 1992a).

In contrast to the effect of full agonists, repeated dosing with bretazenil did not result in tolerance to its anticonvulsant activity in rodents (Haigh and Freely, 1988; Auta et al., 1994) or changes in BZ receptor binding or $GABA_A R$

function (Schoch et al., 1993). In addition, bretazenil showed less frequent and less severe precipitated withdrawal reactions compared to alprazolam after prolonged administration to mice and monkeys (Schoch et al., 1993).

Initial clinical studies demonstrated the anxiolytic efficacy of bretazenil in both generalized anxiety disorder (225 patients) and panic disorder (24 patients); minimal sedative effects were seen at therapeutic doses (*see* Haefely et al., 1990). In a study comparing bretazenil with diazepam and alprazolam, all measures of abuse potential were lower with the former compound (Busto et al., 1994).

5.2.2. Abecarnil

Although abecarnil is commonly regarded as a partial agonist, there is persuasive evidence that, unlike bretazenil, this β-carboline analog can act as a full agonist in some test situations. Overall, abecarnil exhibited greater affinity (sub nanomolar) than diazepam for rat brain BZ sites (Stephens et al., 1993; Ozawa et al., 1994a) and showed approximately a fivefold higher affinity for cerebellar BZ receptors, compared to those found in spinal cord, suggesting some selectivity for BZ1 receptors (Stephens et al., 1990; Ozawa et al., 1994a). Through its action at BZ sites, abecarnil induced potent and efficacious (often equivalent to full agonists) anxiolytic effects in classical conflict tests in rodents, as well as ethologically derived models in rodents and primates (Stephens et al., 1990; Jones et al., 1994; Ozawa et al., 1994a). The compound was also an effective anticonvulsant in many, but not all, animal models of chemically or electrically induced seizures, and was protective in genetic models of epilepsy (Turski et al., 1990).

Despite its potent anxiolytic and anticonvulsant properties, abecarnil produced only slight effects in most tests of sedation, ataxia, muscle coordination, and cognitive function (Stephens et al., 1990; Ozawa et al., 1994a,b), and only weakly potentiated the depressant actions of ethanol and barbiturates (Stephens et al., 1990; Ozawa et al., 1994a). Upon repeated administration, tolerance did not develop to the anxiolytic or anticonvulsant effects of abecarnil (Löscher et al., 1990; Ozawa et al., 1994b). In addition, the withdrawal syndrome observed in mice, cats, dogs, and baboons, after abecarnil discontinuation or challenge with flumazenil was substantially reduced or absent, compared to BZs, suggesting a low dependence potential for the β-carboline (Löscher et al., 1990; Löscher 1993; Sannerud et al., 1992, 1993; Steppuhn et al., 1992; Serra et al., 1993).

Much of the pharmacological profile of abecarnil is consistent with that expected of a drug acting as a partial agonist at BZ receptors (cf bretazenil). This includes the virtual lack of CNS depressant properties (even at receptor occupancies approaching 100%) and minimal tolerance and dependence liability. Moreover, abecarnil can partially antagonize the sedative and ataxic actions of diazepam in rodents (Stephens et al., 1990; Ozawa et al., 1994a) and requires higher fractional receptor occupancy than diazepam to produce equivalent anticonvulsant activity in several animal seizure models (Turski et al., 1990). These and other observations (see Stephens et al., 1990; Osawa et al., 1994a) illustrate the partial agonist nature of abecarnil. However, it is also clear that in certain biochemical and behavioral tests (see Serra et al., 1993; Stephens et al., 1993) abecarnil behaves in a way that is more characteristic of a full agonist. For example, in shock conflict and elevated plus maze models of anxiety, abecarnil achieved its anxiolytic effect at levels of fractional receptor occupancy that were the same or lower than those at which BZs produced similar activity (Stephens et al. 1990; Jones et al., 1993). Although this profile of differing intrinsic activity between the various tests cannot at present be accounted for in detail, it is consistent with data from studies on recombinant $GABA_ARs$ which indicate that abecarnil possesses full agonist activity at some receptors ($\alpha1$ or $\alpha3\beta x\gamma2$) and is a partial agonist at others ($\alpha2$ or $\alpha5\beta x\gamma2$) (Knoflach et al., 1993; Pribilla et al., 1993). In terms of affinity for the different receptors, abecarnil binds with a rank order of potency of $\alpha1 > \alpha5 > \alpha3$ ($\beta x\gamma2$). The degree of selectivity shown here by abecarnil for $\alpha1$- over $\alpha3$-containing $GABA_ARs$ (about 30-fold) is comparable to that of the prototypical BZ1 ligand zolpidem, although the latter agent lacks the affinity of abecarnil for $\alpha5$-containing subtypes (see Sieghart, 1995). Considered as a whole, these findings suggest that abecarnil may achieve its selective pharmacological profile through a unique combination of differential affinity and/or modulatory efficacy at different subtypes of $GABA_ARs$. On the agonist through antagonist to inverse agonist continuum (Fig. 1), abecarnil would appear to lie somewhere between diazepam and bretazenil.

Only one study assessing the anxiolytic efficacy of abecarnil in patients ($n = 129$) has been published in full (Ballenger et al., 1991), although several thousand subjects are known to have taken the drug (see Spencer and Benfield, 1995). In the trial reported by Ballenger and colleagues, abecarnil (3–9 mg/d) was significantly more effective than placebo and produced few serious adverse events. However, at the top dose range tested (15–30 mg/d), the drug produced a high incidence of CNS side effects, most prominent of which was sedation. This initial assessment suggests that, in humans, the separation between therapeutic and untoward effects of abecarnil may not be as great as that predicted from studies using animal models; it will be of great interest to see how the drug performs in a wider patient population. In a small study in 14 healthy volunteers with a history of sedative drug abuse, abecarnil appeared to have less abuse potential than alprazolam (Mumford et al., 1995).

5.3. BZ Receptor Antagonists

Flumazenil (Ro 15-1788) is the prototypical specific BZ receptor antagonist. It has high affinity for BZ binding sites throughout the brain (Haefely et al., 1983) and also for recombinant GABA$_A$Rs constituted from $\alpha 1$, $\alpha 2$, $\alpha 3$, or $\alpha 5$ ($\beta x \gamma 2/3$) subunit combinations (*see* Sieghart, 1995) (i.e., it is not selective for BZ1 or BZ2 receptors). In numerous animal models, flumazenil has been shown to potently antagonize the acute central effects of BZ receptor agonists, partial agonists, and inverse agonists (including all of the other agents discussed in Section 5.) (*see* Haefely et al., 1983; Brogden and Goa, 1991). In vivo data to illustrate BZ receptor occupancy by flumazenil in human brain have been generated using positron emission tomography (PET) (Persson et al., 1985; Samson et al., 1985; Mindus et al., 1986). As an antagonist, flumazenil generally has no physiological effects in its own right, but weak agonist or inverse agonist properties can sometimes be demonstrated (in animals and in humans), depending on the test situation (*see* Malizia and Nutt, 1995).

Flumazenil is generally well-tolerated and enjoys widespread clinical utility, principally for the reversal of BZ-induced sedation/anesthesia in patients undergoing diagnostic or surgical procedures, and also in the treatment of overdose with BZs (Brogden and Goa 1991). Possible additional therapeutic uses are still at the exploratory stage and include reversal of acute ethanol intoxication and treatment of anxiety, epilepsy, and hepatic encephalopathy (Brogden and Goa, 1991; Malizia and Nutt, 1995). Of particular interest are recent attempts to determine whether flumazenil can diminish BZ tolerance and dependence (*see* Malizia and Nutt, 1995). These studies are based on two concepts founded on data from animals: First, that BZ tolerance and withdrawal may result from an alteration in the sensitivity of the BZ receptor, so that agonists lose their efficacy and inverse agonists become more efficacious (Nutt et al., 1992); and second, that by resetting the BZ receptor to its original state, flumazenil may be able to minimize overall withdrawal and reverse tolerance (*see* Malizia and Nutt, 1995). An obvious difficulty in using flumazenil for this purpose in a clinical setting is that the antagonist would be likely to precipitate withdrawal, at least in the short term (Malizia and Nutt, 1995).

The availability of carbon 11-labeled flumazenil for PET studies has provided an increasingly utilized tool for investigating the pathophysiological role of BZ receptors in a variety of human neuropsychiatric and neurological disorders (Malizia and Nutt, 1995). Most work has been done in the area of epilepsy, and several studies have now shown reductions in BZ receptor density in the foci of patients with partial/temporal lobe seizures (Savic et al., 1988; Henry et al., 1993).

5.4. Inverse Agonists

The search for endogenous ligands that physiologically subserve BZ receptors in the brain resulted in the isolation of the ethyl and methyl esters of β-carboline-3-carboxylic acid (β-CCE and β-CCM, respectively) from human urine (Braestrup et al., 1980). Although subsequently shown to be extraction artifacts, these agents proved to have high affinity for central BZ sites (Braestrup et al., 1980) and became the prototypes for a new class of compounds (mostly β-carboline derivatives, such as FG 7142 and DMCM), now described as inverse agonists. Upon binding to BZ receptors, inverse agonists had the opposite functional effects to classical agonists and decreased the action of GABA at GABA$_A$Rs (Hunkeler et al., 1981; Obata et al., 1988). Both partial (e.g., β-CCE and FG 7142) and full (e.g., DMCM) inverse agonists have been identified based on their lesser or greater abilities to inhibit GABA function, respectively (Obata et al., 1988; Gardner, 1989).

Some β-carbolines, including β-CCE and β-CCM, exhibit binding affinities for BZ receptors in cerebellum several times higher than for those in hippocampus and other brain regions (Sieghart, 1989), suggesting a degree of selectivity for the BZ1 subtype. This is consistent with studies using recombinant GABA$_A$Rs showing that β-CCM has a preference for α1- over α2- or α3βxγ2 subunit combinations (*see* Sieghart, 1995). The type of γ subunit present in recombinant receptors plays a crucial role in the functional response to β-carbolines. Thus, DMCM acts as an inverse agonist at γ2-containing receptors, but as a partial agonist at receptors containing γ1 subunits (Puia et al., 1991).

Inverse agonists produced a spectrum of activating behaviors, which included anxiogenic, proconvulsant, or frankly convulsant effects in several animal species (Braestrup et al., 1983; Skolnick et al., 1984) and severe anxiety in humans (Dorow et al., 1983). Moreover, these agents appeared to improve age- and/or scopolamine-impaired cognitive processing in rodents (Jensen et al., 1987; Forster et al., 1995). A fascinating phenomenon has been described following repeated administration of partial inverse agonists. In contrast to the well known tolerance to BZ agonists (*see* Section 5.1.), repetitive dosing of the acutely proconvulsant agent FG 7142 led to a progressively increasing sensitivity to its own effect, so that the compound eventually produced overt behavioral seizures (Little et al., 1984). The underlying basic mechanisms of this so-called kindling effect are still poorly understood and often inconsistent changes in the function of the GABA$_A$R complex have been reported (*see* Schneider and Stephens, 1988). It is apparent, however, that kindling induced by FG 7142 and tolerance to BZ agonists are not manifestations of the same process (Schneider and Stephens, 1988).

Therapeutic opportunities for inverse agonists would appear to be some-what limited because of the propensity of these agents to lower seizure threshold, especially after repeated administration. However, a very weak inverse agonist that is devoid of proconvulsant activity may be of potential value for enhancing memory function.

5.5. BZ1 Receptor Selective Compounds

The existence of central BZ receptor subtypes (*see* Section 5.), and knowledge of their differing distributions throughout the brain (*see* Section 2.), affords the possibility that subtype selective compounds may exhibit enhanced therapeutic profiles over BZ agonists. The greatest progress from efforts to capitalize on this idea has been the discovery of several non-BZ compounds that interact preferentially (but not entirely selectively) with BZ1 sites. Among this group are β-CCE (see Section 5.4.), CL 218,872 (an anxiolytic agent with sedative liability in animals), and, perhaps of most interest, the imidazopyridine derivatives zolpidem and alpidem (Squires et al., 1978; Arbilla et al., 1985; Langer and Arbilla, 1988a,b; Sieghart, 1989; Gillard et al., 1991; Sieghart and Schlerka, 1991; Sanger et al., 1993). These latter agents have been consistently shown to bind with higher affinity (typically 4–11-fold) to BZ receptors in cerebellum than in structures such as hippocampus and spinal cord, thereby highlighting their preferential action at BZ1 receptors (Benavides et al., 1987, 1993; Langer and Arbilla, 1988a,b). In fact, zolpidem and alpidem can differentiate three BZ binding sites labeled with [^{3}H]flumazenil in rat brain tissue for which they have high, intermediate, or very low affinity (Benavides et al., 1993). Comparison of the relative affinities of these agents for the three binding components with those for recombinant GABA_A Rs suggests that the high, intermediate, and very low affinity sites correspond to GABA_A Rs containing α1 (BZ1 sites), α2, or α3 (BZ2: zolpidem-sensitive sites) and α5 subunits (BZ2: zolpidem-insensitive sites), respectively (Pritchett and Seeburg, 1990; Sieghart 1995). In accord with this observation, the distribution of [^{3}H]zolpidem binding sites in rat brain largely parallels the localization of mRNAs encoding the α1, β2, and γ2 subunits of GABA_A Rs (Duncan et al., 1995). Differences have been seen in the extent to which cortical binding of [^{3}H]zolpidem and [^{3}H]alpidem is modulated by GABA, Cl$^-$ ions, and pentobarbital, a finding taken to suggest that alpidem interacts with a conformation of the GABA_A/BZ1 receptor complex distinct from that recognized by zolpidem (Arbilla et al., 1993). Alpidem also has additional high affinity for peripheral-type BZ receptors (Langer and Arbilla, 1988b).

In terms of functional activity, many studies indicate that zolpidem acts as a full agonist (relative to BZs) (Arbilla et al., 1985; Puia et al., 1991; Ruano et al., 1993; Wafford et al., 1993; Lüddens et al., 1994) and alpidem behaves as a partial agonist (with moderate intrinsic activity) (Perrault et al., 1993; but *see* Puia et al., 1991) at BZ1 receptors. Certainly, in vivo, zolpidem and alpidem have very distinctive behavioral profiles, both from each other, and also from BZs.

The relative activity of zolpidem in a battery of rodent models, was characterized as sedative >> anticonvulsant > myorelaxant activity (all effects were reversed by flumazenil); the relative activity of BZs was anxiolytic = anticonvulsant > myorelaxant ≥ sedative (Depoortere et al., 1986; Perrault et al., 1990). The rank order for zolpidem is in accord with the finding that lower BZ site occupancy is required for the sedative action (35%) of this drug, compared to those needed for anticonvulsant/myorelaxant effects (48–56%) (Benavides et al., 1987). The strong sedative action of zolpidem appeared to mask an anxiolytic action (Depoortere et al., 1986). The most potent actions of alpidem were in models of seizures and anxiety (although the spectrum of activity was narrower than that of BZs), with little propensity for producing muscle relaxation (Zivkovic et al., 1990; Perrault et al., 1993; Sanger et al., 1993). The anxiolytic and anticonvulsant properties were fully blocked by flumazenil illustrating that central, and not peripheral, BZ receptors mediate these effects (Zivkovic et al., 1990; Arbilla et al., 1993). Following repeated administration, tolerance did not develop to the anticonvulsant and/or sedative properties of alpidem (Perrault et al., 1993) and zolpidem (Perrault et al., 1992). Moreover, these agents were less prone to cause withdrawal than BZs, upon cessation of chronic dosing or challenge with flumazenil (Perrault et al., 1992, 1993; Sanger et al., 1993; Schoch et al., 1993).

Zolpidem is currently marketed as a sedative-hypnotic. The compound shortens sleep latency, prolongs total sleep time, and has the advantage over BZs of inducing a relatively normal sleep pattern. It is well-tolerated, having little effect on memory and a low propensity for causing withdrawal (Langtry and Benfield, 1990). Alpidem has undergone clinical trials involving several thousand patients with various forms of anxiety. Overall, these studies have shown that the compound is comparable in efficacy to BZs, but with an improved adverse event profile (Legris et al., 1993; Panchera et al., 1993). Longer-term studies suggest that tolerance and withdrawal do not occur (Chevalier et al., 1993; Lader, 1993). Unfortunately, recent reports of alpidem-induced hepatic dysfunction (speculatively attributed to its high affinity for peripheral-type BZ receptors) has led to its suspension (Potokar and Nutt, 1994).

5.6. Zopiclone and Suriclone

The first non-BZ compounds reported to interact with the BZ receptor were the cyclopyrrolones (Blanchard et al., 1979), first exemplified by zopiclone and followed by suriclone. Most studies have shown that these agents competitively displace [^{3}H]flumazenil and [^{3}H]flunitrazepam binding in rodent brain tissue with moderate (IC$_{50}$ 20–40 nM) or high affinity (IC$_{50}$ $\cong$ 1 nM), respectively (Blanchard et al., 1979; Doble et al., 1992; Concas et al., 1994; but *see* Trifiletti and Snyder, 1984). However, it has been demonstrated that the mode of binding of [^{3}H]suriclone, and of radiolabeled BZs to the GABA$_A$R complex, differs in several potentially important respects. Unlike BZ agonist binding, suriclone binding was not enhanced by GABA, Cl$^-$ ions, or barbiturates, and was unaffected by temperature (Blanchard and Julou, 1983; Julou et al., 1985; Zundel et al., 1985; Malgouris et al., 1995). Moreover, in rat membranes photolabeled with flunitrazepam, subsequent reversible binding of BZs was abolished, but the binding of suriclone remained largely intact (Doble et al., 1992). In order to rationalize these data, it has been proposed that cyclopyrrolones and BZs interact with two distinct, perhaps adjacent or overlapping, binding domains and, as a consequence, evoke different confirmational states of the GABA$_A$R complex, which are reflected in the pharmacological differences observed in vivo *(see below)* (Doble et al., 1992, 1995). As yet, there is no evidence from studies using recombinant GABA$_A$Rs to suggest that suriclone or zopiclone can discriminate BZ receptor subtypes, since, like BZ agonists (*see* Section 5.1.), they showed comparable affinities for receptor isoforms containing α1, α2, α3, or α5 subunits (Doble et al., 1992; Faure-Halley et al., 1993). This is consistent with findings in native tissue where the cyclopyrrolones exhibit equivalent affinity for BZ1 and BZ2 receptors (Julou et al., 1985; Doble et al., 1992; Concas et al., 1994; Malgouris et al., 1995). In terms of functional activity at BZ receptors, zopiclone and suriclone have been classified as full agonists (*see* Doble et al., 1992) although the former agent has been described as a partial agonist by some authors (Concas et al., 1994).

The behavioral profiles for zopiclone and suriclone were remarkably similar, ranging from anxiolytic/anticonvulsant properties to sedative/muscle relaxant activity with increasing doses (Julou et al., 1985; Perrault et al., 1990; Doble et al., 1992). The anxiolytic effects, which were of the same magnitude as those of diazepam in both shock-conflict and neophobic models, were abolished by flumazenil (Julou et al., 1985; Doble et al., 1992, 1995). An hypnotic action for zopiclone was also demonstrated in several species using electroencephalographic techniques (Doble et al., 1992, 1995). The separation between doses producing muscle relaxant and anxiolytic/ anticonvulsant effects was considered to be slightly greater for the cyclopyrrolones than for BZs (Julou et al., 1985; Doble et al., 1992). However, a much clearer distinction in the properties of these two chemical classes became apparent following repeated dosing. In contrast to BZs, there was little or no indication of the development of tolerance (e.g., loss of anticonvulsant efficacy) or withdrawal symptoms (e.g., enhanced susceptibility to seizures when challenged by partial inverse agonists) after long-term administration of either zopiclone or suriclone in rodents and primates (Piot et al., 1990; Yanganita, 1993; Doble et al., 1995).

Both cyclopyrrolones have been studied in man, especially zopiclone which is now available as a sedative-hypnotic. This agent has been demonstrated to be a safe and effective sleep-inducer, while leaving sleep architecture relatively unchanged. It has minimal residual effects (e.g., sedation, morning-after amnesia) upon waking and does not cause physical dependence after continued use (Musch and Maillard, 1990; Kerr et al., 1995). A different therapeutic target was pursued for suriclone, namely, generalized anxiety disorder. Several studies showed the compound to produce equivalent anxiolytic efficacy with reduced sedative effects, compared to BZs. The most prominent adverse events tended to be dose-related neurological symptoms, such as dizziness (Julou et al., 1985; Ansseau et al., 1991).

6. The Interaction of Barbiturates with GABA$_A$Rs

Depressant barbiturates, such as pentobarbitol and phenobarbital, have dual actions to facilitate GABA$_A$R-mediated Cl$^-$ conductance. In electrophysiological studies, these agents enhance the actions of GABA by increasing the average channel open time (Study and Barker, 1981; Macdonald and Olsen, 1994); in addition, at high (anesthetic) concentrations, they directly increase channel openings, even in the absence of GABA (Bormann, 1988; Inomata et al., 1988). This latter property highlights an important distinction from BZs, which have no such direct effects on channel openings (*see* Section 5.1.), a difference that probably contributes to the relatively low toxicity of the BZs, compared to the barbiturates.

Further information on the allosteric interactions of barbiturates with GABA$_A$Rs has been obtained in studies showing that they enhance the affinity of [^{3}H]GABA, [^{3}H]muscimol, and [^{3}H]flunitrazepam binding, and inhibit [^{35}S]TBPS binding, in a manner that correlates with their rank order of potency as anesthetics and hypnotics (Olsen, 1982; Squires et al., 1983). These findings suggest the importance of GABA$_A$Rs in mediating the pharmacological actions of barbiturates and also demonstrate that their site(s) of action must be different from those of BZs, GABA, or the cage convulsants. This has been further illustrated using recombinant GABA$_A$Rs, in which only α and β subunits are required for barbiturate action (unlike for BZs, in which an additional γ subunit is needed), although it is possible that all subunits may have binding sites for these agents (*see* Sieghart, 1995; McKernan and Whiting, 1996).

The barbiturates enjoyed a long period of extensive use as sedative hypnotic drugs. However, except for a few specialized uses, such as in emergency treatment of convulsions, they have been largely replaced by the much safer BZs. Compared to BZs, barbiturates have a lower therapeutic index, particularly regarding depression of cardiorespiratory function, are more prone to tolerance development (both pharmacokinetic and pharmacodynamic), and the liability for abuse is greater (Hobbs et al., 1996).

7. The Interaction of Neuroactive Steroids with $GABA_A Rs$

It was in 1984, that electrophysiological studies provided the first evidence that a steroid, in this case the synthetic anesthetic alphaxalone, could potentiate $GABA_A R$-mediated responses (Harrison and Simmonds, 1984). Several structurally related endogenous steroids (e.g., 5α-pregnan-3α-ol-20-one and 5α-pregnan-3α,21-diol-20-one, metabolites of progesterone and deoxycorticosterone, respectively) have since been shown to have similar rapid nongenomic effects (Callachan et al., 1987; Peters et al., 1988). The ability of these substances to allosterically modulate $GABA_A Rs$ has been further confirmed, using numerous other electrophysiological and biochemical techniques (*see* Paul and Purdy, 1992; Gee et al., 1995; Lambert et al., 1995). These findings, together with the realization that the brain can synthesize *de novo* certain steroids (primarily in glia) (Baulieu et al., 1987), led to speculation that so-called neuroactive steroids[a] may be endogenous modulators of central $GABA_A Rs$ (Majewska, 1992; Paul and Purdy, 1992). Synthesis of neuroactive steroids in the brain is thought to be regulated by peripheral-type BZ receptors located on glial mitochondria (Mukhin et al., 1989).

In addition to enhancing GABA-evoked Cl⁻ currents, agents such as alphaxalone directly open the Cl⁻ channel at high concentrations (Callachan et al., 1987; Peters et al., 1988). This dual action is reminiscent of the properties of barbiturates (*see* Section 6.), but detailed pharmacological analyses of steroid-barbiturate (and steroid-BZ) interactions clearly demonstrate a distinct steroid recognition site on $GABA_A Rs$ (Gee, 1988; Lambert et al., 1995). Regionally specific responses have been obtained to neuroactive steroids in both binding assays (Lan and Gee, 1991) and autoradiography studies (Sapp et al., 1992), suggesting that they may have selective actions at $GABA_A R$ subtypes. Evaluation of the effects of these compounds in recombinant

---

[a]Neuroactive steroids refers to those natural or synthetic steroids with well-described actions in altering (either increasing or decreasing) neuronal membrane excitability, irrespective of whether they are synthesised in brain (Paul and Purdy, 1992).

GABA$_A$Rs has produced a somewhat confusing picture. Overall, it would appear that they do not exhibit an absolute receptor subunit selectivity (unlike BZs), although their actions tend to be subtly influenced by subunit composition (Paul and Purdy, 1992; Gee et al., 1995; Lambert et al., 1995). The precise site of action of those naturally occurring steroids that act as noncompetitive antagonists at GABA$_A$Rs (e.g., pregnenolone sulfate), is apparently even less well understood (Paul and Purdy, 1992; Gee et al., 1995; Lambert et al., 1995).

Behaviorally, many of the neuroactive steroids that enhance GABA$_A$R function produce anxiolytic, anticonvulsant, sedative-hypnotic, and anesthetic activity (both in animals and in humans); conversely, those that act as antagonists at GABA$_A$Rs are excitatory and sometimes induce seizures (Majewska, 1992; Gee et al., 1995; Lambert et al., 1995). Unfortunately, the separation between doses required for anxiolytic/anticonvulsant and sedative effects is often rather poor. However, certain pregnandiols induce only a modest potentiation of GABA-evoked Cl⁻ currents and in animal models exhibit an improved therapeutic ratio, thus highlighting a potential future strategy for therapeutically exploiting the steroid recognition site on GABA$_A$Rs (Lambert et al., 1995).

In terms of possible pathophysiological roles, it has been suggested that because endogenous steroids bidirectionally modulate the function of GABA$_A$Rs and affect neuronal excitability, aberrant synthesis of centrally active steroids may contribute to a myriad of psychophysiological phenomena, including anxiety, depression, stress, and seizures. Certainly, conditions such as Cushing's disease (characterized by overstimulation of adrenal steroids) and Addison's disease (adrenal insufficiency) are associated with many neuropsychiatric manifestations (Majewska, 1992).

8. The Interaction of Ethanol with GABA$_A$Rs

Alcohol (ethanol) is one of the most widely used (and abused) recreational drugs. It is now recognized that the therapeutic value of this agent for CNS disorders is extremely limited and that chronic ingestion of excessive amounts can lead to major social and medical (e.g., high risk of dependence) problems (Hobbs et al., 1996; O'Brien, 1996). Many pharmacological actions of ethanol are similar to those produced by BZs and barbiturates, including anxiolytic, anticonvulsant, ataxic, and sedative-hypnotic effects. Several research groups have now confirmed that at pharmacologically relevant concentrations (10–100 mM), alcohol can augment GABA$_A$-ergic responses at behavioral, electrophysiological, and biochemical levels (*see* Korpi, 1994, for review). This provides persuasive evidence that at least some of the neuropharmacological effects of ethanol are mediated at GABA$_A$Rs, although the precise site and mode of action remains somewhat controversial. For example, ethanol does not alter the binding of [^{3}H]GABA or [^{3}H]BZs to rat brain membranes, and only appears to allosterically inhibit [^{35}S]TBPS binding at relatively high concentrations ($\geq$ 100 mM) (*see* Korpi, 1994; Sieghart, 1995).

There are indications that modulation of GABA$_A$-ergic function by ethanol varies between brain regions; it has been suggested that this differential sensitivity may be caused by the expression of different receptor subunits (Givens and Breese, 1990). In certain recombinant GABA$_A$Rs, alcohol potentiation is dependent on the alternatively spliced long form of the γ2 subunit (γ2L) (Wafford et al., 1991). The γ2L subunit carries an extra consensus sequence for protein kinase C (Whiting et al., 1990); it is possible that the hypnotic action of ethanol is associated with changes in the phosphorylation of this subunit. Other studies have shown that the nature of the α subunit variant can influence sensitivity to a high concentration (100 mM) of ethanol (independently of the γ2 spliced form), with the α6 subunit being slightly favored over the α1 subunit (Lüddens and Korpi, 1995). The partial inverse agonist Ro 15-5413, an imidazobenzodiazepine compound that binds with high affinity to recombinant GABA$_A$Rs containing the α6 subunit (Lüddens et al., 1990), has been reported to reverse the motor incoordination and ataxia induced by excessive ethanol consumption (Suzdak et al., 1986). Moreover, in rat strain lines selected for high or low sensitivity to ethanol, differences were observed in the binding of [^{3}H]Ro 15-4513 in the cerebellum (virtually the sole locus for α6 subunits in brain) (Uusi-Oukari and Korpi, 1990).

9. The Interaction of Other Classes of Compounds with GABA$_A$Rs

Numerous other agents interact directly with the GABA$_A$R complex; some of the most interesting examples are presented in Table 2.

10. GABA$_A$R Subtypes, Partial Agonism, and Behavior

A recent review has suggested that there are approximately eight major GABA$_A$R subtypes within mammalian brain, each with distinctive regional and cellular distributions (McKernan and Whiting 1996; Table 1). Almost half of all brain GABA$_A$Rs consist of the α1 subunit in combination with the β2 and γ2 subunits; a further 35% of the total are composed of the α2β3γ2 or α3β*x*γ2/3 subtypes (McKernan and Whiting, 1996). These two large populations correspond to the BZ1 and BZ2 receptors originally defined by

Table 2
Other Classes of Direct Modulators of GABA$_A$Rs

Compound/ chemical class	Activity	Mode/site of action
Avermectin B1α	Antihelminthic, insecticidal	Binding site not identical with those of GABA, BZs, barbiturates, or TBPS[a]
Ro 5-4864	Convulsant	Inhibits GABA$_A$R function via an action at a unique low affinity binding site (K_D 250 nM)[a]
Zn^{++}	Endogenous modulator	Binds to a divalent cation site and inhibits GABA$_A$R function[a]
Chlormethiazole/ propofol and halothane	Anxiolytic, anticonvulsant, sedative hypnotic/general anesthetics	Potentiate GABA-activated Cl$^-$ currents at low concentrations and directly open the Cl$^-$ channel at high concentrations; their site(s) of action remain to be determined but appear to be distinct from other known GABA$_A$R modulators[a]
Loreclazole	Anticonvulsant, anxiolytic	Acts at a novel binding site that is solely selective for recombinant GABA$_A$Rs containing β2 or β3 subunits over those constituted from the β1 subunit[a,b]
Dihydroimidazo- quinoxalines	Not known	In recombinant GABA$_A$Rs, the prototypical agent U-93631, accelerated the decay of GABA-induced Cl$^-$ currents without changing their amplitude; interacts with a novel binding site arising from a common sequence among α1, β2, and γ2 subunits[a,c]
Pyrido[2,3-*b*] indoles	Anxiolytic	Enhance GABA-Cl$^-$ currents in recombinant GABA$_A$Rs possibly via an action at β1 and γ2 subunits[d,e]

[a]*See* Sieghart, 1995 for further details.
[b]Wafford et al., 1994.
[c]Dillon et al., 1993.
[d]Blackburn et al., 1995.
[e]Unpublished observations.

radioligand binding studies before cloning of the GABA$_A$R gene family commenced (*see* Section 5.). Our understanding of the function of BZ1 (and, by inference, BZ2) receptors in the familiar pharmacological effects of BZs has been aided by the discovery of zolpidem and alpidem. These agents have reasonable selectivity for BZ1 sites, and in particular, have very low affinity for BZ2 receptors constituted from α5 subunits (*see* Sections 5. and 5.5.).

From the information discussed earlier in this chapter and now summarized in Table 3, the following tentative conclusions can be made. (1) Selec-

Table 3
BZ Receptor Agonists: Comparison of Affinity/Intrinsic Activity
at BZ Receptor Subtypes with In Vivo Properties

	Relative affinities for BZ1[a] and BZ2[b] receptors	Intrinsic activity	Rank order of in vivo actions[c,d]
Benzodiazepines (e.g., diazepam)	BZ1 = BZ2	A	AX ≥ AC > S ≥ MR
Bretazenil	BZ1 = BZ2	PA	AX, AC >> S, MR
Abecarnil	BZ1 > BZ2(α5) > BZ2(α3)	PA (A α1,α3)	AX ≥ AC > S > MR
Zolpidem	BZ1 > BZ2(α2,α3) >> BZ2(α5)	A	S > AX > AC >> MR
Alpidem	BZ1 > BZ2(α3) > BZ2(α5)	PA	AX, AC > S >> MR
Zopiclone/ suriclone	BZ1 = BZ2	A	AX, AC > S > MR

[a] ≡ α1βxγ2.
[b] ≡ α2,α3,α5βxγ2.
[c] Derived from effects with increasing doses (variations can be seen dependent on the test systems used).
[d] With the exception of BZs, all agents have minimal tolerance and dependence liability.
A, full agonist; AC, anticonvulsant; AX, anxiolytic; MR, muscle relaxant; PA, partial agonist; S, sedative.
See text for references.

tivity for BZ1 receptors markedly reduces the propensity of drugs to produce muscle relaxation; this implicates an important role for BZ2 receptors in controlling muscle tone. In keeping with this opinion, BZ2 receptors are found in the motor neurons of the spinal cord, where they could well be implicated in control of motor coordination (McKernan and Whiting, 1996). (2) Similarly, the minimal potential for zolpidem to induce tolerance and dependence upon chronic dosing suggests that BZ2 receptors may also underlie these particular liabilities for BZs. (3) A high degree of intrinsic activity at BZ1 sites (cf zolpidem) is associated with a sedative-hypnotic action. (4) BZ1 subtype selective partial agonists (cf alpidem) produce anticonvulsant or anxiolytic activity in the absence of behavioral depression. Conversely, partial inverse agonists with selectivity for these sites (e.g., β-CCE) are anxiogenic and proconvulsant. These findings illustrate a potential role of BZ1 sites in pathways modulating anxiety and seizure states. (5) BZ2 receptors are likely to be involved in the anxiolytic and anticonvulsant actions of BZs since the BZ1 selective partial agonist alpidem exhibits a much-reduced spectrum of activity, compared to BZs in animal models of anxiety and seizures. Furthermore, in higher levels of intrinsic activity at BZ1 receptors, as seen for zolipidem, result in the occurrence of sedative actions ahead of anxiolytic effects, i.e., the opposite profile to BZs.

These statements are very speculative, particularly regarding attempts to define a functional role for BZ2 receptors in the absence of any selective ligands for this subtype. Another factor that needs consideration when undertaking this type of analysis is that, besides the importance of subtype selectivity, the behavioral outcome of a given drug is also determined by the level of intrinsic activity at the various BZ receptors. For example, favorable behavioral profiles, compared to classical BZs, have been observed for agents with partial agonist properties at all BZ receptor subtypes (cf bretazenil, Table 3). To add to an already complex situation, abecarnil (Table 3) acts as a partial agonist only at some subtypes ($\alpha2$- and $\alpha5$-containing receptors) and as a full agonist at others ($\alpha1$- and $\alpha3$-containing receptors), but still exhibits advantages over BZs.

The experience with abecarnil and zolpidem suggests it may be beneficial in terms of reducing BZ-like side effects, to limit either efficacy or affinity at BZ receptors constituted from $\alpha5$ subunits (Möhler et al., 1995). The majority of $\alpha5$-containing receptors are located in hippocampus and have been hypothesized to mediate the amnestic properties of BZs (Benavides et al., 1993; Faure-Halley et al., 1993). The recent discovery of imidazobenzodiazepine ligands that bind selectively to $\alpha5$-containing BZ receptors, should help test this hypothesis (Zhang et al., 1995).

The $\alpha4$ or $\alpha6$ subunit-containing $GABA_ARs$ are generally insensitive to BZs, such as diazepam. Receptors containing the $\alpha6$ subunit are of particular interest, because they are expressed almost exclusively in granule cells in the cerebellum (Lüddens et al., 1990). It has been proposed, though not yet proven, that these receptors are functionally involved in mediating the ataxic effects of alcohol (Lüddens et al., 1990; see Section 8.). The least-characterized members of the $GABA_AR$ family are those containing the $\alpha4$ subunit. Other than evidence for their localization in thalamus and hippocampal dentate gyrus, little is known about this particular $GABA_AR$ subtype (McKernan and Whiting, 1996).

11. Future Outlook

$GABA_ARs$ have already proven to be the primary target for some of the most widely used psychotropic drugs of modern medicine, principally the BZs. Within the last decade, molecular biology has provided unequivocal proof of the existence in brain of multiple subtypes of $GABA_ARs$. This has led to considerable speculation that it may be possible to target various $GABA_ARs$, in the expectation of providing a new generation of drugs with improved (or even additional) therapeutic properties, compared to BZs. To some extent, this has been achieved in the design of agents with selectivity (although limited) for BZ1 receptors. However, in order for the potential of this concept to become fully realized, much effort will initially be required to firmly establish roles for the individual GABA$_A$R subtypes at both physiological and, ultimately, behavioral levels. Several approaches can be taken to help achieve this difficult goal. For example, the use of recently developed subunit-selective antisera, in tandem with lesions of specific pathways in the brain, might reveal associations between GABA$_A$R subtypes and known neuronal pathways. Alternatively, the application of novel molecular biological technologies, such as antisense and transgenics, might also be useful to manipulate the expression of individual subunits, the effects of which can be determined using biochemical, electrophysiological, or behavioral techniques. The future of research on GABA$_A$Rs and their modulators promises to be very exciting.

References

Allan, A. M., Baier, L. D., and Zhang, X. (1992) Effects of lorazepam tolerance and withdrawal on GABA$_A$ receptor-operated chloride channels. *J. Pharmacol. Exp. Ther.* **261**, 295–402.

Angelotti, T. and Macdonald, R. L. (1993) Assembly of GABA$_A$ receptor subunits: $\alpha_1\beta_1$ and $\alpha_1\beta_1\gamma_{2S}$ subunits produce unique ion channels with dissimilar single-channel properties. *J. Neurosci.* **13**, 1429–1440.

Anholt, R. R., De Souza, E. B., Oster-Granite, M. L., and Snyder, S. H. (1985) Peripheral-type benzodiazepine receptors: autoradiographic localisation in whole-body sections of neonatal rats. *J. Pharmacol. Exp. Ther.* **233**, 517–526.

Ansseau, M., Olie, J-P., Von Frenckell, R., Jourdain, G., Stehle, B., and Guillet, P. (1991) Controlled comparisons in the efficacy and safety of four doses of suriclone, diazepam and placebo in generalised anxiety disorder. *Psychopharmacology* **104**, 439–443.

Arbilla, S., Benavides, J., Scatton, B., Tan, S., and Langer, S. Z. (1993) The mechanism of action of alpidem, in *Imidazopyridines and Anxiety Disorders: A Novel Experimental and Therapeutic Approach* (Bartholini, G., Garreau, M., Morselli, P. L., and Zivkovic, B., eds.), Raven, New York, pp. 61–67.

Arbilla, S., Depoortere, H., George, P., and Langer, S. Z. (1985) Pharmacological profile of zolpidem at benzodiazepine receptors and electrocorticogram in rats. *Naunyn Schmiedeberg's Arch. Pharmacol.* **330**, 248–251.

Auta, J., Giusti, P., Guidotti, A., and Costa, E. (1994) Imidazenil, a partial positive allosteric modulator of GABA$_A$ receptors, exhibits low tolerance and dependence liabilities in the rat. *J. Pharmacol. Exp. Ther.* **270**, 1262–1269.

Ballenger, J. C., McDonald, S., Noyes, R., Rickelo, K., Sussman, N., Woods, S., Patin, J., and Singer, J. (1991) The first double blind, placebo-controlled trial of a partial benzodiazepine agonist abecarnil (ZK 112-119) in generalised anxiety disorder. *Psychopharmacol. Bull.* **27**, 171–179.

Baulieu, E.-E., Robel, P., Vatier, O., Haug, A., Le Gascogne, C., and Bourreau, E. (1987) Neurosteroids: pregnenolone and dehydroepiandrosterone in the rat brain, in *Recep-*

tor-Receptor Interaction, a New Intramembrane Integrative Mechanism (Fuxe, K. and Agnati, L. F., eds.), MacMillan, Basingstoke, UK, pp. 89–104.

Benavides, J., Peny, B., Dubois, A., Perrault, G., Morel, E., Zivkovic, B., and Scatton, B. (1987) In vivo interaction of zolpidem with central benzodiazepine (BZD) binding sites (as labeled by [^{3}H]Ro 15-1788) in the mouse brain. Preferential affinity of zolpidem for the ω_1 (BZD$_1$) subtype. *J. Pharmacol. Exp. Ther.* **245,** 1033–1041.

Benavides, J., Peny, B., Ruano, D., Vitorica, J., and Scatton, B. (1993) Comparative autoradiographic distribution of central ω (benzodiazepine) modulatory site subtypes with high, intermediate and low affinity for zolpidem and alpidem. *Brain Res.* **604,** 240–250.

Blackburn, T. P., Davies, D. T., Forbes, I. T., Hayward, C. J., Johnson, C. N., Martin, R. T., Piper, D. C., Thomas, D. R., Thompson, M., Upton, N., and Ward, R. W. (1995) Isosteric replacement of the indole nucleus by benzothiophene in a series of pyrido[2,3-*b*]indoles with potential anxiolytic activity. *Bioorg. Med. Chem. Lett.* **5,** 2589–2592.

Blanchard, J. C., Boireau, A., Garret, C., and Julou, L. (1979) *In vitro* and *in vivo* inhibition by zopiclone of benzodiazepine binding to rodent brain receptors. *Life Sci.* **24,** 2417–2420.

Blanchard, J. C. and Julou, L. (1983) Suriclone—a new cyclopyrrolone derivative recognising receptors labelled by benzodiazepines in rat hippocampus and cerebellum. *J. Neurochem.* **40,** 601–607.

Bormann, J. (1988) Electrophysiology of GABA$_A$ and GABA$_B$ receptor subtypes. *Trends Neurosci.* **11,** 112–116.

Bowery, N. G., Collins, J. F., and Hill, R. G. (1976) Bicyclic phosphorous esters that are potent convulsants and GABA antagonists. *Nature (Lond.)* **261,** 601–603.

Braestrup, C. (1977) Benzodiazepine receptors in rat brain. *Nature (Lond.)* **266,** 732–734.

Braestrup, C. and Nielsen, M. (1983) Benzodiazepine receptors, in *Handbook of Psychopharmacology*, vol. 17 (Iversen, L. L., Iversen, S. D., and Snyder, S. H., eds.), Plenum, New York, pp. 285–384.

Braestrup, C., Nielsen, M., Honore, T., Jensen, I. H., and Petersen, E. N. (1983) Benzodiazepine receptor ligands with positive and negative efficacy. *Neuropharmacology* **22,** 1451–1457.

Braestrup, C., Nielsen, M., and Olsen, C. E. (1980) Urinary and brain β-carboline- 3-carboxylates as potent inhibitors of brain benzodiazepine receptors. *Proc. Natl. Acad. Sci. USA* **77,** 2288–2292.

Braestrup, C., Schmeichen, R., Neef, G., Nielsen, M., and Petersen, E. N. (1982) Interaction of convulsive ligands with benzodiazepine receptors. *Science (Wash., DC)* **216,** 1241–1243.

Brogden, R. N. and Goa, K. L. (1991) Flumazenil: a reappraisal of its pharmacological properties and therapeutic efficacy as a benzodiazepine antagonist. *Drugs* **42,** 1061–1089.

Brooks-Kayal, A. R. and Pritchett, D. B. (1993) Developmental changes in human γ-aminobutyric acid$_A$ receptor subunit composition. *Annals of Neurol.* **34,** 687–693.

Busto, U., Kaplan, H. L., Zawertailo, L., and Sellers, E. M. (1994) Pharmacologic effects and abuse liability of bretazenil, diazepam and alprazolam in humans. *Clin. Pharmacol. Ther.* **55,** 451–463.

Callachan, H., Cottrell, G. A., Hather, N. Y., Lambert, J. J., Nooney, J. M., and Peters, J. A. (1987) Modulation of the GABA$_A$ receptor by progesterone metabolites. *Proc. R. Soc. London Ser.* **231,** 359–369.

Charney, D.S. and Woods, S.W. (1989) Benzodiazepine treatment of panic disorder: a comparison of alprazolam and lorazepam. *J. Clin. Psychiatry* **50**, 418–423.

Chevalier, S. F., Mendelwicz, J., and Coupez, R. (1993) Safety and efficacy of alpidem, in *Imidazopyridines in Anxiety Disorders: A Novel Experimental and Therapeutic Approoch* (Bartholini, G., Garreau, M., Morselli, P.L., and Zivkovic, B., eds.), Raven, New York, pp. 193–199.

Concas, A., Serra, M., Atsoggiu, T., and Biggio, G. (1988) Foot-shock stress and anxiogenic β-carbolines increase t-[^{35}S]butylbicyclophosphorothionate binding in the rat cerebral cortex, an effect opposite to anxiolytic and γ-aminobutyric acid mimetics. *J. Neurochem.* **51**, 1868–1876.

Concas, A., Serra, M., Santoro, G., Maciocco, E., Cuccheddu, T., and Biggio, G. (1994) The effect of cyclopyrrolones on GABA_A receptor function is different from that of benzodiazepines. *Naunyn Schmiedebergs Arch. Pharmacol.* **350**, 294–300.

Costa, E. and Guidotti, A. (1991) Minireview: diazepam binding inhibitor (DBI): a peptide with multiple biological actions. *Life Sci.* **49**, 325–344.

Costa, E., Guidotti, A., Mao, C. C., and Suria, A. (1975) New concepts on the mechanism of action of the benzodiazepines. *Life Sci.* **17**, 167–186.

Depoortere, B., Zivkovic B., Lloyd, K. G., Sanger, D. J., Perrault, G., Langer, S. Z., and Bartholini, G. (1986) Zolpidem, a novel nonbenzodiazepine hypnotic. I. Neuropharmacological and behavioural effects. *J. Pharmacol. Exp. Ther.* **237**, 649–658.

Dillon, G. H., Im, W. B., Carter, D. B., and McKinley, D. D. (1995) Enhancement by GABA of the association rate of picrotoxin and *tert*-butylbicyclophosphorothionate to the rat cloned $\alpha_1\beta_2\gamma_2$ GABA_A receptor subtype. *Br. J. Pharmacol.* **115**, 539–545.

Dillon, G. H., Im, H. K., Hamilton, B. J., Carter, D. B., Gammill, R. B., Judge, T. M., and Im, W. B. (1993) U-93631 causes rapid decay of γ-aminobutyric acid-induced chloride currents in recombinant rat γ-aminobutyric acid type A receptors. *Mol. Pharmacol.* **44**, 860–864

Doble, A., Canton, T., Malgouris, C., Stutzmann, J. M., Piot, O., Bardone, M. C., Pauchet, C., and Blanchard, J. C. (1995) The mechanism of action of zopiclone. *Eur. Psychiatry* **10 (Suppl. 3)**, 117–128.

Doble, A., Canton, T., Piot, O., Zundel, J. L., Stutzmann, J. M., Cotrel, C., and Blanchard, J. C. (1992) The pharmacology of cyclopyrrolone derivatives acting at the GABA_A/benzodiazepine receptors, in *GABAergic Synaptic Transmission: Molecular, Pharmacological and Clinical Aspects* (Biggio, G., Concas, A., and Costa, E., eds.), Raven, New York, pp. 407–418.

Dorow, R., Horowski, R., Paschelke, G., Amin, M., and Braestrup, C. (1983) Severe anxiety induced by FG 7142, a β-carboline ligand for benzodiazepine receptors. *Lancet* **II**, 98–99.

Dubois, A., Benavides, J., Peny, B., Duverger, D., Fage, D., Gotti, B., MacKenzie, E. T., and Scatton, B. (1988) Imaging of primary and remote ischaemic and excitotoxic brain lesions. An autoradiographic study of peripheral type benzodiazepine binding sites in the rat and cat. *Brain Res.* **445**, 77–90.

Duncan, G. E., Breese, G. R., Criswell, H. E., McCowan, T. J., Herbert, J. S., Devaud, L. L., and Morrow, A. L. (1995) Distribution of [^{3}H]zolpidem binding sites in relation to messenger RNA encoding the α_1, β_2 and γ_2 subunits of GABA_A receptors in rat brain. *Neuroscience* **64**, 1113–1128.

Edgar, P. P. and Schwarz, R. D. (1992) Functionally relevant γ-aminobutyric acid_A receptors: equivalence between receptor affinity (K_D) and potency (EC_{50})? *Mol. Pharmacol.* **41**, 1124–1129.

Facklam, M., Schoch, P., Bonetti, E. P., Jenck, F., Martin, J. R., Moreau, J. L., and Haefely, W. E. (1992a) Relationship between benzodiazepine receptor occupancy and functional effects in vivo of four ligands of differing intrinsic efficacies. *J. Pharmacol. Exp. Ther.* **261**, 1113–1121.

Facklam, M., Schoch, P., and Haefely, W. (1992b) Relationship between benzodiazepine receptor occupancy and potentiation of γ-aminobutyric acid-stimulated chloride flux in vitro of four ligands of differing intrinsic efficacies. *J. Pharmacol. Exp. Ther.* **261**, 1106–1112.

Faure-Halley, C., Graham, D., Arbilla, S., and Langer, S. Z. (1993) Expression and properties of recombinant $\alpha_1\beta_2\gamma_2$ and $\alpha_5\beta_2\gamma_2$ forms of the rat GABA$_A$ receptor. *Eur. J. Pharamacol.* **246**, 283–287.

File, S.E. (1985) Tolerance to the behavioural actions of benzodiazepines. *Neurosci. Biobehav. Rev.* **9**, 113–122.

File, S. E. and Pellow, S. (1987) Behavioural pharmacology of minor tranquilisers. *Pharmac. Ther.* **35**, 265–290.

Forster, M. J., Prather, P. L., Patel, S. R., and Lal, H. (1995) The benzodiazepine receptor inverse agonist RO 15-3505 reverses recent memory deficits in aged mice. *Pharmacol. Biochem. Behav.* **51**, 557–560.

Fritschy, J. M., Paysan, J., Enna, A., and Möhler, H. (1994) Switch in the expression of rat GABA$_A$-receptor subtypes during postnatal development: an immunohistochemical study. *J. Neurosci.* **14**, 5302–5324.

Fuchs, K., Möhler, H., and Sieghart, W. (1988) Various proteins from rat brain, specifically and irreversibly labeled by [^{3}H]flunitrazepam, are distinct α-subunits of the GABA benzodiazepine receptor complex. *Neurosci. Lett.* **90**, 314–319.

Gallager, D. W., Lakoski, J. M., Gonsales, S. F., and Rauch, S. L. (1984) Chronic benzodiazepine treatment decreases postsynaptic GABA sensitivity. *Nature* **308**, 74–77.

Gardner, C. R. (1989) Interpretation of the behavioural effects of benzodiazepine receptor ligands. *Drugs of the Future* **14**, 51–67.

Gee, K.W. (1988) Steroid modulation of the GABA/benzodiazepine receptor linked chloride ionophore. *Mol. Neurobiol.* **2**, 291–317.

Gee, K. W., Lawrence, L. J., and Yamamura, H. J. (1986) Modulation of the chloride ionophore by benzodiazepine receptor ligands: influence of γ-aminobutyric acid and ligand efficacy. *Mol. Pharmacol.* **30**, 218–225.

Gee, K. W., McCauley, L. D., and Lan, N. C. (1995) A putative receptor for neurosteroids on the GABA$_A$ receptor complex: the pharmacological properties and therapeutic potential of epalons. *Crit. Rev. Neurobiol.* **9**, 207–227.

Gillard, N. P., Quirk K., Ragan, C. I., and McKernan, R. M. (1991) [^{125}I]Iodoclonazepam, a specific high affinity radioligand for the identification of BZ$_1$ and BZ$_2$ sites in rat brain. *Eur. J. Pharmacol.* **195**, 407–409.

Giusti, P. and Arban, R. (1993) Physiological and pharmacological bases for the diverse properties of benzodiazepines and their congeners. *Pharmacol. Res.* **27**, 201–215.

Giusti, P., Ducic, I., Puia, G., Arban, R., Walser, A., Guidotti, A., and Costa, E. (1993) Imidazenil: a new partial positive allosteric modulator of γ-aminobutyric acid (GABA) action at GABA$_A$ receptors. *J. Pharmacol. Exp. Ther.* **266**, 1018–1028.

Givens, B. S. and Breese, G. R. (1990) Site-specific enhancement of γ-aminobutyric acid mediated inhibition of neural activity by ethanol in the rat medial septal area. *J. Pharmacol. Exp. Ther.* **254**, 528–538.

Günther, U., Benson, J., Benke, D., Fritschy, J.-M., Reyes, G., Knoflach, F., Crestani, F.,

Aguzzi, A., Arigoni, M., Lang, Y., Bluethmann, H., Möhler, H., and Lüscher, B. (1995) Benzodiazepine-insensitive mice generated by targeted disruption of the γ_2 subunit gene of γ-aminobutyric acid type A receptors. *Proc. Natl. Acad. Sci.* **92**, 7745–7753.

Haefely, W. (1989) Pharmacology of the allosteric modulation of GABA$_A$ receptors by benzodiazepine receptor ligands, in *Allosteric Modulation of Amino Acid Receptors: Therapeutic Implications* (Barnard, E. A., and Costa, E., eds.), Raven, New York, pp. 47–69.

Haefely, W., Bonetti, E. P., Burkard, W. P., Cumin, R., Laurent, J.-P., Möhler, H., Pieri, L., Polc, P., Richards, J. G., Schaffner, R., and Scherschlicht, R. (1983) Benzodiazepine antagonists, in *The Benzodiazepines: From Molecular Biology to Clinical Practice* (Costa, E., ed.), Raven, New York, pp. 137–146.

Haefely, W., Kuskar, A., Möhler, H., Pieri, L., Polc, P., and Schaffner, R. (1975) Possible involvement of GABA in the central actions of benzodiazepines. *Adv. Biochem. Psychopharmacol.* **14**, 131–152.

Haefely, W., Kyburz, E., Gerecke, M., and Möhler, H. (1985) Recent advances in the molecular pharmacology of benzodiazepine receptors and in the structure-activity relationships of their agonists and antagonists, in *Advances in Drug Research*, vol. 14 (Testa, B., ed.) Academic, London, pp. 165–322.

Haefely, W., Martin, J. R., and Schoch, P. (1990) Novel anxiolytics that act as partial agonists at benzodiazepine receptors. *Trends Pharmacol. Sci.* **11**, 452–456.

Haigh, J. R. M. and Freely, M. (1988) RO 16-6028, a benzodiazepine receptor partial agonist, does not exhibit anticonvulsant tolerance in mice. *Eur. J. Pharmacol.* **147**, 283–285.

Harrison, N. L. and Simmonds, M. A. (1984) Modulation of the GABA receptor complex by a steroid anaesthetic. *Brain Res.* **323**, 287–292.

Henry, T. R., Frey, K. A., Sakellares, J. C., Gilman, S., Koeppe, R. A., Brunberg, J. A., Ross, D. A., Berent, S., Young, A. B., and Kuhl, D. E. (1993) In vivo cerebral metabolism and central benzodiazepine-binding in temporal lobe epilepsy. *Neurology* **43**, 1998–2006.

Hobbs, R. W., Rall, T. W., and Verdon, T. A. (1996) Hypnotics and sedatives; ethanol, in *Goodman and Gilman's The Pharmacological Basis of Therapeutics*, 9th ed. (Hardman, J. G. and Limbard, L. E., eds.), McGraw-Hill, New York, pp. 361–396.

Hollister, L. E., Muller-Oerlinghausen, B., Rickels, K., and Shader, R. I. (1993) Clinical use of benzodiazepines. *J. Clin. Psychopharmacol.* **13 (Suppl. 1)**, 1–169.

Hunkeler, W., Möhler, H., Piere, L., Polc, P., Bonetti, E. P., Cumin, R., Schaffner, R., and Haefely, W. (1981) Selective antagonists of benzodiazeopines. *Nature (Lond.)* **290**, 514–516.

Im, W. B. and Blakeman, D. P. (1991) Correlation between γ-aminobutyric acid$_A$ receptor ligand-induced changes in t-butylbicyclophosphoro-[^{35}S]thionate binding and ^{36}Cl$^-$ uptake in rat cerebrocortical membranes. *Mol. Pharmacol.* **39**, 394–398.

Inomata, N., Tokutomi, N., Oyama, Y., and Akaike, N. (1988) Intracellular picrotoxin blocks pentobarbital-gated Cl$^-$ conductance. *Neurosci. Res.* **6**, 72–75.

Jensen, L. H., Stephens, D. N., Sarter, M., and Petersen, E. N. (1987) Bidirectional effects of β-carbolines and benzodiazepines on cognitive processes. *Brain Res. Bull.* **19**, 359–364.

Jones, G. H., Schneider, C., Schneider, H. H., Seidler, J., Cole, B. J., and Stephens, D. N. (1994) Comparison of several benzodiazepine receptor ligands in two models of anxiolytic activity in the mouse: an analysis based on fractional receptor occupancies. *Psychopharmacology* **114**, 191–199.

Julou, L., Blanchard, J. C., and Dreyfus, J. F. (1985) Pharmacological and clinical studies of cyclopyrrolones: zopiclone and suriclone. *Pharmacol. Biochem. Behav.* **23**, 653–659.

Kardos, J. and Cash, D. J. (1990) $^{36}Cl^-$ flux measurements and desensitization of the γ-aminobutyric acid$_A$ receptor. *J. Neurochem.* **55**, 1095–1099.

Karobath, M., Placheta, P., Lippitsch, M., and Krogsgaard-Larsen, P. (1979) Is stimulation of benzodiazepine receptor binding mediated by a novel GABA receptor? *Nature (Lond.)* **278**, 748,749.

Kerr, J. S., Dawe, R. A., Parkin, C., and Hindmarch, I. (1995) Zopiclone in elderly patients: efficacy and safety. *Human Psychopharmacol.* **10**, 221–229.

Klepner, C. A., Lippa, A. S., Benson, D. I., Sabo, M. C., and Beer, B. (1979) Resolution of two biochemically and pharmacologically distinct benzodiazepine receptors. *Pharmacol. Biochem. Behav.* **11**, 457–462.

Knoflach, F., Drescher, U., Scheurer, L., Malherbe, P., and Möhler, H. (1993) Full and partial agonism displayed by benzodiazepine receptor ligands at recombinant γ-aminobutyric acid$_A$ receptor subtypes. *J. Pharmacol. Exp. Ther.* **266**, 385–391.

Korpi, E.R. (1994) Role of GABA$_A$ receptors in the actions of alcohol and alcoholism: recent advances. *Alcohol and Alcoholism* **29**, 115–129.

Lader, M. H. (1993) Withdrawal symptoms and rebound with anxiolytic drugs, in *Imidazopyridines in Anxiety Disorders: A Novel Experimental and Therapeutic Approach* (Bartholini, G., Garreau, M., Morselli, P. L., and Zivkovic, B., eds.), Raven, New York, pp. 227–233.

Lader, M. H. (1994) Benzodiazepines: a risk-benefit profile. *CNS Drugs* **1**, 377–387.

Lader, M. H. and File, S. H. (1987) The biological basis of benzodiazepine dependence. *Psychological Med.* **17**, 593–547.

Lambert, J. J., Belelli, D., Hill-Venning, C., and Peters, J. A. (1995) Neurosteroids and GABA$_A$ receptor function. *Trends Pharmacol. Sci.* **16**, 295–303.

Lan, N. C. and Gee, K. W. (1991) GABA$_A$ receptor complex in rat frontal cortex and spinal cord show differential responses to steroid modulation. *Am. Soc. Pharm. Exp. Ther. Mol. Pharmacol.* **40**, 995–999.

Langer, S. Z. and Arbilla, S. (1988a) Limitations of the benzodiazepine receptor nomenclature: a proposal for a pharmacological classification as omega receptor subtypes. *Fund. Clin. Pharmacol.* **2**, 159–170.

Langer, S. Z. and Arbilla, S. (1988b) Imidazopyridines as a tool for the charactersiation of benzodiazepine receptors: a proposal for a pharmacological classification as omega receptors. *Pharmacol. Biochem. Behav.* **29**, 763–766.

Langtry, H. D. and Benfield, P. (1990) Zolpidem. A review of its pharmacodynamic and pharmacokinetic properties and therapeutic potential. *Drugs* **40**, 291–313.

Legris, P., George, Y., and Boval, P. (1993) A comparative study of alpidem versus buspirone, in *Imidazopyridines in Anxiety Disorders: A Novel Experimental and Therapeutic Approach* (Bartholini, G., Garreau, M., Morselli, P.L., and Zivkovic, B., eds.) Raven, New York, pp. 183–192.

Leonard, B. E. (1993) Commentary on the mode of action of benzodiazepines. *J. Psychiatr. Res.* **27 (Suppl. 1)**, 193–207.

Lippa, A. S., Coupet, J., Greenblatt, E. N., Klepner, C. A., and Beer, B. (1979) A synthetic nonbenzodiazepine ligand for benzodiazepine receptors: a probe for investigating neuronal substrates of anxiety. *Pharmacol. Biochem. Behav.* **11**, 99–106.

Little, H. J., Nutt, D. J., and Taylor, S. C. (1984) Acute and chronic effects of benzodiazepine receptor ligand FG 7142: proconvulsant properties and kindling. *Br. J. Pharmacol.* **83,** 951–958.

Löscher, W. (1993) Abecarnil shows reduced tolerance development and dependence potential in comparison to diazepam: animal studies. *Psychopharmacol. Ser.* **11,** 96–112.

Löscher, W., Hönack, D., Scherkl, R., Hashem, A., and Frey, H. H. (1990) Pharmacokinetics, anticonvulsant efficacy and adverse effects of the β-carboline abecarnil, a novel ligand for benzodiazepine receptors, after acute and chronic administration in dogs. *J. Pharmacol. Exp. Ther.* **225,** 541–548.

Löscher, W. and Schmidt, D. (1988) Which animal models should be used in the search for new antiepileptic drugs? A proposal based on experimental and clinical considerations. *Epilepsy Res.* **2,** 145–181.

Lüddens, H. and Korpi, E. R. (1995) Biological function of GABA$_A$/benzodiazepine receptor heterogeneity. *J. Psychiat. Res.* **29,** 77–94.

Lüddens, H., Korpi, E. R., and Seeburg, P. H. (1995) GABA$_A$/benzodiazepine receptor heterogeneity: neurophysiological implications. *Neuropharmacology* **34,** 245–254.

Lüddens, H., Pritchett, D. B., Köhler, M., Killisch, I., Keinänen, K., Monyer, H., Sprengel, R., and Seeburg, P. H. (1990) Cerebellar GABA$_A$ receptor selective for a behavioural alcohol antagonist. *Nature (Lond.)* **346,** 648–651.

Lüddens, H., Seeburg, P. H., and Korpi, E. R. (1994) Impact of β and γ variants on ligand binding properties of γ-aminobutyric acid type A receptors. *Mol. Pharmacol.* **45,** 810–814.

Macdonald, R. L. and Olsen, R. W. (1994) GABA$_A$ receptor channels. *Ann. Rev. Neurosci.* **17,** 569–602.

Macdonald, R. L. and Twyman, R. E. (1992) Kinetic properties and regulation of GABA$_A$ receptor channels, in *Ion Channels*, vol. 3 (Narahashi, T., ed.), Plenum, New York, pp. 315–343.

Majewska, M. D. (1992) Neurosteroids: endogenous bimodal modulators of the GABA$_A$ receptor. Mechanism of action and physiological significance. *Prog. Neurobiol.* **38,** 379–395.

Malgouris, C., Perrot, F., Dupuis, M., Kiosseff, T., Daniel, M., Blanchard, J. C., and Doble, A. (1995) Autoradiographic distribution of [^{3}H]-suriclone binding sites in rat brain. *Drug Dev. Res.* **34,** 336–343.

Malizia, A. L. and Nutt, D. J. (1995) The effects of flumazenil in neuropsychiatric disorders. *Clin. Neuropharmacol.* **3,** 215–232.

Marks, J. (1983) The benzodiazepines—for good or evil. *Neuropsychobiology* **10,** 115–126.

McKernan, R. M. and Whiting, P. J. (1996) Which GABA$_A$-receptor subtypes really occur in the brain. *Trends Neurosci.* **19,** 139–143.

Miller, L. G., Greenblatt, D. J., Barnhill, J. G., and Shader, R. I. (1988) Tolerance is associated with benzodiazepine receptor down-regulation and decreased γ-aminobutyric acid$_A$ receptor function. *J. Pharmacol. Exp. Ther.* **246,** 170–176.

Miller, L. G., Woolverton, S., Greenblatt, D. J., Lopez, F., Roy, R. B., and Shader, R. I. (1989) Chronic benzodiazepine administration. IV. Rapid tolerance and receptor down regulation associated with alprazolam administration. *Biochem. Pharmacol.* **38,** 3773–3777.

Mindus, P., Ehrin, E., Eriksson, L., Fardre, L., and Hedstrom, C. G. (1986) Central benzodiazepine receptor binding studies with ^{11}C labelled Ro 15-1788 and positron emission tomography. *Pharmacopsychiatry* **19,** 2,3.

Möhler, H., Knoflach., F., Paysan, J., Motejlek, K., Benke, D., Lüscher, B., and Fritschy, J. M. (1995) Heterogeneity of GABA_A-receptors: cell-specific expression, pharmacology and regulation. *Neurochem. Res.* **20**, 631–636.

Möhler, H. and Okada, T. (1977) Benzodiazepine receptor: demonstration in the central nervous system. *Science* **198**, 849–851.

Möhler, H. and Richards, J. G. (1981) Agonist and antagonist benzodiazepine receptor interaction in vitro. *Nature (Lond.)* **294**, 763–765.

Mukhin, A. G., Papadopoulos, V., Costa, E., and Krueger, K. E. (1989) Mitochondrial benzodiazepine receptors regulate steroid biosynthesis. *Proc. Natl. Acad. Sci. USA* **86**, 9813–9816.

Mumford, G. K., Rush, C. R., and Griffiths, R. R. (1995) Abecarnil and alprazolam in humans: behavioural, subjective and reinforcing effects. *J. Pharmacol. Exp. Ther.* **272**, 570–580.

Musch, B. and Maillard, F. (1990) Zopiclone, the third generation hypnotic: a clinical overview. *Int. Clin. Psychopharmacol.* **5**, 147–158.

Nutt, D. J., Smith, C. F., Bennett, R., and Jackson, H. C. (1992) Investigations on the "set-point" theory of benzodiazepine receptor function, in *GABAergic Synaptic Transmission* (Biggio, G., Concas, A., and Costa, E., eds.), Raven, New York, pp. 419–429.

Obata, T., Morelli, M., Concas, A., Serra, M., and Yamamura, H. I. (1988) Modulation of GABA-stimulated chloride flux into membrane vesicles from rat cerebral cortex by benzodiazepines and nonbenzodiazepines, in *Chloride Channels and Their Modulation by Neurotransmitters and Drugs* (Biggio, G. and Costa, E., eds.), Raven, New York, pp. 175–187.

O'Brien, C.P. (1996) Drug addiction and drug abuse, in *Goodman and Gilman's The Pharmacological Basis of Therapeutics*, 9th ed. (Hardman, J. G.and Limbard, L. E., eds.), McGraw-Hill, New York, pp. 557–577.

Olsen, R.W. (1982) Drug interactions at the GABA receptor-ionophore complex. *Ann. Rev. Pharmacol. Toxicol.* **22**, 245–277.

Olsen, R. W., Bergmann, M. O., Van Ness, P. C., Lummis, S. C., Watkins, A. E., Napias, C., and Greenlee, D. V. (1981) γ-Aminobutyric acid receptor binding in mammalian brain. Heterogeneity of binding sites. *Mol. Pharmacol.* **19**, 217–227.

Olsen, R. W. and Snowman, A. M. (1983) [³H]Bicuculline methochloride binding to low-affinity γ-aminobutyric acid receptor sites. *J. Neurochem.* **41**, 1653–1663.

Olsen, R. W. and Tobin, A. J. (1990) Molecular biology of GABA_A receptors. *FASEB J.* **4**, 1469–1480.

Owen, R. T. and Tyrer, P. (1983) Benzodiazepine dependence. *Drugs* **25**, 385–398.

Ozawa, M., Nakada, Y., Sugimachi, K., Yabuuchi, F., Akai, T., Mizuta, E., Kuno, S., and Yamaguchi, M. (1994a) Pharmacological characterisation of the novel anxiolytic β-carboline in rodents and primates. *Jpn. J. Pharmacol.* **64**, 179–187.

Ozawa, M., Sugimachi, K., Nakada-Kometani, Y., Akai, T., and Yamaguchi, M. (1994b) Chronic pharmacological activities of the novel anxiolytic β-carboline abecarnil in rats. *J. Pharmacol. Exp. Ther.* **269**, 457–462.

Panchera, P., Bressa, G. M., and Borghi, C. (1993) Double-blind randomised studies on the therapeutic action of alpidem in generalised anxiety disorders, in *Imidazopyridines in Anxiety Disorders: A Novel Experimental and Therapeutic Approach* (Bartholini, G., Garreau, M., Morselli, P. L., and Zivkovic, B., eds.), Raven, New York, pp. 155–164.

Parola, A. L., Yarnamura, H. I., and Laird, H. E., II (1993) Minireview: peripheral-type benzodiazepine receptors. *Life. Sci.* **52,** 1329–1342.

Paul, S. M. and Purdy, R. H. (1992) Neuroactive steroids. *FASEB J.* **6,** 2311–2322.

Paysan, J., Bolz, J., Möhler, H., and Fritschy, J. M. (1994) GABA_A receptor α_1 subunit, an early marker for area specification in developing rat cerebral cortex. *J. Comp. Neurol.* **350,** 133–149.

Perrault, G., Morel, E., Sanger, D. J., and Zivkovic, B. (1990) Differences in pharmacological profiles of a new generation of benzodiazepine and non-benzodiazepine hypnotics. *Eur. J. Pharmacol.* **187,** 487–494.

Perrault, G., Morel, E., Sanger, D. J., and Zivkovic, B. (1992) Lack of tolerance and physical dependence upon repeated treatment with the novel hypnotic zolpidem. *J. Pharmacol. Exp. Ther.* **263,** 290–303.

Perrault, G., Morel, E., Sanger, D. J., and Zivkovic, B. (1993) Repeated treatment with alpidem, a new anxiolytic, does not induce tolerance or physical dependence. *Neuropharmacology* **32,** 855–863.

Persson, A., Ehrin, E., Eriksson, L., Fardre, L., Hedstrom, C. G., Litton, J. A., Mindus, P., and Sedvall, G. (1985) Imaging of [^{11}C]-labelled Ro 15- 1788 binding to benzodiazepine receptors in the human brain by positron emission tomography. *J. Psychiatr. Res.* **19,** 609–622.

Peters, J. A., Kirkness, E. F., Callachan, H., Lambert, J. J., and Turner, A. J. (1988) Modulation of the GABA_A receptor by depressant barbiturates and pregnane steroids. *Br. J. Pharmacol.* **94,** 1257–1269.

Petursson, H. and Lader, M. H. (1981) Benzodiazepine dependence. *Br. J. Addict.* **76,** 133–145.

Piot, O., Betschart, J., Stutzmann, J. M., and Blanchard, J. C. (1990) Cyclopyrrolones, unlike some benzodiazepines, do not induce physical dependence in mice. *Neurosci. Lett.* **117,** 140–143.

Polc, P. (1988) Electrophysiology of benzodiazepine receptor ligands: multiple mechanisms and sites of action. *Prog. Neurobiol.* **31,** 349–424.

Potokar, J. and Nutt, D. J. (1994) Anxiolytic potential of benzodiazepine partial agonists. *CNS Drugs* **1,** 305–315.

Pribilla, I., Neuhaus, R., Huba, R., Hillmann, M., Turner, J. D., Stephens, D. N., and Schneider, H. H. (1993) Abecarnil is a full agonist at some, and a partial agonist at other recombinant GABA_A receptor subtypes. *Psychopharmacology Ser.* **11,** 50–61.

Pritchett, D. B., Lüddens, H., and Seeburg, P. H. (1989a) Type I and type II GABA_A-benzodiazepine receptors produced in transfected cells. *Science (Wash. DC)* **245,** 1389–1392.

Pritchett, D. B. and Seeburg, P. H. (1990) γ-Aminobutyric acid_A receptor α_5-subunit creates novel type II benzodiazepine receptor pharmacology. *J. Neurochem.* **54,** 1802–1804.

Pritchett, D. G., Sontheimer, H., Shivers, B. D., Ymer, S., Kettenmann, H., Schofield, P. R., and Seeburg, P. H. (1989b) Importance of a novel GABA_A receptor subunit for benzodiazepine pharmacology. *Nature* **338,** 582–585.

Puia, G., Ducic, I., Vicini, S., and Costa, E. (1992) Molecular mechanisms of the partial allosteric modulatory effects of bretazenil at γ-aminobutyric acid type A receptor. *Proc. Natl. Acad. Sci.* **89,** 3620–3624.

Puia, G., Vicini, S., Seeburg, P. H., and Costa, E. (1991) Influence of recombinant γ-aminobutyric acid_A receptor subunit composition on the action of allosteric modulators of γ-aminobutyric acid-gated Cl⁻ currents. *Mol. Pharments. Mol. Pharmacol.* **39**, 691–696.

Richards, J. G., Schoch, P., and Haefely, W. (1991) Benzodiazepine receptors: new vistas. *Semin. Neurosci.* **3**, 191–203.

Rickels, K. and Schweizer, E. E. (1987) Current pharmacotherapy of anxiety and panic, in *Psychopharmacology, The Third Generation of Progress* (Meltzer, H. Y., ed.), Raven, New York, pp. 1193–1203.

Ruano, D., Benavides, J., Machado, A., and Vitorica, J. (1993) Regional differences in the enhancement by GABA of [^{3}H]zolpidem binding to ω_1 sites in rat brain membranes and sections. *Brain Res.* **600**, 134–140.

Samson, Y., Hantraye, P., Baron, J. C., Soussaline, F., and Maziere, M. (1985) Kinetics and displacement of [^{11}C] Ro 15-1788, a benzodiazepine antagonist studied in human brain *in vivo* by positron tomography. *Eur. J. Pharmacol.* **110**, 247–251.

Sanger, D. J., Perrault, G., Morel, E., Joly, D., and Zivkovic, B. (1993) The psychopharmacological profile of alpidem, in *Imidazopyridines in Anxiety Disorders: A Novel Experimental and Therapeutic Approach* (Bartholini, G., Garreau, M., Morselli, P. L., and Zivkovic, B., eds.), Raven, New York, pp. 73–84.

Sannerud, C. A., Ator, N. A., and Griffiths, R. R. (1992) Behavioural pharmacology of abecarnil in baboons: self-injection, drug discrimination and physical dependence. *Behav. Pharmacol.* **3**, 507–516.

Sannerud, C. A., Ator, N. A., and Griffiths, R. R. (1993) Behavioural pharmacology of abecarnil in baboons: reduced dependence and abuse potential. *Psychopharmacol. Ser.* **11**, 113–119.

Sapp, D. W., Witte, U., Turner, D. M., Longoni, B., Kokka, N., and Olsen, R. W. (1992) Regional variation in steroid anaesthetic modulation of [^{35}S]TBPS binding to γ-aminobutyric$_A$ receptors in rat brain. *Am. Soc. Pharm. Exp. Ther. Mol. Pharmacol.* **262**, 801–808.

Savic, I., Persson, A., Roland, P., Pauli, S. Sedvall, G., and Widen, L. (1988) In vivo demonstration of reduced benzodiazepine receptor binding in human epileptic foci. *Lancet* **2**, 863–866.

Schneider, H. H. and Stephens, D. N. (1988) Co-existence of kindling induced by β-carboline, FG 7142 and tolerance to diazepam following chronic treatment in mice. *Eur. J. Pharmacol.* **154**, 35–45.

Schoh, P., Moreau, J. L., Martin, J. R., and Haefely, W. E. (1993) Aspects of benzodiazepine receptor structure and function with relevance to drug tolerance and dependence. *Biochem. Soc. Symp.* **59**, 121–134.

Schousboe, A. and Redburn, D. A. (1995) Modulatory actions of γ-aminobutyric acid (GABA) on GABA type A receptor subunit expression and function. *J. Neurosci. Res.* **41**, 1–7.

Segal, M. and Barker, J. L. (1984) Rat hippocampal neurones in culture: properties of GABA activated Cl⁻ ion conductance. *J. Neurophysiol.* **55**, 500–515.

Serra, M., Ghiani, C. A., Motzo, C., and Biggio, G. (1993) Pharmacological evidence for full agonist activity of abecarnil at certain GABA$_A$ receptors. *Pharmacol. Ser.* **11**, 62–78.

Serra, M., Ghiani, C. A., Motzo, C., Cuccheddu, T., Floris, S., Giusti, P., and Biggio, G. (1994) Imidazenil, a new partial agonist of benzodiazepine receptors, reverses the inhibitory action of isoniazid and stress on γ-aminobutyric acid$_A$ receptor function. *J. Pharmacol. Exp. Ther.* **269**, 32–38.

Sieghart, W. (1989) Multiplicity of GABA_A-benzodiazepine receptors. *Trends Pharmacol. Sci.* **10**, 407–411.

Sieghart, W. (1995) Structure and pharmacology of γ-aminobutyric acid_A receptor subtypes. *Pharmacol. Rev.* **47**, 181–234.

Sieghart, W. and Schlerka, W. (1991) Potency of several type I-benzodiazepine receptor ligands for inhibition of [³H]flunitrazepam binding in different rat brain tissues. *Eur. J. Pharmacol.* **197**, 103–107.

Skolnick, P., Crawley, J. N., Glowa, J. R., and Paul, S. M. (1984) β-Carboline-induced anxiety states. *Psychopathology* **17**, 52–60.

Smith, G. B. and Olsen, R. W. (1995) Functional domains of GABA_A receptors. *Trends Pharmacol. Sci.* **16**, 162–167

Spencer, C. M. and Benfield, P. (1995) Abecarnil in generalised anxiety disorder: an initial appraisal of its clinical potential. *CNS Drugs* **3**, 69–82.

Squires, R. F., Benson, D. I., Braestrup, C., Coupet, J., Klepner, C. A., Myers, V., and Beer, B. (1979) Some properties of brain specific benzodiazepine receptors: new evidence for multiple receptors. *Pharmacol. Biochem. Behav.* **10**, 825–830.

Squires, R. F. and Braestrup, C. (1977) Benzodiazepine receptors in rat brain. *Nature (Lond.)* **266**, 732–734.

Squires, R. F., Casida, J. E., Richardson, M., and Saederup, E. (1983) [³⁵S]-*t*-butylbicyclophosphorothionate binds with high affinity to brain specific sites coupled to γ-aminobutyric acid_A and ion recognition sites. *Mol. Pharmacol.* **23**, 326–336.

Stephens, D. N., Schneider, H. H., Kehr, W., Andrews, J. S., Rettig, K. J., Turski, L., Schmiechen, R., Turner, J. D., Jensen, L. H., Petersen, E. N., Honore, T., and Hansen, J. B. (1990) Abecarnil, a metabolically stable, anxioselective β-carboline acting at benzodiazepine receptors. *J. Pharmacol. Exp. Ther.* **253**, 334–343.

Stephens, D.N., Turski, L., Hillman, M., Turner, J. D., Schneider, H. H., and Yamaguchi, M. (1992) What are the differences between abecarnil and conventional benzodiazepine anxiolytics? in *GABAergic Synaptic Transmission* (Biggio, G., Concas, A., and Costa, E., eds.), Raven, New York, pp. 395–405.

Stephens, D. N., Turski, L., Jones, G. H., Steppuhn, K. G., and Schneider, H. H. (1993) Abecarnil: a novel anxiolytic with mixed full agonist/partial agonist properties in animal models of anxiety and sedation. *Psychopharmacol. Ser.* **11**, 79–95.

Stephenson, F. A., Duggan, M. J., and Pollard, S. (1990) The γ₂-subunit is an integral component of the γ-aminobutyric acid_A receptor, but the α₁ polypeptide is the principal site of the agonist benzodiazepine photoaffinity labeling reaction. *J. Biol. Chem.* **265**, 21,160–21,165.

Steppuhn, K. G., Schneider, H. H., Turski, L., and Stephens, D. N. (1992) Long-term treatment with abecarnil does not induce diazepam-like dependence in mice. *J. Pharmacol. Exp. Ther.* **264**, 1395–1400.

Study, R. E. and Barker, J. L. (1981) Diazepam and (–)pentobarbital: fluctuation analysis reveals different mechanisms for potentiation of γ-aminobutyric acid responses in cultured central neurones. *Proc. Natl. Acad. Sci. USA* **78**, 7180–7184.

Supavilai, P. and Karobath, M. (1984) [³⁵S]*t*-butylbicyclophosphorothionate binding sites are constituents of the γ-aminobutyric acid benzodiazepine receptor complex. *J. Neurosci.* **4**, 1193–1200.

Suzdak, P. D., Glowa, J. R., Crawley, J. N., Schwartz, R. D., Skolnick, P., and Paul, S. M. (1986) A selective imidazobenzodiazepine antagonist of ethanol in the rat. *Science (Wash. DC)* **234**, 1243–1247.

Thiebot, M.-H. and Soubrie, P. (1983) Behavioural pharmacology of the benzodiazepines, in *The Benzodiazepines: From Molecular Biology to Clinical Practice* (Costa, E., ed.), Raven, New York, pp. 67–92.

Trifiletti, R. R. and Snyder, S. H. (1984) Anxiolytic cyclopyrrolones zopiclone and suriclone bind to a novel site linked allosterically to benzodiazepine receptors. *Mol. Pharmacol.* **26,** 458–469.

Turski, L., Stephens, D.N., Jensen, L.H., Petersen, E. N., Meldrum, B. S., Patel, S., Bondo Hansen, J., Löscher, W., Schneider, H. H., and Schmiechen, R. (1990) Anticonvulsant action of the β-carboline abecarnil: studies in rodents and baboon, *Papio papio. J. Pharmacol. Exp. Ther.* **253,** 344–352.

Uusi-Oukari, M., and Korpi, E. R. (1990) Diazepam sensitivity of the binding of an imidazobenzodiazepine, [^{3}H]Ro 15-4513, in cerebellar membranes from two rat lines developed for high and low alcohol sensitivity. *J. Neurochem.* **54,** 1980–1987.

Wafford, K. A., Bain, C. J., Quirk, K., McKernan, R. M., Wingrove, P. B., Whiting, P. J., and Kemp, J. A. (1994) A novel allosteric modulatory site on the $GABA_A$ receptor β subunit. *Neuron* **12,** 775–782.

Wafford, K. A., Burnett, D. M., Leidenheimer, N. J., Burt, D. R., Wang, J. B., Kofuji, P., Dunwiddie, T. V., Harris, R. A., and Sikola, J. M. (1991) Ethanol sensitivity of the $GABA_A$ receptor expressed in *Xenopus* oocytes requires 8 amino acids contained in the γ_2L-subunit. *Neuron* **7,** 27–33.

Wafford, K. A., Whiting, P. J., and Kemp, J. A. (1993) Differences in affinity of benzodiazepine receptor ligands at recombinant γ-aminobutyric acid$_A$ receptor subtypes. *Mol. Pharmacol.* **43,** 240–244.

Whiting, P., McKernan, R. M., and Iversen, L. L. (1990) Another mechanism for creating diversity in γ-aminobutyrate type A receptors: RNA splicing directs expression of two forms of γ_2 subunit one of which contains a protein kinase C phosphorylation site. *Proc. Natl. Acad. Sci. USA* **87,** 9966–9970.

Wisden, W., Laurie, D. J., Monyer, H., and Seeburg, P. H. (1992) The distribution of 13 $GABA_A$ receptor subunit mRNAs in the rat brain. I. Telencephalon, diencephalon, mesencephalon. *J. Neurosci.* **12,** 1040–1062.

Woods, J. H., Katz, J. L., and Winger, G. (1987) Abuse liability of benzodiazepines. *Pharmacol. Rev.* **39,** 251–392.

Woods, J. H., Katz, J. L., and Winger, G. (1992) Benzodiazepines: use, abuse and consequences. *Pharmacol. Rev.* **44,** 151–347.

Wu, Y., Rosenberg, H. C., and Chiu, T. H. (1995) Rapid down-regulation of [^{3}H]zolpidem binding to rat brain benzodiazepine receptors during flurazepam treatment. *Eur. J. Pharmacol.* **278,** 125–132.

Yanganita, T. (1993) Dependence potential of zopiclone studied in monkeys. *Pharmacology* **27 (Suppl. 2),** 216–227.

Zhang, P., Lin., U., McKernan, R., Wafford, K., and Cook, J. M. (1995) Studies of novel imidazobenzodiazepine ligands at $GABA_A$/BzR subtypes: effect of C(3) substituents on receptor subtype selectivity. *Med. Chem. Res.* **5,** 487–495.

Zivkovic, B., Morel, E., Joly, D., Perrault, G., Sanger, D. J., and Lloyd, K. G. (1990) Pharmacological and behavioural profile of alpidem as an anxiolytic. *Pharmacopsychiatry* **23,** 108–113.

Zundel, J. L., Blanchard, J. C., and Julou, L. (1985) Partial chemical characterisation of cyclopyrrolones ([^{3}H]-suriclone) and benzodiazepines ([^{3}H]-flunitrazepam) binding sites differences. *Life Sci.* **36,** 2247–2255.

CHAPTER 5

The Interaction
of Intravenous Anesthetic Agents
with Native
and Recombinant GABA$_A$ Receptors

An Electrophysiological Study

Jeremy J. Lambert, Delia Belelli,
Marco Pistis, Claire Hill-Venning,
and John A. Peters

1. Introduction

The γ-aminobutyric acid type-A (GABA$_A$) receptor is a ligand-gated, anion-selective, ion channel that exists as a pentameric complex of structurally homologous subunits (Sieghart, 1995; Smith and Olsen, 1995). Four families of subunit, termed α, β, δ, and γ, whose members may co-assemble to create GABA$_A$ receptors with differential biophysical and pharmacological properties, are currently recognized (Burt and Kamatchi, 1991; Macdonald and Angelotti, 1993; Whiting et al., 1995). GABA$_A$ receptor isoforms mediate the majority of the inhibitory action of GABA within the central nervous system (CNS), the activation of postsynaptically located GABA$_A$ receptors resulting in an increase in membrane conductance, predominantly to chloride ions, which shunts the influence of excitatory neurotransmitters, such as glutamate (Mody et al., 1994).

GABA$_A$ receptor-mediated inhibition represents a key process in which information transfer within the CNS can be modulated by therapeutic agents. Facilitation of GABA-ergic transmission by drugs from diverse chemical classes can produce a broad spectrum of behavioral effects that include

The GABA Receptors Eds.: S. J. Enna and N. G. Bowery
Humana Press Inc., Totowa, NJ

anxiolytic, anticonvulsant, sedative, and most profoundly, general anesthetic actions (Sieghart, 1995). The latter is remarkable because it represents the common end-point of the physiological and pharmacological actions of structures that vary from simple, chemically inert gases to complex steroidal agents that display exquisite structure-activity requirements for the induction of general anesthesia (Phillipps, 1975; Franks and Lieb, 1994; Lambert et al., 1995; Little, 1996). Against this background, it has become increasingly difficult to continue to support a unitary theory of general anesthesia; yet, the fact remains that the majority of clinically useful anesthetics at relevant concentrations, and most experimental anesthetics, share the common feature of potentiating the actions of GABA at the $GABA_A$ receptor (Tanelian et al., 1993; Franks and Lieb, 1994). While not dismissing the importance of alternative ion channel targets as mediators of anesthetic action, positive allosteric modulation of the $GABA_A$ receptor, in addition to being well documented, has the simplistic appeal of being a logical mechanism by which the various components of the anesthetic state might be achieved.

Recent electrophysiological studies suggest that, at least for some GABA-ergic synapses within the CNS, the concentration of synaptically released GABA is sufficient to saturate a relatively small number of postsynaptically located $GABA_A$ receptors, which respond rapidly and efficiently to occupation by the transmitter (Mody et al., 1994; cf Frerking et al., 1995). These features place a number of limitations on the mechanisms by which the many anesthetic agents that are known to exert a positive allosteric influence upon the $GABA_A$ receptor can act to augment fast inhibitory neurotransmission within the CNS. In particular, prolongation of the duration of inhibitory postsynaptic currents (IPSCs) to achieve a temporal summation of inhibitory tone, rather than an augmentation of IPSC peak amplitude, would appear to be the most relevant variable (Harrison et al., 1987a; Jones and Harrison, 1993).

If it is accepted that the modulation of $GABA_A$ receptor-mediated inhibition is likely to contribute to general anesthesia, it is clearly relevant to question whether all $GABA_A$ receptor isoforms are uniformly sensitive to anesthetic action, or whether subunit composition exerts a substantial influence. The issue assumes importance because the differential distribution of $GABA_A$ receptor subunits within the CNS (Whiting et al., 1995) might help to explain regional variations in sensitivity to anesthetics. Moreover, the identification of subunit combinations that respond differentially to general anesthetic agents (Harris et al., 1995) can be expected to provide clues about protein domains that contribute to anesthetic binding pockets. A burgeoning literature addressing the role of subunit composition in the allosteric modulation of recombinant $GABA_A$ receptor isoforms makes it timely to survey the extent of developments in this field. In reviewing the literature and comparing the actions of these anesthetics on recombinant receptors composed of different subunits, the following should be born in mind: The magnitude of GABA potentiation produced by these agents is dependent upon the control concentration of GABA applied relative to the maximal response produced by GABA (e.g., Harris et al., 1995; Belelli et al., 1996). As the affinity of GABA for recombinant receptors is dependent upon their subunit composition (Ebert et al., 1994), the control concentration of GABA utilized must be titrated to the receptor being studied (e.g., EC_{10} concentration; *see* Belelli et al., 1996) for meaningful comparison of anesthetic action to be made across different $GABA_A$ receptors. Furthermore, it cannot be assumed that all subunits, injected or transfected into cell lines or *Xenopus laevis* oocytes, are uniformly expressed. Indeed, recent evidence suggests that certain combinations are retained in the endoplasmic reticulum and are not expressed on the cell surface (Connolly et al., 1996).

The present review focuses upon intravenous anesthetics drawn from several different chemical classes, including barbiturate (pentobarbitone), pregnane steroid (alphaxalone, 5α-pregnan-3α-ol-20-one), alkylphenol (propofol), and imidazole (etomidate) compounds (*see* Fig. 1). The actions of these agents upon both native and recombinant $GABA_A$ receptors will be addressed, together with recent indications that the positive allosteric regulation by certain of these agents may extend to the related anion-selective, ligand-gated channel, the strychnine-sensitive glycine receptor.

2. Barbiturates

Investigations that began over 50 years ago first suggested that anesthetic barbiturates may act to enhance neuronal inhibition (Eccles and Malcolm, 1946; Eccles et al., 1963). Subsequently, several electrophysiological studies have demonstrated that, among other actions, depressant barbiturates act as positive allosteric modulators of the $GABA_A$ receptor to enhance GABA-mediated inhibition (e.g., Nicoll, 1975; Barker and Mathers, 1981; Schulz and Macdonald, 1981). Complementary neurochemical approaches have established that anesthetic barbiturates potentiate GABA-stimulated [$^{36}Cl^-$] flux in rat brain synaptosomes and enhance the binding of $GABA_A$ receptor agonists (e.g., [^3H]muscimol) and benzodiazepines (e.g., [^3H]flunitrazepam) to, and displace the binding of, noncompetitive antagonists (e.g., [^{35}S]TBPS) from vertebrate brain membrane homogenates (e.g., Olsen et al., 1986; Ticku and Rastogi, 1986; Olsen, 1988, Sieghart, 1995).

Analysis of the power spectra of GABA-induced current fluctuations, recorded from mouse spinal neurons in culture in the presence and absence of

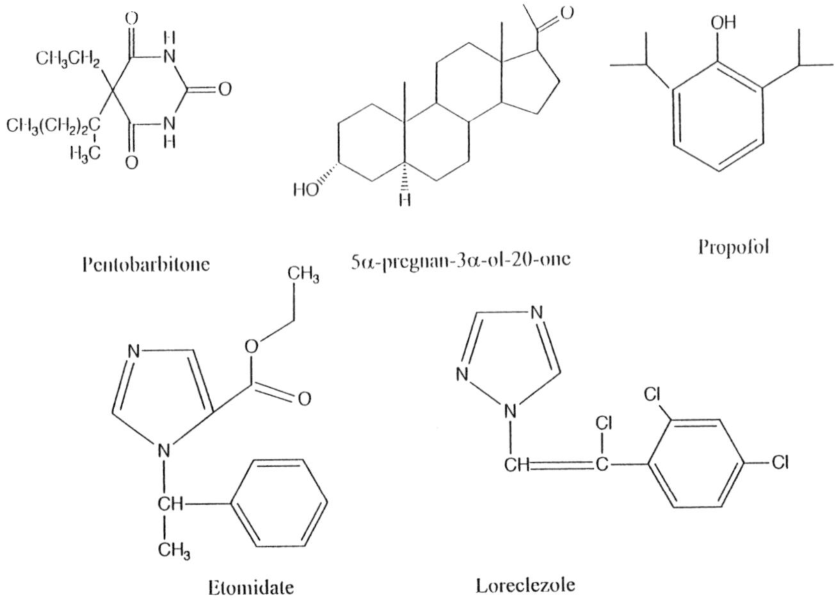

Pentobarbitone   5α-pregnan-3α-ol-20-one   Propofol

Etomidate   Loreclezole

Fig. 1. The diverse chemical structures of the iv anesthetic agents described here. The structure of the anticonvulsant loreclezole is shown for comparison with the anesthetic etomidate.

depressant barbiturates, suggested their enhancement of agonist function may be caused primarily by prolongation of the mean channel open duration, with little or no influence on the frequency of channel opening, or single channel conductance (Study and Barker, 1981). A subsequent kinetic analysis utilizing patch-clamp techniques demonstrated that GABA-gated chloride channels of mouse spinal neurons may exist in three distinct open states (Macdonald et al., 1989). The introduction of modulatory concentrations of phenobarbitone or pentobarbitone did not prolong all single channel openings *per se*, but instead increased the probability that the channel will enter a naturally occurring open state of relatively long duration (Macdonald et al., 1989).

What are the consequences of this modulation of channel kinetics for GABA-ergic neurotransmission? Several studies have reported that clinically relevant concentrations of barbiturates dramatically prolong the decay time of GABA receptor-mediated inhibitory postsynaptic currents (IPSCs) recorded from brain slices and synaptically coupled neurons grown in cell culture (Barker and McBurney, 1979; Segal and Barker, 1984; Gage and Robertson, 1985; Holland et al., 1990; De Koninck and Mody, 1994). Electrically evoked IPSCs result from the release of GABA from several synaptic boutons. Unless this release is completely synchronous, the influence of modulatory drugs upon IPSC rise and decay times and peak amplitude cannot simply be employed to infer the underlying kinetic mechanism(s) (Mody et al., 1994). The application of the patch-clamp technique to in vitro brain slices (pretreated with tetrodotoxin and ionotropic glutamate receptor antagonists) has allowed miniature (m) IPSCs to be recorded from neuronal cell bodies with a preserved natural synaptic architecture. Quantal analysis and the low current variance associated with the peak of the synaptic response suggest that such events result from the saturation of a small number of receptors by high concentrations of GABA (Mody et al., 1994). Recordings performed under these conditions have recently been made from dentate gyrus granule cells of the rat hippocampus (De Koninck and Mody, 1994). Given the lack of a barbiturate effect upon channel opening frequency (Macdonald et al., 1989), together with the proposed saturation of the postsynaptic receptors during the synaptic event, it was not surprising that pentobarbitone (50 μM) had little or no influence upon the amplitude, or rise time, of the mIPSC (De Koninck and Mody, 1994). However, consistent with its action on GABA channel gating kinetics (Macdonald et al., 1989), pentobarbitone dramatically prolonged the mIPSC decay time (De Koninck and Mody, 1994).

The application of nonstationary fluctuation analysis to the mIPSC permits the determination of the single-channel properties of synaptic $GABA_A$ receptors (Mody et al., 1994; De Koninck and Mody, 1994). Reinforcing the results of current fluctuation and single channel studies, pentobarbitone was found to have no effect upon single-channel conductance, or the number of channels activated by GABA, but to dramatically alter the open-channel kinetics (De Koninck and Mody, 1994). Such an effect provides a powerful molecular mechanism to enhance synaptic transmission, even under conditions in which, at the peak of the synaptic event, the synaptic $GABA_A$ receptor population may be saturated by neurotransmitter. It is pertinent to note that the majority of electrophysiological studies, examining the influence of anesthetics upon $GABA_A$ receptor function, quantify the actions of such compounds to potentiate the amplitude of currents induced by submaximal concentrations of GABA. The recent demonstration that the fast timecourse of mIPSCs can be reproduced by rapidly (<1mS) applying saturating concentrations of GABA onto excised outside-out membrane patches, containing a few $GABA_A$ receptors, may provide an experimental model that mimics anesthetic action in vivo more closely (Maconochie et al., 1994; Puia et al., 1994; Jones and Westbrook, 1996).

It has long been known that, at concentrations higher than those required for the enhancement of $GABA_A$ receptor-mediated responses, depressant barbiturates, such as pentobarbitone, directly activate the receptor-channel complex (Nicoll, 1975; Barker and Ransom, 1978; Nicoll and Wojtowicz, 1980). Acting upon voltage-clamped neurons, or paraneurons maintained in culture, pentobarbitone induces a current response that has been described to vary linearly with membrane potential (Akaike et al., 1987), or to display slight outward (Akaike et al., 1985; Peters et al., 1988) or inward (Robertson, 1989) rectification. As for potentiation of GABA, direct activation of the receptor complex is stereoselective, the order of potency being (–)-pentobarbitone > (±)-pentobarbitone > (+)-pentobarbitone (Huang and Barker, 1980; Akaike et al., 1985; ffrench-Mullen et al., 1993). On the basis of pH-induced alterations in the effectiveness of pentobarbitone, it has been suggested that the neutral species is responsible for agonism (Robertson, 1989).

At very high concentrations (≥ 1 mM), pentobarbitone has been reported to elicit complex current responses in which a transient peak current, succeeded by a decline to a plateau, is terminated by the redevelopment of the current response upon washout of the barbiturate (Akaike et al., 1987; Peters et al., 1988; Robertson, 1989; Uchida et al., 1996). It has been suggested that the decay of the current to a plateau might reflect blockade of the chloride ionophore by high concentrations of pentobarbitone. Upon washout, the dissociation of pentobarbitone from the channel, combined with activation of the receptor complex by pentobarbitone prebound to the higher-affinity agonist site, could conceivably account for the redevelopment of the current response (Akaike et al., 1987).

The direct effects of pentobarbitone described above are susceptible to antagonism by picrotoxin (Akaike et al., 1987; Robertson, 1989) or bicuculline (Peters et al., 1988; Robertson, 1989; Uchida et al., 1996) and to potentiation by pregnane steroids or benzodiazepine agonists (Peters et al., 1988). The competitive GABA$_A$ receptor antagonist SR95531 has recently been reported to be ineffective in blocking responses evoked by pentobarbitone from rat hippocampal neurons (Uchida et al., 1996). It has been suggested that bicuculline sterically hinders the binding of both GABA and pentobarbitone to distinct sites *(see* Section 2.1.2.*)*, but SR95531 occludes only the binding of GABA (Uchida et al., 1996). However, it has also been claimed that the direct agonist action of pentobarbitone on human recombinant GABA$_A$ receptors composed of α, β, and γ subunits is sensitive to neither bicuculline nor SR95531 (Thompson et al., 1996; *see* Section 2.1.2.). Surprisingly little information is available concerning the direct effects of pentobarbitone at the single channel level. Fluctuation analysis applied to GABA$_A$ receptor-mediated currents, recorded from mouse spinal neurons, suggests GABA and pentobarbitone to gate channels with similar conductances. The apparent open time of the pentobarbitone-evoked channels was estimated to be approx five times longer than those evoked by GABA (Mathers and Barker, 1980).

As described above, voltage-clamp recordings have revealed multiple effects of pentobarbitone acting at native GABA$_A$ receptors, including potentiation, direct activation, and a putative blockade of the associated chloride channel. These phenomena are also evident at recombinant GABA$_A$ receptors.

2.1. Modulation of Recombinant Receptors

Both the potentiating and direct agonist actions of pentobarbitone are readily reproduced with recombinant receptors expressed in cell lines or *Xenopus laevis* oocytes (Fig. 2A,B).

2.1.1. Potentiation

Studies utilizing recombinant GABA$_A$ receptors reveal that pentobarbitone does not exhibit a strict subunit preference. This is clearly illustrated by experiments performed upon homomeric receptors. The expression of either α or β subunits in cell lines, or *Xenopus laevis* oocytes, results in the formation of recombinant receptors which are either insensitive to, or only modestly activated, by GABA (e.g., Blair et al., 1988; Pritchett et al., 1988; Sigel et al., 1990; Sanna et al., 1995a,b; Krishek et al., 1996). Despite this limitation, in those studies in which a functional response to GABA has been obtained, pentobarbitone produced a clear potentiation of the agonist-evoked current (Blair et al., 1988; Pritchett et al., 1988; Joyce et al., 1993; Sanna et al., 1995a), demonstrating that an allosteric binding site for barbiturate potentiation is present on homomeric receptors formed from either subunit. Indeed, recent evidence indicates a barbiturate allosteric site to be present on a much more primitive GABA receptor. A cDNA *(Rdl)* encoding a GABA receptor from *Drosophila melanogaster* has been isolated and, upon expression in *Xenopus* oocytes, forms functional, homomeric GABA-gated chloride channels (ffrench-Constant et al., 1993; Chen et al., 1994), which are positively modulated by pentobarbitone (Chen et al., 1994; Belelli et al., 1996). The predicted amino acid sequence of the *Drosophila* subunit exhibits little overall homology to α, β, γ, or δ subfamilies of GABA receptor subunits. A dendrogram analysis suggests this invertebrate receptor had branched before the separation of the five established GABA receptor channel subunit families; yet, it is clear that it shares with the vertebrate α or β subunits a binding site for the modulatory actions of pentobarbitone (Tyndale et al., 1995).

Electrical signals mediated by the strychnine-sensitive, glycine-activated chloride channel have been reported to be insensitive to, or only modestly enhanced by, barbiturates (Barker and Ransom, 1978; Akaike et al.,

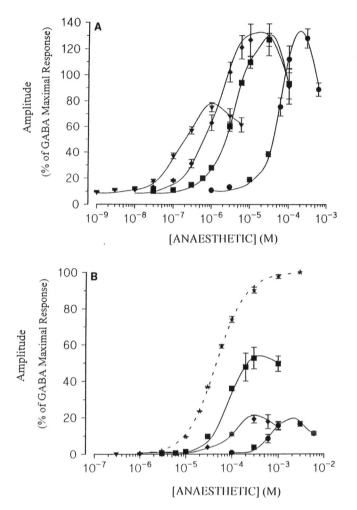

Fig. 2. A comparison of the GABA modulatory and direct agonist actions of four structurally distinct general anesthetic agents. All data were obtained from *Xenopus laevis* oocytes voltage-clamped at –60mV and expressing human α1β2γ2L recombinant receptors (thought to be a dominant receptor subunit combination in vivo). **(A)** The graph illustrates the relationship between anesthetic concentration and the enhancement of GABA (EC_{10} concentration of agonist)-evoked currents (expressed relative to the maximal current induced by GABA) for 5α3α (▼), etomidate (◆), propofol (■), and pentobarbitone (●). The anesthetic EC_{50} calculated for the data are: 5α3α = 177 ± 2 nM; etomidate = 1.2 ± 0.1 µM; propofol = 3.8 ± 0.2 µM and pentobarbitone 55 ± 4 µM (n = 4). Hence the neurosteroid is approximately 300-fold more potent than pentobarbitone for this receptor subunit combination. Note also that the maximal effect produced by 5α3α is less than for the other anesthetics. **(B)** The graph illustrates relationships between the concentration of anesthetic and the

1985). In agreement, we have recently demonstrated that relatively high concentrations of pentobarbitone are not inert and can enhance glycine-evoked chloride currents recorded from *Xenopus* oocytes expressing mammalian $\alpha 1$ and β glycine receptor subunits (Pistis et al., 1996; Fig. 3). Hence, a binding site for this anesthetic, although less effective than for the $GABA_A$ receptor, is also presented by this related amino acid receptor chloride channel.

Although the stoichiometry of pentameric native $GABA_A$ receptors remains conjectural, the majority of endogenous receptors are thought to consist of at least three distinct subunits (McKernan and Whiting, 1996). For such ternary subunit combinations, the GABA-potentiating actions of pentobarbitone are little influenced by the subtype of β subunit present within the oligomeric complex $\alpha 1$ βx $\gamma 2S$ (where $x = 1–3$; Hadingham et al., 1993; Thompson et al., 1996). Although not investigated systematically, the presence of a δ subunit also appears to have little influence on the potentiation of GABA-evoked responses by this barbiturate (Saxena and Macdonald, 1994). Furthermore, unlike the benzodiazepines, the presence of a γ subunit is not a prerequisite for enhancement of GABA responses by pentobarbitone; indeed the coexpression of the $\gamma 2L$ subunit with the $\alpha 1$ and $\beta 1$ subunits results in a reduced maximal effect of the barbiturate as compared with the $\alpha 1$ $\beta 1$ binary subunit combination (Horne et al., 1993). The influence of the subtype of α subunit in the tertiary combination αx β $\gamma 2S$ (where $x = 1, 3, 4, 5,$ or 6) on the potentiation of GABA-evoked currents by pentobarbitone has been investigated in some detail (Thompson et al., 1996; Wafford et al., 1996). Those studies revealed that, although the nature of the α subunit has little influence on the potency with which pentobarbitone enhances GABA, it is an important regulator of the maximal increase produced, with $\alpha 6$- or $\alpha 4$-containing receptors being particularly efficacious in this regard (Thompson et al., 1996; Wafford et al., 1996).

Little is known concerning the location of the barbiturate modulatory site on the $GABA_A$ receptor. Intracellularly applied barbiturates appear inert in relation to both GABA modulation and the direct activation of the receptor-channel complex (Akaike et al., 1985, 1987; Lambert et al., 1990). As such

---

magnitude of the direct current (in the absence of GABA) produced, expressed relative to the maximal current induced by GABA. The symbols are those of Fig. 2A. For comparison, the GABA-concentration response curve (w) is also illustrated. For this receptor subunit combination the relative agonist EC_{50} and maximum current produced (E_{max}), respectively, are: propofol = 70 ± 1 μM, $53 \pm 6\%$; etomidate 130 ± 2 μM, $19 \pm 2\%$; pentobarbitone 604 ± 85 μM, $17 \pm 1\%$. Note that because of the small magnitude of the neurosteroid-induced current ($\sim 0.5\%$ of the GABA maximum), no EC_{50} could be calculated.

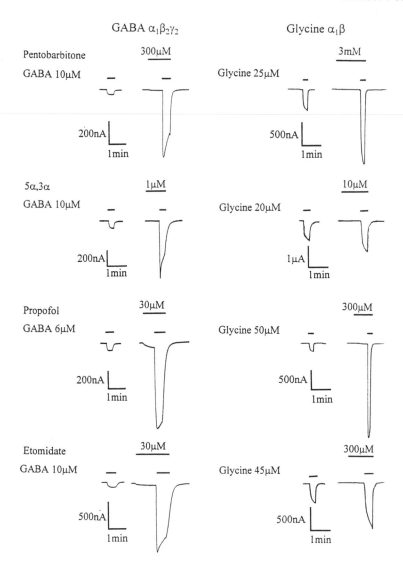

Fig. 3. A comparison of the positive allosteric actions of general anesthetics on recombinant GABA$_A$ (a1b2g2L) and glycine (a1b) receptors expressed in *Xenopus laevis* oocytes. All anesthetics tested here were selective for GABA$_A$ receptors over glycine receptors. However, note that although less sensitive, propofol and pentobarbitone produce a large maximal enhancement of the glycine-evoked current. By contrast, the maximal effect of etomidate on the glycine-evoked current is modest; 5a3a produces little or no enhancement. All oocytes utilized were voltage-clamped at –60 mV, and in each case an appropriate concentration (EC$_{10}$) of agonist was applied.

compounds are highly lipophilic, it would appear unlikely that the anesthetic modulation of $GABA_A$ receptor function occurs as a consequence of a perturbation of the membrane structure surrounding the receptor protein, or the occupation of a hydrophobic region of the $GABA_A$ receptor protein bounded by membrane lipid. Although the possibility remains that barbiturates may exert differential effects at the exo- and cytofacial leaflets of the plasma membrane, the weight of evidence is consistent with an extracellularly located binding site for the anesthetic on the $GABA_A$ receptor protein itself.

The pronounced influence of receptor subunit composition upon benzodiazepine pharmacology, and the subsequent use of domain exchange and site-directed mutagenesis, has led to the identification of amino acid residues on the α and γ subunits, which may contribute to a benzodiazepine-binding pocket located between these subunits (Smith and Olsen, 1995; Galzi and Changeux, 1995; Luddens et al., 1995). The lack of an absolute subunit specificity for pentobarbitone described above would seem to preclude this approach in better defining this barbiturate modulatory site. However, the insensitivity of the retinal ρ1 subunit (which, upon expression, forms functional homomeric GABA-gated chloride channels) to barbiturate modulation, may offer an alternative approach for the future (Cutting et al., 1991).

2.1.2. Direct Activation

The pentobarbitone agonist site on the receptor is similarly obscure, although the recent identification of recombinant receptors, which exhibit differential GABA-mimetic responses to this anesthetic, may provide some useful pointers *(see below)*. Both electrophysiological and radioligand binding experiments have long suggested that the binding sites that mediate activation by GABA and pentobarbitone are distinct, a view confirmed by recent mutagenesis studies. Point mutations introduced into the extracellular N-terminal domain of the rat β2 subunit, co-expressed with rat α1 and γ2 subunits, were found to cause large increases in the EC_{50} for both GABA and muscimol, but produced no corresponding change of the EC_{50} for pentobarbitone (Amin and Weiss, 1993). For oocytes expressing the ternary combination αx, βy γ2S (where x = 1, 3, 4, 5, or 6 and y = 1, 2, or 3), the direct effects of pentobarbitone appear to be influenced by both the α and β subunit subtypes (Thompson et al., 1996; Wafford et al., 1996). In particular, the introduction of either an α6 or an α4 subunit dramatically affects the magnitude of the pentobarbitone-induced current. As described above, GABA-evoked currents recorded from α4-containing receptors (α4 β1 γ2S) are greatly potentiated by pentobarbitone. Nevertheless, at this heterooligomeric assembly, even relatively high concentrations of this anesthetic (1 mM) induce only modest (6% of the GABA maximum) direct currents (cf $\alpha1$ $\beta1$ $\gamma2S = 31\%$). A comparison with $\alpha6$-containing receptors is particularly striking; pentobarbitone produces direct current responses that even exceed those evoked by saturating concentrations of GABA (147% of the GABA maximum; Thompson et al., 1996; Wafford et al., 1996). These observations are consistent with the hypothesis that the pentobarbitone modulatory and activation sites are distinct, a notion supported by results obtained with the invertebrate *Rdl* receptor, which, in functional assays, exhibits only the modulatory site (Chen et al., 1994; Belelli et al., 1996).

For the ternary subunit combinations αx βy $\gamma2S$ (where $x = 1$ or 6, $y = 1$, 2, or 3), the subtype of β subunit exerts only a subtle influence on either potency, or the magnitude of the direct activation induced by pentobarbitone, with a modest preference exhibited for $\beta2$ or $\beta3$ over $\beta1$ (Thompson et al., 1996). However, experiments utilizing homomeric receptors advocate the β subunit as an important locus in the agonist action of pentobarbitone. The human $\beta1$ GABA$_A$ subunit expressed in *Xenopus* oocytes assembles into spontaneously open homooligomeric chloride selective channels, which are only weakly (and inconsistently) gated by GABA, but strongly activated (relative to GABA) by either pentobarbitone or the intravenous anesthetic propofol (Sanna et al., 1995a,b). Such findings have been confirmed and extended, utilizing the mouse $\beta1$ subunit expressed in either oocytes or HEK293 cells (Krishek et al., 1996). In that study, the homooligomeric receptor was completely insensitive to three GABA$_A$ receptor agonists, but was activated by pentobarbitone and propofol. Spontaneously open channels, inferred from outward current responses recorded from whole cells in response to picrotoxin, Zn^{++} or penicillin G were additionally directly resolved in outside-out membrane patches excised from oocytes (Krishek et al., 1996). A notable feature of the latter study was the unusually high potency of pentobarbitone as an agonist ($EC_{50} \cong 6$ μM). Much lower potencies are commonly reported for the direct effect of pentobarbitone upon a variety of heterooligomeric GABA$_A$ receptor complexes (Belelli et al., 1996; Thompson et al., 1996; *see* Fig. 2B). It would appear that the human and mouse $\beta1$ subunits possess a barbiturate binding site coupled to the chloride ionophore, though whether the pentobarbitone-induced current represents the opening of additional ion channels, or modulation of constitutively active ionophores, remains to be addressed. Similar experiments upon homooligomeric receptors assembled from bovine $\beta1$ subunits that do not display spontaneous openings but are activated by GABA$_A$ receptor agonists (Krishek et al., 1996), may prove useful in this respect. In any event, the observation that $\beta1$ subunits of mouse, human, and rat (Sigel et al., 1989; Sanna et al., 1995a; Krishek et al., 1996) form spontaneously active channels, but those of bovine origin do not, warrants further investigation.

Oocytes preinjected with cRNA encoding mouse $\alpha 1$, $\gamma 2S$, or δ subunits or $\alpha 1$ $\gamma 2S$, or $\alpha 1$ δ binary combinations, are insensitive to GABA, pentobarbitone or picrotoxin (Cestari et al., 1996). Although these observations could be construed to reinforce the importance of the β subunit in the action of pentobarbitone, it is difficult to control for lack of functional expression, a clear possibility in the light of recent investigations (Connolly et al., 1996). However, mouse $\beta 2$ or $\beta 3$ subunits, when expressed in oocytes, do form functional homomeric receptors, which are activated by pentobarbitone (Cestari et al., 1996) and, additionally, by the intravenous anesthetics etomidate and propofol. For the $\beta 3$ receptor construct, such barbiturate-activated currents were blocked by picrotoxin and zinc and enhanced by lanthanum. Whether or not these receptors were spontaneously active is not explicitly stated (Cestari et al., 1996). However, by contrast to the human $\beta 1$ subunit, and, indeed to the results of Krishek et al. (1996) discussed above, the mouse $\beta 1$ subunit expressed by Cestari et al. appeared insensitive to pentobarbitone. This discrepancy seems unlikely to be explained by differential expression of the $\beta 1$ homooligomer in the two studies, because in both cases a picrotoxin-induced outward current was present.

In conclusion, the allosteric actions of pentobarbitone do not exhibit an absolute subunit specificity, although the magnitude of the enhancement of GABA-evoked responses by this anesthetic is much greater for $\alpha 4$ and $\alpha 6$ subunit-containing receptors. Studies with invertebrate and vertebrate recombinant receptors confirm the long-held view (based on anesthetic concentration–response relationships) that the pentobarbitone agonist site is distinct from the modulatory site. The nature of the α subunit subtype within the heterooligomeric receptor can greatly influence the magnitude of the pentobarbitone-induced response, with the β subtype exerting only a modest impact. Interestingly, homomeric α receptors and receptors composed of two subunits (excluding β subunits) are insensitive to the agonist actions of this barbiturate. This apparent contradiction may be explained by suggesting that within heteromeric receptors, which are more representative of native GABA$_A$ receptors, the agonist action of pentobarbitone is primarily dependent upon the β subunit, but this interaction is additionally influenced by the α subtype. Indeed, the benzodiazepine binding pocket has been proposed to be located between the interfaces of the α and γ subunits (Smith and Olsen, 1995). For the barbiturates, perhaps analogous sites reside between the α and β subunits. However, it must be emphasized that these studies with recombinant receptors do not distinguish between an effect of subunit composition on binding, or transduction, or both.

3. Neurosteroids

Certain naturally occurring pregnane steroids have long been known to produce rapid and, presumably, nongenomic, sedative, and anesthetic effects (e.g., Selye, 1941). The observation that alphaxalone (a synthetic anesthetic pregnane steroid), like pentobarbitone, caused a prolongation of inhibition, recorded from neurons of guinea pig olfactory slices (Scholfield, 1980), suggested that such steroids may act to modulate transmission mediated by $GABA_A$ receptors. Subsequently, Harrison and Simmonds (1984) demonstrated that alphaxalone potentiated $GABA_A$ receptor-mediated responses, recorded extracellularly from slices of the rat cuneate nucleus, but the behaviorally inert isomer, betaxalone, was inactive in this respect. The structural similarity of alphaxalone to certain endogenous steroids raised the tantalizing prospect that a crucial component of central inhibition might be subject to regulation by such compounds. These studies provided the catalyst for numerous electrophysiological and biochemical investigations that have clearly identified certain naturally occurring steroids to be among the most potent of known positive allosteric modulators of the $GABA_A$ receptor (Lambert et al., 1995). Furthermore, the possibility of an endogenous modulatory role for such steroids in physiological or pathophysiological states has been strengthened by the recent observation that the brain itself is capable of synthesizing these neurosteroids (reviewed in Lambert et al., 1995). Here, we will restrict discussion to their molecular mechanism and possible site of action.

The potent positive allosteric interaction of alphaxalone with the $GABA_A$ receptor, observed with extracellular recording techniques, was readily confirmed in voltage-clamp experiments performed on neuronal and paraneuronal cells in culture (Barker et al., 1987; Cottrell et al., 1987). Parallel studies extended this action to certain endogenous steroids and established a strict structure-activity relationship in which the progesterone metabolites 5α-pregnan-3α-ol-20-one (5α3α) and 5β-pregnan-3α-ol-20-one (5β3α), and the deoxycorticosterone metabolite 5α-pregnane-3α-21-diol-20-one (THDOC), were found to exceed alphaxalone in their potency (Majewska et al., 1986; Callachan et al., 1987; Harrison et al., 1987b; Peters et al., 1988). Compared to barbiturates, such steroids are much more potent allosteric regulators (Fig. 2A), with aqueous concentrations as low as 1–3 nM producing a clear enhancement of GABA-evoked currents (Woodward et al., 1992; Belelli et al., 1996). The behavioral effects of these steroids are stereoselective and this is mirrored in their interaction with the $GABA_A$ receptor. Hence, 3β-hydroxy isomers are inactive, but the orientation of steroid A/B ring fusion is not a crucial determinant of either GABA modulatory or behavioral activity, although the *cis* (5α) configuration tends to be favored over *trans* (5β) (Harrison and Simmonds, 1984; Cottrell et al., 1987; Harrison et al., 1987b; Peters et al., 1988; Gee et al., 1988; Turner et al., 1989; Hawkinson et al., 1994). The aforementioned steroids are not water soluble, and this feature has hindered their clinical development (Carl et al., 1994). However, the water soluble steroidal anesthetics minaxolone [2β-ethoxy-11α-dimethylamino-5α-pregnan-3α-ol-20-one], ORG20599 [(2β,3α,5α)-21-chloro-2-(4-morphinyl) pregnan-20-one], and ORG 21465 [(2β,3α,5α)-3-hydroxy-2-(2,2-dimethylmorpholin-4-yl) pregnane-11,20-dione] have recently been shown to exhibit potent activity at the GABA$_A$ receptor (Lambert et al., 1991; Hill-Venning et al., 1994a, 1996; Gemmell et al., 1995).

When investigated on inhibitory transmission between synaptically coupled rat hippocampal neurons maintained in cell culture, alphaxalone, 5α3α, and THDOC all produced a barbiturate-like prolongation of the IPSC, with little or no effect on the IPSC rise time or amplitude (Harrison et al., 1987a,b). Recently, similar observations have been made for THDOC on mIPSCs (determined in the presence of tetrodotoxin), recorded from rat hippocampal dentate granule cells and cerebellar Purkinje cells in brain slices (Cooper et al., 1995). As for pentobarbitone, such an effect is compatible with a steroid-induced increase of the mean channel open time of the GABA receptor. Analysis of the influence of alphaxalone on the power spectra produced by GABA-induced current fluctuations, recorded from spinal neurons, provided further, albeit indirect, support for this putative molecular mechanism (Barker et al., 1987). Subsequent patch-clamp studies utilizing bovine chromaffin cells revealed that the steroids 5α3α and 5β3α dramatically change the kinetic behavior of the GABA$_A$ receptor in the absence of an obvious effect upon single channel conductance (Callachan et al., 1987; Lambert et al., 1987; Hill-Venning et al., 1994b). The GABA$_A$ receptors of bovine chromaffin cells exhibit multiple interconverting single channel conductance states (Peters et al., 1989; Hill-Venning et al., 1994b). This feature has precluded any meaningful quantitative analysis of neurosteroid modulation of these receptors. However, in the case of mouse spinal neurons in culture, a single main conductance state often predominates. As mentioned in Section 2., analysis of these channels reveals three kinetically distinct open states (Macdonald et al., 1989; Twyman and Macdonald, 1992; Macdonald and Olsen, 1994). The neuroactive steroids appear to act primarily by promoting the relative frequency of occurrence of the two longest-lived open states (Twyman and Macdonald, 1992). In this respect, their molecular mechanism resembles that of the barbiturates. However, the neuroactive steroids additionally increased the frequency of single channel openings (Twyman and Macdonald 1992). Whether this represents a direct activation of the GABA$_A$ receptor-channel complex by the steroid (Callachan et al.,

1987; Cottrell et al., 1987), or a true enhancement of GABA-activated channel openings similar to that produced by the benzodiazepines (Vicini et al., 1987; Rogers et al., 1994), remains to be determined.

At concentrations that exceed those required to produce a substantial enhancement of GABA-evoked currents (≥ 300 nM), steroids such as $5\alpha 3\alpha$, $5\beta 3\alpha$, and alphaxalone directly activate the GABA$_A$ receptor channel complex to produce current responses that demonstrate slight outward rectification (Cottrell et al., 1987; Callachan et al., 1987; Robertson, 1989). On isolated outside-out membrane patches, these neuroactive steroids induce single channel openings with a conductance and reversal potential similar to those evoked by GABA (Cottrell et al., 1987; Callachan et al., 1987). Such steroid-induced single-channel or whole-cell currents are enhanced by diazepam or phenobarbitone and are blocked by bicuculline or picrotoxin, confirming the involvement of the GABA$_A$ receptor in this effect (Cottrell et al., 1987; Callachan et al., 1987; Barker et al., 1987; Robertson, 1989). Although these direct effects are relatively small, compared to those induced by pentobarbitone or propofol (Belelli et al., 1996; Hill-Venning et al., 1996; *see* Fig. 2B), they occur at much lower concentrations. Moreover, in neurons that express the GABA$_A$ receptor at high density, such as rat hippocampal neurons in cell culture, the steroid-induced conductance increase is of sufficient magnitude to shunt the neuronal input resistance to a level where depolarizations evoked by glutamate receptor activation fall below the threshold for action potential discharge (Lambert et al., 1990). It is conceivable that this modest, but relatively potent direct effect of the neuroactive steroids, could contribute to the behavioral actions of these compounds.

3.1. Modulation of Recombinant Receptors

3.1.1. Potentiation and Direct Activation

The effects of neurosteroids in inhibiting [^{35}S]TBPS binding and enhancing GABA-stimulated chloride uptake are dependent upon the brain region examined (Gee et al., 1995; Olsen and Sapp, 1995), suggesting steroid receptor heterogeneity. This proposal is supported by the influence of binary combinations of steroids on the binding of [^{35}S]TBPS and the benzodiazepine [^{3}H]flunitrazepam to rat brain membranes (Prince and Simmonds, 1993; McCauley et al., 1994, 1995) and the differential effects of THDOC on mIPSCs, recorded from rat hippocampal dentate granule cells and cerebellar Purkinje cells (Cooper et al., 1995). In the above studies, the composition of the native GABA$_A$ receptors is heterogeneous, and the phenomena observed may reflect the existence of receptors with distinctive affinities for the neuroactive steroids. However, studies of steroidal regulation of recombinant GABA$_A$ receptor isoforms designed to test this possibility have produced a rather confusing picture. In the interests of clarity, the present discussion will be mainly restricted to functional (electrophysiological) studies.

Recordings from transiently transfected HEK293 cells, and outside-out membrane patches derived from them, demonstrate both the modulatory and GABA-mimetic effects of steroids to be preserved on human $\alpha1\beta1\gamma2L$, $\alpha1\beta1$, or $\beta1$ receptors with no evidence of subunit selectivity (Puia et al., 1990). As noted for pentobarbitone and propofol (Sanna et al., 1995a), both the modulatory and agonist site for the neuroactive steroids appear to be represented on the homooligomeric $\beta1$ subunit. When expressed in *Xenopus* oocytes, the human $\beta1$ GABA$_A$ receptor is reported to mediate only a modest GABA-mimetic effect in response to alphaxalone, and in some cases, no current response was detected (Sanna et al., 1995a). Mouse $\beta1$ subunits, similarly expressed, are also refractory to direct activation by $5\beta3\alpha$ (Krishek et al., 1996). These discrepancies may reflect differences in experimental protocol or expression systems. Alternatively, the small magnitude of the steroid-induced current (relative to responses evoked by GABA, pentobarbitone, or propofol, which has been noted for both native and recombinant GABA$_A$ receptors; Hill-Venning et al., 1996; Belelli et al., 1996; *see* Fig. 2B) may have compromised the detection of steroid agonist activity in the oocyte model. In the case of native GABA$_A$ receptors, the potentiation of GABA by neuroactive steroids results mainly from modulation of open channel kinetics (Twyman and Macdonald, 1992). By contrast, acting at recombinant receptors, $5\alpha3\alpha$ had little effect on the open channel burst duration, but appeared to produce, at least superficially, a benzodiazepine-like increase in the frequency of GABA$_A$ receptor channel openings (Rogers et al., 1994; Puia et al., 1990). The modulation of channel kinetics by barbiturates was consistent across native and recombinant receptors (Macdonald et al., 1989; Puia et al., 1990). These results may suggest that the steroid modulatory site, although present, is incorrectly coupled to its effector mechanism in the recombinant receptors. It would be of interest to extend these studies to include recombinant receptors composed of subunits that may be more closely representative of native receptors (McKernan and Whiting, 1996).

As noted in Section 2.1.1., the majority of native GABA$_A$ receptors are thought to be heteropentamers composed of three distinct subunit types (McKernan and Whiting, 1996). Although not investigated extensively, the subtype of β subunit does not appear to influence the neurosteroid modulatory action as $\alpha1\beta x\gamma2$ receptors (where x = 1, 2, or 3), when expressed in *Xenopus laevis* oocytes, are equally sensitive to the allosteric actions of the pregnane steroids (Hadingham et al., 1993). Indeed, $5\alpha3\alpha$ potentiates GABA-evoked currents recorded from oocytes expressing only the binary subunit combination $\alpha1,\gamma2$, demonstrating that the presence of a β subunit is not a prerequisite for steroid modulation (D. Belelli, unpublished observations). The majority of reports agree that, in contrast to the benzodiazepines, the presence of a γ subunit is not required for steroid modulation of GABA-evoked currents (Puia et al., 1990, Shingai et al., 1991, Hill-Venning et al., 1991). Alphaxalone is reported to have no effect on GABA-evoked currents recorded from Chinese hamster ovary (CHO) cells transfected with rat $\alpha 1\beta 2$ or, $\alpha 1\beta 3$ subunits, although a direct agonist action of the steroid was evident (Valeyev et al., 1993). The subtype of γ subunit expressed in the ternary combination $\alpha 1\beta 1\gamma x$ (where $x = 1$, 2, or 3) does appear to influence neurosteroid modulation of the $GABA_A$ receptor. Hence, the enhancement of GABA-evoked currents recorded from HEK293 cells expressing the $\alpha 1\beta 1\gamma 1$ combination was much greater than that found for either the $\alpha 1\beta 1\gamma 2L$ or $\alpha 1\beta 1\gamma 3$ recombinant receptors (Puia et al., 1993).

To date, no clear consensus has emerged from electrophysiological studies investigating the role of the subtype of α subunit. In *Xenopus* oocytes expressing the $\alpha 1$, $\alpha 2$, or $\alpha 3$ subunits as a ternary combination with the $\beta 1$ and $\gamma 2$ subunits, the potentiation of GABA-evoked currents by $5\alpha 3\alpha$ was greater for those receptors that contained the $\alpha 1$ subunit (Shingai et al., 1991). By contrast, other studies have not detected a differential interaction between this steroid and receptors composed from $\alpha x\beta 1\gamma 2$ subunits expressed in oocytes (where $x = 1$–3; Lambert et al., 1996) or HEK293 cells (where $x = 1$–3 and 5; Puia et al., 1993). HEK293 cells expressing the $\alpha 6\beta 1\gamma 2$ subunit combination are reported to exhibit a reduced neurosteroid modulatory effect (Puia et al., 1993). However, in *Xenopus* oocytes, the maximal enhancement of the GABA-evoked current, mediated by the $\alpha 6$ subunit co-expressed with $\beta 1$ and $\gamma 2$ subunits was found to be approximately twice that of the other combinations tested ($\alpha 1$, $\alpha 2$, or $\alpha 3\beta 1\gamma 2$) (Lambert et al., 1996). The latter observation is in agreement with the results of both radioligand binding (Korpi and Luddens, 1993) and autoradiographic (Olsen and Sapp, 1995) studies. As the $\alpha 6$ subunit is confined to the granule cells of the cerebellum (Laurie et al., 1992), an area of the CNS important for motor coordination, these observations may be relevant to the behavioral effects of the anesthetic steroids. Although relatively high concentrations of pentobarbitone and propofol can enhance glycine-evoked currents, the effects of $5\alpha 3\alpha$ on this related inhibitory amino acid receptor channel are either minimal or absent (Fig. 3).

4. Propofol

Propofol (2, 6-diisopropylphenol) is a widely utilized general anesthetic agent. This neurodepressant is reported to enhance inhibitory synaptic transmission in the feline spinal cord (Lodge and Anis, 1984), and to potentiate

GABA-induced depolarizations in slices of rat olfactory cortex (Collins, 1988), suggesting an interaction with the $GABA_A$ receptor channel complex. Voltage-clamp and patch-clamp studies on paraneurons and central neurons in culture indicate that clinically relevant concentrations of propofol allosterically regulate the activity of the $GABA_A$ receptor (Hales and Lambert, 1991). Such observations have subsequently been confirmed in a number of complementary studies (Hara et al., 1993, 1994; Orser et al., 1994; Zimmerman et al., 1994; Adodra and Hales, 1995). Potentiation of GABA-evoked responses by propofol is associated with a parallel rightward shift of the GABA concentration-response curve (Hara et al., 1994; Orser et al., 1994), indicating an apparent increase in the affinity of GABA.

Interaction studies suggest the site of action of propofol to be distinct from that of either benzodiazepines or neuroactive steroids, but some degree of overlap with the barbiturate site has been reported (Lambert and Hales, 1991; Hara et al., 1993). Modulatory concentrations of propofol greatly increase the open probability of GABA-activated ion channels (Hales and Lambert, 1991; Orser et al., 1994). There is little effect on the open time duration *per se*, but the frequency of channel events is apparently increased (Orser et al., 1994). However, in the latter study, the influence of propofol on the GABA channel burst duration was not determined and the possibility remains that, as for barbiturates (Macdonald et al., 1989), this is a prime molecular mechanism; this is a view reinforced by visual inspection of published single channel records (*see* Hales and Lambert, 1991).

The effects of propofol on inhibitory synaptic transmission have been determined under voltage-clamp conditions, using mouse hippocampal neurons in culture (Orser et al., 1994). Propofol produced a concentration-dependent prolongation of the mIPSC decay, with little effect on mIPSC amplitude, actions reminiscent of those of the barbiturates and neurosteroids (Orser et al., 1994).

At concentrations generally greater than those required for allosteric modulation, the application of propofol to GABA-sensitive cells directly elicits a chloride-mediated current (Hales and Lambert, 1991; Hara et al., 1993; Orser et al., 1994). Such propofol-induced currents are potentiated by diazepam, and antagonized by bicuculline and zinc, and hence arise from the direct activation of the $GABA_A$ receptor channel complex by the anesthetic (Hales and Lambert, 1991; Hara et al., 1993; Adodra and Hales, 1995). On outside-out membrane patches, propofol induces single channels of an amplitude similar, or identical, to those activated by GABA (Hales and Lambert, 1991; Orser et al., 1994). Mirroring the propofol-induced, whole-cell current, such single channel events are reduced in frequency by the co-application of bicuculline (Hales and Lambert, 1991).

At relatively high concentrations, the washout of propofol is associated with a rebound current (Orser et al., 1994; Adodra and Hales, 1995), as described for pentobarbitone above. Such responses presumably result from the rapid dissociation of propofol from a low-affinity inhibitory site, to reveal the additional current that may result from the residual occupancy of a higher-affinity agonist site by the anesthetic, though other interpretations are possible (Adodra and Hales, 1995).

Propofol is a highly lipophilic molecule and, in principle, could disturb $GABA_A$ receptor channel function indirectly, by perturbing the membrane surrounding the inhibitory receptor protein. However, both the modulatory and the GABA-mimetic effect of propofol exhibit a clear membrane asymmetry, activity being apparent only when the drug is applied extracellularly (Hales and Lambert, 1991). Similar observations have been made for neuroactive steroids and barbiturates (Lambert et al., 1990) and suggest extracellularly located, presumably protein, binding sites for these agents.

4.1. Modulation of Recombinant Receptors

4.1.1. Potentiation

Both the GABA modulatory and the GABA-mimetic actions (*see* Section 4.1.2.) of propofol are well-represented on recombinant receptors and for a variety of expression systems (Hill-Venning et al., 1991; Jones et al., 1995; Sanna et al., 1995a,b; Cestari et al., 1996; Krishek et al., 1996; Wafford et al., 1996; *see* Fig. 2). Such experiments demonstrate that the GABA-modulatory actions of propofol are evident for ternary subunit receptor combinations ($\alpha\beta\gamma2$), for binary combinations ($\alpha\beta$, $\alpha\gamma2$, $\beta2$, $\gamma2$), and, indeed, for homomeric receptors composed of β subunits alone (Hill-Venning et al., 1991; Sanna et al., 1995a,b; Jones et al., 1995; Belelli et al., 1996; Wafford et al., 1996). GABA-evoked currents recorded from oocytes expressing invertebrate *(Rdl)* homomeric receptors are enhanced by propofol with an EC_{50} and maximal effect similar to that reported for mammalian recombinant receptors (Belelli et al., 1996). The potentiating actions of positive allosteric modulators are dependent upon the control concentration of GABA applied relative to the maximal response for this agonist (Harris et al., 1995; Belelli et al., 1996). However, the affinity of GABA for the recombinant receptor is dependent upon the subunit composition of the receptor (Ebert et al., 1994). Collectively, these observations confound absolute comparisons of propofol potency and efficacy across receptors of varied subunit composition (Sanna et al., 1995b), unless the control GABA concentration is titrated to the receptor under investigation. A recent study (Wafford et al., 1996) utilizing such appropriate agonist concentrations has investigated the influence of the α isoform on the GABA-modulatory actions of propofol ($\alpha x\beta\gamma2$, where

$x = 1, 4,$ or 6). Propofol did not discriminate across these α isoforms, but pentobarbitone produced a much greater maximal effect for $\alpha4$- and $\alpha6$- than for $\alpha1$-containing receptors, suggesting that the pentobarbitone and propofol modulatory sites are distinct (Wafford et al., 1996).

Experiments performed with mouse spinal neurons in culture demonstrated that, in addition to acting at the $GABA_A$ receptor, propofol at higher concentrations may enhance the activity of the related glycine-activated chloride channel (Hales and Lambert, 1991), although the glycine-evoked current recorded from rat hippocampal neurons in culture appeared to be unaffected (Hara et al., 1993, 1994). We have recently investigated the actions of this anesthetic on glycine-evoked responses recorded from oocytes expressing mammalian $\alpha1\beta$ glycine receptors (Pistis et al., 1996). Here, propofol produced a large (to approximately the maximum response produced by a saturating concentration of glycine) concentration-dependent potentiation of glycine-evoked currents with an EC_{50} for propofol of 28 μM (Pistis et al., 1996; *see* Fig. 3). By comparison, under identical recording conditions, propofol enhanced GABA-evoked currents (to the GABA maximum) from oocytes expressing human $\alpha3\beta1\gamma2L$ receptors with an EC_{50} of 3 μM. Hence, the propofol modulatory site is represented on the glycine receptor although approximately 10-fold higher concentrations of the anesthetic are required to produce an equivalent effect, compared to the $GABA_A$ receptor.

4.1.2. Direct Activation

The direct activation of the $GABA_A$ receptor by relatively high concentrations of propofol is readily reproduced for recombinant $GABA_A$ receptors (*see* Fig. 2B). For homomeric β $GABA_A$ receptors expressed in oocytes, propofol, like pentobarbitone, induces a relatively large current response, which is antagonized by picrotoxin (Sanna et al., 1995a,b; Krishek et al., 1996; Cestari et al., 1996). The coexpression of the β subunit with other subunits (α and γ) appears to reduce the magnitude of the propofol-induced current (relative to GABA). Emphasizing the importance of the β subunit, the coexpression of α and $\gamma2S$ subunits produces a receptor which, although sensitive to the allosteric actions of propofol, is inert regarding the agonist effect of propofol (Sanna et al., 1995b). Similarly, only the propofol modulatory site is represented on the invertebrate *Rdl* recombinant receptor (Belelli et al., 1996). For ternary subunit receptors, the isoform of the α subunit may also influence the agonist effect of propofol. A comparison of $\alpha6$, $\alpha1$, and $\alpha4\beta\gamma2S$ receptors demonstrated a relatively large direct effect for $\alpha6$-containing receptors, which was much reduced for $\alpha1$, and minimal or absent for $\alpha4$-containing receptors (Wafford et al., 1996). This profile is identical to that determined for pentobarbitone and suggests that these anesthetics may share a common agonist binding site, although they may have different modulatory sites (*see* Sections 2.1.1. and 2.1.2. and Wafford et al., 1996).

5. Etomidate

Etomidate is an intravenous general anesthetic that is utilized in clinical practice as an induction agent, partly as a consequence of its cardiovascular stability (Janssen et al., 1975; Ebert et al., 1992). Early electrophysiological studies suggesting a GABA-mimetic action of this anesthetic demonstrated etomidate to induce a concentration-dependent and bicuculline-sensitive depolarization of hemisected spinal cord or superior cervical ganglia in vitro (Evans and Hill, 1978). Furthermore, a positive allosteric interaction with the $GABA_A$ receptor was suggested by the observation that etomidate enhances GABA-ergic inhibition in hippocampal slices (Ashton and Wauquier, 1985; Proctor et al., 1986). Voltage-clamp experiments, utilizing both recombinant and native $GABA_A$ receptors, have confirmed low concentrations of etomidate to potentiate GABA-evoked currents, and higher concentrations to be GABA-mimetic (Robertson, 1989; Belelli et al., 1996; Yang and Uchida, 1996). Furthermore, as for pentobarbitone and propofol, GABA-mimetic concentrations of the anesthetic are often associated with a brief increase of the etomidate-induced current upon washout of the anesthetic (Robertson, 1989). Such washout currents have been attributed to the unbinding of the anesthetic from a low-affinity site associated with the chloride channel (Robertson, 1989).

Radioligand binding studies provide additional support for a GABA modulatory action of etomidate. Etomidate enhances the binding of [^{3}H]GABA (Thyagarajan et al., 1983) and [^{3}H]diazepam (Ashton et al., 1981; Thyagarajan et al., 1983) to rat brain membrane homogenates, and allosterically inhibits the binding of [^{35}S]TBPS (Olsen et al., 1986; Ticku and Rastogi, 1986). At the single channel level, relatively low concentrations of etomidate ($\sim$8 μM) have no effect upon the elementary conductance of $GABA_A$ receptors of rat hippocampus, but produce a prolongation of the GABA-activated channel open time and increase the frequency of GABA channel opening (Yang and Uchida, 1996).

The influence of etomidate on inhibitory neurotransmission has been determined by utilizing synaptically-coupled hippocampal neurons in culture. In that system, GABA modulatory concentrations of etomidate ($\sim$8 μM) prolonged the decay of mIPSCs (recorded in the presence of tetrodotoxin), but enhanced their amplitude (Yang and Uchida, 1996). Although the latter effect may be consistent with an anesthetic-induced increase in the probability of the channel being activated by GABA, it is difficult to reconcile with the saturation of $GABA_A$ receptors by neurotransmitter, which is proposed to occur during the synaptic event (mIPSC) (*see* Mody et al., 1994). Of course, the dynamics of neurotransmitter release and synaptic architecture may be different for brain slices and neuronal cells in culture. Alternatively, if the recorded mIPSC results from the release of GABA from more than one synaptic bouton, despite the presence of tetrodotoxin, and such release is not perfectly synchronous, then the effects of etomidate on channel kinetics (Yang and Uchida, 1996) might be anticipated to produce an enhanced mIPSC current amplitude (Mody et al., 1994).

5.1. Modulation of Recombinant Receptors

5.1.1. Potentiation and Direct Activation

Utilizing the *Xenopus laevis* oocyte expression system, we have recently investigated the influence of the isoform of the β and α subunit upon the modulatory actions of etomidate (Hill-Venning et al., 1995; *see* Figs. 2 and 4). In qualitative agreement with its actions on native receptors, etomidate potentiated GABA-evoked currents mediated by all the human recombinant $GABA_A$ receptors tested ($\alpha x\beta y\gamma 2L$; where $x = 1, 2, 3$, and 6, $y = 1$ and 2), although the characteristics of this interaction were dependent on both the α and β subunit isoforms. For all β2-containing receptors tested, the calculated EC_{50} for etomidate varied little (0.6–1.2 μ*M*) with the α subunit isoform (α = 1, 2, 3, and 6) (*see* Table 1). However, the substitution of the β2 for the β1 subunit produced a 9–12-fold increase of the EC_{50} (~6–11 μ*M*; *see* Table 1) for this anesthetic for all α isoforms tested. For α1, α2, and α6, the magnitude of the potentiation of GABA-evoked currents produced by etomidate was greater for β2- than for the corresponding β1-containing receptors (Table 1). This difference was most marked for the α6β1γ2L compared to α6β2γ2L receptors, where etomidate maximally enhanced GABA-evoked currents to ~30% and ~170% of the maximum response to GABA, respectively (Table 1; Fig. 4). The potency of etomidate is clearly influenced by the isoform of the β subunit, but the magnitude of the effect is dictated by both the subtype of the β and α subunit. By comparison, the modulatory actions of pentobarbitone and propofol were little affected by the β subunit isoform, suggesting the etomidate binding site to be distinct from that for these anesthetics (Belelli and Hill-Venning, unpublished observations). In agreement, GABA-evoked currents, recorded from oocytes expressing the invertebrate *Rdl* receptor are enhanced by pentobarbitone and propofol, but not by etomidate (Chen et al., 1994; Belelli et al., 1996). The role of the γ subunit on the GABA modulatory actions of etomidate has not been systematically investigated, although a comparison of receptors composed of α1β1 and α1β1γ2s subunits (expressed in HEK 293 cells) demonstrates that the γ2 subunit is not essential for activity, but may influence the nature of the perturbation of GABA-activated channel kinetics by the anesthetic (Uchida et al., 1995).

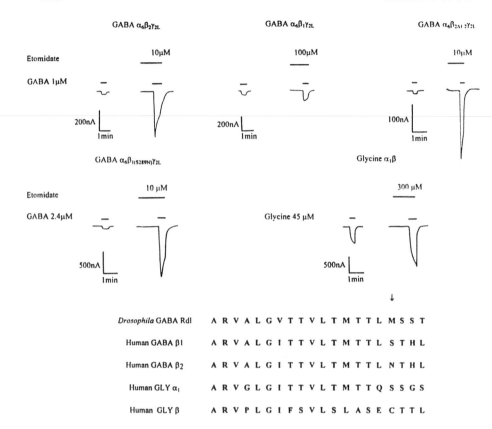

Fig. 4. The positive allosteric actions of etomidate are subunit dependent.**Top panel:** The maximum potentiation of GABA-evoked currents produced by etomidate is much greater for the α6β2γ2L than for the α6β1γ2L subunit combination. The coexpression of the α6 and γ2L subunits with a chimeric β subunit construct (containing the N terminal extracellular domain of the b1 subunit and the transmembrane M1–M4 to carboxyl tail region of the β2 subunit) restores the actions of this anesthetic. **Middle panel:** Similarly, the action of etomidate is present on a α6β1(S289N)γ2L construct, where a point mutation of the β1 serine to the β2 asparagine residue has been introduced. The glycine-evoked current (α1 contains a serine, β a cysteine in this equivalent position) is only modestly enhanced by this anesthetic. **Bottom panel:** Alignment of the primary amino acid sequences (single letter code) of the putative M2 region of related inhibitory amino acid receptor subunits. The position of the residue, which influences etomidate action, is indicated by the arrow. All records illustrated are taken from experiments utilizing *Xenopus laevis* oocytes voltage-clamped at –60 mV (D. Belelli, C. Hill-Venning, J. J. Lambert, J. A. Peters, K. A. Wafford, and P. J. Whiting, unpublished observations; and Hill-Venning et al. 1995).

Table 1

A Comparison of the Etomidate EC$_{50}$ and E$_{max}$ for the Modulatory and Direct Agonist Actions of This Anesthetic Across Different Recombinant GABA$_A$ Receptors Expressed in *Xenopus laevis* Oocytes

Subunit Combination	ETOMIDATE Modulation EC$_{50}$	Modulation E$_{max}$	Agonist EC$_{50}$	Agonist E$_{max}$
α1β2γ2	1.2 ± 0.1 μM	127 ± 12%	130 ± 2.4 μM	19 ± 2%
α1β1γ2	10.8 ± 1.1 μM	79 ± 2%	N.D.	4 ± 1% (1 mM)
α2β2γ2	0.9 ± 0.1 μM	107 ± 1%	50.1 ± 2.8 μM	27 ± 8%
α2β1γ2	6.3 ± 3.1 μM	65 ± 3%	N.D.	5 ± 1% (1 mM)
α3β2γ2	1.0 ± 0.1 μM	88 ± 6%	107.6 ± 3.9 μM	9 ± 1%
α3β1γ2	8.1 ± 0.9 μM	75 ± 8%	N.D.	~3%
α6β2γ2	0.6 ± 0.04 μM	169 ± 14%	22.2 ± 1.4 μM	51 ± 15%
α6β1γ2	7.4 ± 0.6 μM	28 ± 2%	N.D.	~6% (3 mM)

N.D. = not determined because of the small magnitude of the etomidate-induced current. The number in parenthesis is the maximum concentration of etomidate that induced the small direct current for the b1-containing receptors. The E$_{max}$ is expressed as a percentage of the maximum response to GABA. All data were obtained from oocytes voltage-clamped at –60 mV (from Hill-Venning et al. 1995).

The GABA-mimetic action of etomidate, reported for native $GABA_A$ receptors is also highly dependent upon the β subunit. Indeed, a recent report has demonstrated that etomidate, like propofol and pentobarbitone, can directly activate homomeric β2 or β3 (murine) receptors expressed in *Xenopus* oocytes (Cestari et al., 1996). The etomidate agonist site is clearly represented on the β subunit. The majority of native receptors are thought to be composed of at least three distinct subunits (McKernan and Whiting, 1996). For such recombinant receptors, the β isoform had a clear effect on the GABA-mimetic actions of etomidate. For receptors containing the β2 subunit, clear agonist effects of etomidate were evident; these were either minimal or absent for β1-containing receptors (Table 1). The β isoform, in addition to affecting the GABA modulating properties of etomidate also greatly influences the GABA-mimetic action of this anesthetic. For β2-containing receptors, the EC_{50} for the direct activation of the $GABA_A$ receptor channel complex by etomidate was influenced by the α isoform (range ~22–130 μM; α1- and α6-containing receptors, respectively); by contrast, the GABA-modulatory effect was not (Table 1). Additionally, for β2-containing receptors, the magnitude of the etomidate-induced current is dependent upon the α subtype (e.g., maximal effect = 9 and 51% of the maximum response to GABA for the α3- and α6-containing receptors, respectively; *see* Table 1).

The α6 subunit is expressed exclusively in the granule cells of the cerebellum (e.g., McKernan and Whiting 1996). A strain of rats have been identified that exhibit pronounced ataxia and postural impairment to benzodiazepines (Korpi et al., 1993). Genetic analysis of such rats has revealed a point mutation of their α6 subunit that confers a high affinity for benzodiazepines to such α6-containing receptors compared to wild type α6 receptors which are insensitive to classical benzodiazepines (Korpi et al., 1993). Collectively, these results suggest that $GABA_A$ receptors that contain the α6 subunit may play an important role in cerebellar motor control and its perturbation by drugs. Given the differential interaction of etomidate with the α6-containing receptors, these effects may contribute to the behavioral actions of this anesthetic. The application of whole-cell clamp techniques to cerebellar slices will provide a better understanding of the role of the α6 subunit in the inhibitory circuitry of the cerebellum (Puia et al., 1994; Kaneda et al., 1995). Clearly, it would be of interest to investigate the modulation of granule cell mIPSCs by etomidate, to observe whether the subtype selectivity evident in experiments performed with recombinant receptors has a functional consequence for synaptic transmission.

In preliminary experiments, we have investigated the functional domains of the β subunit, which may impart this differential sensitivity to etomidate (Belelli, D., Lambert, J. J., Peters, J. A., Wafford, K. A., and Whiting, P. J., unpublished observations). For receptors composed of α6 and γ2L subunits, together with a β1/β2 Lys 237-Gly 334 chimera (containing the N terminal region of the β1 subunit and the putative M1 to carboxyl terminal region of the β2 subunit), the effects of etomidate are indistinguishable from α6β2 (wild type) γ2L receptors. This observation suggests that a key region that confers the enhanced activity of etomidate is located distal to the N-terminal extracellular portion of the receptor protein. This profile is reminiscent of the situation for the positive allosteric actions of the anticonvulsant loreclezole (Wingrove et al., 1994). Indeed, the structure of loreclezole is similar to that of etomidate (Fig. 1). Site-directed mutagenesis studies have highlighted the importance of an asparagine residue (for β2 and β3 subunits) located toward the extracellular side of the M2 region of the subunit (Fig. 4), a region thought to form the lining of the associated chloride ion channel (Wingrove et al., 1994). Mutation of this amino acid to a serine residue results in a reduction of the sensitivity to loreclezole; the mutation of the equivalent serine residue of the β1 subunit to an asparagine enhances loreclezole sensitivity. In preliminary experiments, the mutation of this serine to an asparagine residue of the β1 subunit increases the potency and maximal effects of the GABA-modulatory activity of etomidate and enhances the direct agonist actions of the anesthetic (Fig. 4).

The molecular interactions of this general anesthetic with the $GABA_A$ receptor are subunit-specific and are greatly influenced by a single amino acid located near the putative channel forming domain M2. These observations do not support a nonspecific membrane perturbation as the mechanism of anesthetic action. However, whether the asparagine residue contributes to the etomidate binding site, or, in view of its location, influences the transduction process, is not known. Whether the primary influence of this amino acid is on binding affinity, transduction, or both, the recent observation that the positive allosteric actions associated with relatively high concentrations of the β carboline DMCM (Stevenson et al., 1995) are similarly influenced by this residue, highlights this domain as an important modulatory locus for drug action.

The overlap of loreclezole and etomidate does not extend to the *Rdl* invertebrate GABA receptor, where only the former drug is active (Belelli et al., 1996). Furthermore, the mutation of the asparagine residue of the β3 subunit (loreclezole-sensitive) to a methionine residue (the equivalent amino acid in the *Rdl* subunit, which is also loreclezole sensitive) results in a receptor that is loreclezole-insensitive (Stevenson et al., 1995), suggesting a distinct locus or transduction mechanism for loreclezole at invertebrate and vertebrate receptors (Belelli et al., 1996).

The vertebrate glycine receptor α subunit, like the β1 GABA$_A$ subunit, possesses a serine residue at this key position; the glycine β subunit has a cysteine residue (Langosch, 1995). We have recently demonstrated that etomidate can produce a modest potentiation of glycine-evoked currents recorded from *Xenopus* oocytes expressing the α1β glycine receptor subunits (Pistis et al., 1996). Clearly, it would be of interest to determine the influence on etomidate action of mutating the α1 serine residue to an asparagine and then assess whether this domain might play a similar critical role for a related inhibitory amino acid receptor.

6. Conclusion

Intravenous anesthetics are structurally diverse and yet may share a common molecular mechanism of action, namely, the enhancement of fast inhibitory neurotransmission in the CNS by an allosteric interaction with the GABA$_A$ receptor protein. Theoretically, this universal action could arise from a nonspecific perturbation of the neuronal membrane by the anesthetic which, as a consequence, modulates the kinetic behavior of the GABA$_A$ receptor channel complex. This hypothesis is attractive because it provides a mechanism that might explain the apparent lack of a clear structure–activity relationship. However, evidence reviewed here strongly suggests the presence of distinct binding sites on the GABA$_A$ receptor protein for these anesthetics.

Several laboratories are now utilizing recombinant receptors, together with the techniques of domain exchange and site-directed mutagenesis, with the aim of identifying the nature and location of the anesthetic binding sites and key residues required for the perturbation of the receptor-channel transduction process that they produce. Such studies may eventually allow a better understanding of the molecular mechanism that underpins the remarkable behavioral changes that rapidly follow the injection of an intravenous anesthetic.

Acknowledgments

Work from the authors' laboratory reported here was supported by grants from the MRC, MRC (ROPA), Organon Teknika, and the Scottish Epilepsy Society. We thank K. Wafford and J. Yang for providing unpublished material and P. J. Whiting and H. Betz for supplying the GABA$_A$ and glycine subunit cDNAs, respectively.

References

Adodra, S. and Hales, T. G. (1995) Potentiation, activation and blockade of GABA$_A$ receptors of clonal murine hypothalamic GT1-7 neurones by propofol. *Br. J. Pharmacol.* **115,** 953–960.

Akaike, N., Hattori, K., Inomata, N., and Oomura, Y. (1985) γ-Aminobutyric-acid and pentobarbitone-gated chloride currents in internally perfused frog sensory neurones. *J. Physiol.* **360,** 367–386.

Akaike, N., Maruyama, T., and Tokutomi, N. (1987) Kinetic properties of pentobarbitone-gated chloride current in frog sensory neurones. *J. Physiol.* **394,** 85–98.

Amin, J. and Weiss, D. S. (1993) $GABA_A$ receptor needs two homologous domains of the β-subunit for activation by GABA, but not by pentobarbitone. *Nature* **366,** 565–569.

Ashton, D. and Wauquier, A. (1985) Modulation of a GABA-ergic inhibitory circuit in the in vitro hippocampus by etomidate isomers. *Anesth. Analg.* **64,** 975–980.

Barker, J. L., Harrison, N. L., Lange, G. D., and Owen, D. G. (1987) Potentiation of γ-aminobutyric acid-activated chloride conductance by a steroid anesthetic in cultured rat spinal neurones. *J. Physiol.* **386,** 485–501.

Barker, J. L. and McBurney, R. N. (1979) Phenobarbitone modulation of postsynaptic GABA receptor function on cultured mammalian neurons. *Proc. R. Soc. Lond. B.* **206,** 319–327.

Barker, J. L. and Mathers, D. A. (1981) GABA receptors and the depressant action of pentobarbital. *Trends Neurosci.* **4,** 10–13.

Barker, J. L. and Ransom, B. R. (1978) Pentobarbitone pharmacology of mamalian central neurones grown in tissue culture. *J. Physiol.* **280,** 355–372.

Belelli, D., Callachan, H., Hill-Venning, C., Peters, J. A., and Lambert, J. J. (1996) Interaction of positive allosteric modulators with human and *Drosophila* recombinant GABA receptors expressed in *Xenopus laevis* oocytes. *Br. J. Pharmacol.* **118,** 563–576.

Blair, L. A. C., Levitan, E. S., Marshall, J., Dionne, V. E., and Barnard, E. A. (1988) Single subunits of the $GABA_A$ receptor form ion channels with properties of the native receptor. *Science* **242,** 577–579.

Burt, D. R. and Kamatchi, G. L. (1991) $GABA_A$ receptor subtypes: from pharmacology to molecular biology. *FASEB J.* **5,** 2916–2923.

Callachan, H., Cottrell, G. A., Hather, N. Y., Lambert, J. J., Nooney, J. M., and Peters, J. A. (1987) Modulation of the $GABA_A$ receptor by progesterone metabolites. *Proc. R. Soc. Lond. B.* **231,** 359–369.

Carl, P., Høgskilde, S., Lang-Jensen, T., Bach, V., Jacobsen, J., Sorensen, M. B., Grälls, M., and Widlund, L. (1994) Pharmacokinetics and pharmacodynamics of eltanolone (pregnanolone), a new steroid intravenous anaesthetic, in humans. *Acta Anaesthiol. Scand.* **38,** 734–741.

Cestari, I. N., Uchida, I., Li, L., Burt, D., and Yang, J. (1996) The agonist action of pentobarbital on $GABA_A$ β-subunit homomeric receptors. *Neuroreport* **7,** 943–947.

Chen, R., Belelli, D., Lambert, J. J., Peters, J. A., Reyes, A., and Lan, N. C. (1994) Cloning and functional expression of a Drosophila γ-aminobutyric acid receptor. *Proc. Natl. Acad. Sci. USA* **91,** 6069–6073.

Collins, G. C. S. (1988) Effects of the anaesthetic 2,6-diisopropylphenol on synaptic transmission in the rat olfactory cortex slice. *Br. J. Pharmacol.* **95,** 939–949.

Connolly, C. N., Krishek, B. J., McDonald, B. J., Smart, T. G., and Moss, S. J. (1996) Assembly and cell surface expression of hereromeric and homomeric γ-aminobutyric acid type A receptors. *J. Biol. Chem.* **271,** 89–96.

Cooper, E. J., Johnston, G. A. R., and Edwards, F. A. (1995) Differential sensitivity of synaptic GABAergic currents to a neuroactive steroid in brain slices from male rats. *Soc. Neurosci Abs.* **21,** 531.4.

Cottrell, G. A., Lambert, J. J., and Peters, J. A. (1987) Modulation of GABA$_A$ receptor activity by alphaxalone. *Br. J. Pharmacol.* **90,** 491–500.

Cutting, G. R., Lu, L., O'Hara, B., Kasch, L. M., Donovan, D., Schimoda, S., Antonarakis, S. E., Guggino, W. B., Uhl, G. R., and Kazazion, H. H. (1991) Cloning of the GABA p1 cDNA; a novel GABA subunit highly expressed in the retina. *Proc. Natl. Acad. Sci. USA* **88,** 2673–2677.

De Koninck, Y. and Mody, I. (1994) Noise analysis of miniature IPSCs in adult rat brain slices: properties and modulation of synaptic GABA$_A$ receptor channels. *J. Neurophysiol.* **71,** 1318–1335.

Ebert, B., Wafford, K. A., Whiting, P. J., Krogsgaard-Larsen, P., and Kemp, J. A. (1994) Molecular pharmacology of γ-aminobutyric acid type A receptor agonists and partial agonists in oocytes injected with different α, β, and γ receptor subunit combinations. *Mol. Pharmacol.* **46,** 957–963.

Ebert, T. J., Muzi, M., Berens, R., Goff, D., and Kampine, J. P. (1992) Sympathetic responses to induction of anesthesia with propofol or etomidate. *Anesthesiology* **76,** 725–733.

Eccles, J. C., and Malcolm, J. L. (1946) Dorsal root potentials of the spinal cord. *J. Neurophysiol.* **9,** 139–160.

Eccles, J. C., Schmidt, R., and Willis, W. D. (1963) Pharmacological studies on presynaptic inhibition. *J. Physiol.* **168,** 500–530.

Evans, R. H. and Hill, R. G. (1978) GABA-mimetic action of etomidate. *Experentia* **34,** 1325–1327.

ffrench-Constant, R. H., Rocheleau, T. A., Steichen, J. C., and Chalmers, A. E. (1993) A point mutation a *Drosophila* receptor conferes insecticide resistance. *Nature* **363,** 449–451.

ffrench-Mullen, J. M. H., Barker, J. L., and Rogawski, M. A. (1993) Calcium block by (–)-pentobarbital, phenobarbital, and CHEB but not (+)-pentobarbital in acutely isolated hippocampal CA1 neurons: comparison with effects on GABA-activated Cl⁻ current. *J. Neurosci.* **13,** 3211–3221.

Franks, N. P. and Lieb, W. R. (1994) Molecular and cellular mechanisms of general anaesthesia. *Nature* **367,** 607–614.

Frerking, M., Borges, S., and Wilson, M. (1995) Variation in GABA mini amplitude is the consequence of variation in transmitter concentration. *Neuron* **15,** 885–895.

Gage, P. W. and Robertson, B. (1985) Prolongation of inhibitory postsynaptic currents by pentobarbitone, halothane and ketamine in CA1 pyramidal cells in rat hippocampus. *Br. J. Pharmacol.* **85,** 675–681.

Galzi, J. L. and Changeux, J.-P. (1995) Neurotransmitter-gated ion channels as unconventional allosteric proteins. *Current Opinion Struct. Biol.* **4,** 554–565.

Gee, K. W., Bolger, M. B., Brinton, R. E., Coirini, H., and McEwen, B. S. (1988) Steroid modulation of the chloride ionophore in rat brain: structure-activity requirements, regional dependence and mechanism of action. *J. Pharmacol. Exp. Ther.* **246,** 803–812.

Gee, K. W., McCauley, L. D., and Lan, N. C. (1995) A putative receptor for neurosteroids on the GABA$_A$ receptor complex: the pharmacological properties and therapeutic potential of epalons. *Crit. Rev. Neurobiol.* **9,** 207–227.

Gemmell, D. K., Byford, A., Anderson, A., Marshall, R. J., Hill, D. R., Campbell, A. C., Hamilton, N., Hill-Venning, C., Lambert, J. J., and Peters, J. A. (1995) The anaesthetic and GABA modulatory actions of ORG 21465, a novel water soluble steroidal intravenous anaesthetic agent. *Br. J. Pharmacol.* **116,** 443P.

Hadingham, K. L., Wingrove, P. B., Wafford, K. A., Bain, C., Kemp, J. A., Palmer, K. J., Wilson, A. W., Wilcox, A. S., Sikela, J. M., Ragan, C. I., and Whiting, P. J. (1993) Role of the β subunit in determining the pharmacology of human γ-aminobutyric acid type A receptors. *Mol. Pharmacol.* **44,** 1211–1218.

Hales, T. G. and Lambert, J. J. (1991) The actions of propofol on inhibitory amino acid receptors of bovine adrenomedullary chromaffin cells and rodent central neurones. *Br. J. Pharmacol.* **104,** 619–628.

Hara, M., Kai, Y., and Ikemoto, Y. (1993) Propofol activates GABA$_A$ receptor-chloride ionophore complex in dissociated hippocampal pyramidal neurones of the rat. *Anesthesiology* **79,** 781–788.

Hara, M., Kai, Y., Ikemoto, Y. (1994) Enhancement by propofol of the γ-aminobutyric acid$_A$ response in dissociated hippocampal pyramidal neurones of the rat. *Anesthesiology* **81,** 988–994.

Harris, R. A., Mihic, S. J., Dildy-Mayfield, J. E., and Machu, T. K. (1995) Actions of anesthetics on ligand-gated ion channels: role of receptor subunit composition. *FASEB J.* **9,** 1454–1462.

Harrison, N. L., Majewska, M. D., Harrington, J. W., and Barker, J. L. (1987b) Structure-activity relationships for steroid interaction with the γ-aminobutyric acid$_A$ receptor complex. *J. Pharmacol. Exp. Ther.* **241,** 346–353.

Harrison, N. L. and Simmonds, M. A. (1984) Modulation of the GABA receptor complex by a steroid anaesthetic. *Brain Res.* **323,** 287–292.

Harrison, N. L., Vicini, S., and Barker, J. L. (1987a) A steroid anaesthetic prolongs inhibitory postsynaptic currents in cultured rat hippocampal neurons. *J. Neurosci.* **7,** 604–609.

Hawkinson, J. E., Kimbrough, C. L., Belelli, D., Lambert, J. J., Purdy, R. H., and Lan, N. C. (1994) Correlation of neuroactive steroid modulation of [^{35}S]t-butylbicyclo-phosporothionate and [^{3}H]flunitrazepam binding and γ-aminobutyric acid$_A$ receptor function. *Mol. Pharmacol.* **46,** 977–985.

Hill-Venning, C., Belelli, D., Hope, A. G., Peters, J. A., and Lambert, J. J. (1995) Modulation of recombinant GABA$_A$ receptors by the general anaesthetic etomidate is subunit dependent. *Soc. Neurosci. Abs.* **21,** 339.6.

Hill-Venning, C., Belelli, D., Peters, J. A., and Lambert, J. J. (1994b) Electrophysiological studies of neurosteroid modulation of γ-aminobutyric acid type A receptor, in *Neurobiology of Steroids* (deKloet, E. R. and Sutanto, W., eds.), Academic, San Diego, pp. 446–467.

Hill-Venning, C., Callachan, H., Peters, J. A., Lambert, J. J., Gemmell, D. K., and Campbell, A. C. (1994a) Modulation of the GABA$_A$ receptor by Org 20599: a water-soluble pregnane steroid. *Br. J. Pharmacol.* **111,** 183P.

Hill-Venning, C., Peters, J. A., Callachan, H., Lambert, J. J., Gemmell, D. K., Anderson, A., Byford, A., Hamilton, N., Hill, D. R., Marshall, R. J., and Campbell, A. C. (1996) The anaesthetic action and modulation of GABA$_A$ receptor activity by the novel water soluble aminosteroid ORG 20599. *Neuropharmacology* (in press).

Hill-Venning, C., Lambert, J. J., Peters, J. A., and Hales, T. G. (1991) The actions of neurosteroids on inhibitory amino acid receptors, in *Neurosteroids and Brain Function* (Costa, E. and Paul, S. M., eds.), Thieme, New York, 77–85.

Holland, K. D., Canney, D. J., Rothman, S. M., Ferrendelli, J. A., and Covey, D. F. (1990) Physiological modulation of the GABA receptor by convulsant and anti-convulsant barbiturates in cultured rat hippocampal neurons. *Brain Res.* **516,** 147–150.

Horne, A. L., Harkness, P. C., Hadingham, K. L., Whiting, P., and Kemp, J. A. (1993) The influence of the γ_{2L} subunit on the modulation of responses to GABA$_A$ receptor activation. *Br. J. Pharmacol.* **108**, 711–716.

Huang, L.-Y. M. and Barker, J. L. (1980) Pentobarbital: stereoselective actions of (+) and (–) isomers revealed on cultured mammalian neurones. *Science* **207**, 195–197.

Janssen, P. A. J., Niemegeers, J. E., and Marsboom, R. P. H. (1975) Etomidate, a potent non-barbiturate hypnotic. Intravenous etomidate in mice, rats, guinea-pigs, rabbits and dogs. *Arch. Int. Pharmacodyn.* **214**, 92–132.

Jones, M. V. and Harrison, N. L. (1993) Effect of volatile anesthetics on the kinetics of inhibitory post-synaptic currents in cultured hippocampal neurons. *J. Neurophysiol.* **70**, 1339–1349.

Jones, M. V., Harrison, N. L., Pritchett, D., and Hales, T. G. (1995) Modulation of the GABA$_A$ receptor by propofol is independent of the γ subunit. *J. Pharmacol. Exp. Ther.* **274**, 962–968.

Jones, M. V. and Westbrook, G. L. (1996) The impact of receptor desensitization on fast synaptic transmission. *Trends Neurosci.* **19**, 96–101.

Joyce, K. A., Atkinson, A. A., Bermudez, I., Beadle, D. J., and King, L. A. (1993) Synthesis of functional GABA$_A$ receptors in stable insect cell lines. *FEBS Lett.* **335**, 61–64.

Kaneda, M., Farrant, M., and Cull-Candy, S. G. (1995) Whole cell and single channel currents activated by GABA and glycine in granule cells of the cerebellum. *J. Physiol.* **485.2**, 419–435.

Korpi, E. R., Kleingoor, C., Kettenmann, H., and Seeburg, P. H. (1993) Benzodiazepine-induced motor impairment linked to point mutation in cerebellar GABA$_A$ receptor. *Nature* **361**, 356–359.

Korpi, E. R. and Luddens, H. (1993) Regional γ-aminobutyric-acid sensitivity of *t*-butyl-bicyclophoshoro[^{35}S]thionate binding depends on γ-aminobutyric-acid A receptor α6 subunit. *Mol. Pharmacol.* **44**, 87–92.

Krishek, B. J., Moss, S. J., and Smart, T. G. (1996) Homomeric β1 γ-aminobutyric acid$_A$ receptor-ion channels: evaluation of pharmacological and physiological properties. *Mol. Pharmacol.* **49**, 494–504.

Lambert, J. J., Belelli, D., Hill-Venning, C., Callachan, H., and Peters, J. A. (1996) Neurosteroid modulation of native and recombinant GABA$_A$ receptors. *Cell. Mol. Neurobiol.* **16**, 155–174.

Lambert, J. J., Belelli, D., Hill-Venning, C., and Peters, J. A. (1995) Neurosteroids and GABA$_A$ receptor function. *Trends Pharmacol. Sci.* **16**, 295–303.

Lambert, J. J., Hill-Venning, C., Peters, J. A., Sturgess, N. C., and Hales, T. G. (1991) The actions of anesthetic steroids on inhibitory and excitatory amino acid receptors, in *Transmitter Amino Acid Receptors: Structures, Transduction and Models for Drug Development* (Barnard, E. A. and Costa, E., eds.), Thieme, New York, pp. 219–236.

Lambert, J. J., Peters, J. A., and Cottrell, G. A. (1987) Actions of synthetic and endogenous steroids on the GABA$_A$ receptor. *Trends Pharmacol. Sci.* **8**, 224–227.

Lambert, J. J., Peters, J. A., Sturgess, N. C., and Hales, T. G. (1990) Steroid modulation of the GABA$_A$ receptor complex: electrophysiological studies, in *Steroids and Neuronal Activity* (Chadwick, D. and Widdows, K., eds.), Wiley, Chichester, UK, pp. 56–82.

Langosch, D. (1995) Inhibitory glycine receptors, in *Ligand- and Voltage-gated Ion Channels. Handbook of Receptors and Channels* (North, R. A., ed.), CRC, Boca Raton, FL, pp. 291–305.

Laurie, D. J., Seeburg, P. H., and Wisden, W. (1992) The distribution of 13 GABA$_A$ receptor subunit mRNAs in the rat brain II. Olfactory bulb and cerebellum. *J. Neurosci.* **12**, 1063–1076.

Little, H. J. (1996) Has molecular pharmacology contributed to our understanding of the mechanism(s) of general anaesthesia? *Pharmacol. Ther.* **69**, 37–58.

Lodge, D. and Anis, N. A. (1984) Effects of ketamine and three other anaesthetics on spinal reflexes and inhibitions in the cat. *Br. J. Anaesth.* **56**, 1143–1151.

Luddens, H., Korpi, E. R., and Seeburg, P. H. (1995) GABA$_A$/Benzodiazepine receptor heterogeneity: neurophysiological implications. *Neuropharmacology* **34**, 245–254.

Maconochie, D. J., Zemple, J. M., and Steinbach, J. H. (1994) How quickly can GABA$_A$ receptors open? *Neuron* **12**, 61–71.

Macdonald, R. L. and Olsen, R. W. (1994) GABA$_A$ receptor channels. *Ann. Rev. Neurosci.* **17**, 569–602.

Macdonald, R. L., Rogers, C. J., and Twyman, R. E. (1989) Barbiturate regulation of kinetic properties of the GABA$_A$ receptor channel of mouse spinal neurons in culture. *J. Physiol.* **417**, 483–500.

Macdonald, R. L. and Angelotti, T. P. (1993) Native and recombinant GABA$_A$ receptor channels. *Cell Physiol. Biochem.* **3**, 352–373.

Majewska, M. D., Harrison, N. L., Schwartz, R. D., Barker, J. L., and Paul, S. M. (1986) Steroid hormone metabolites are barbiturate-like modulators of the GABA receptor. *Science* **232**, 1004–1007.

Mathers, D. and Barker, J. L. (1980) (−)-Pentobarbital opens ion channels of long duration in cultured mouse spinal neurons. *Science* **209**, 507–509.

McCauley, L. D. and Gee, K. W. (1994) Detection and characterization of epalon receptors: novel recognition sites for neuroactive steroids that modulate the GABA$_A$ receptor complex, in *Neurobiology of Steroids* (deKloet, E. R. and Sutanto, W., eds.), Academic, San Diego, pp. 211–241.

McCauley, L. D., Liu, V., Chen, J. S., Hawkinson, J. E., Lan, N. C., and Gee, K. W. (1995) Selective actions of certain neuroactive pregnanediols at the γ-aminobutyric acid type A receptor complex in rat brain. *Mol. Pharmacol.* **47**, 354–362.

McKernan, R. M. and Whiting, P. J. (1996) Which GABA$_A$ receptor subtypes really occur in the brain? *Trends Neurosci.* **19**, 139–143.

Mody, I., DeKoninck, Y., Otis, T. S., and Soltesz, I. (1994) Bridging the cleft at GABA synapses in the brain. *Trends Neurosci.* **17**, 517–525.

Nicoll, R. A. (1975) Pentobarbital: action on frog motoneurons. *Brain Res.* **96**, 119–123.

Nicoll, R. A. and Wojtowicz, J. M. (1980) The effects of pentobarbital and related compounds on frog motoneurons. *Brain Res.* **191**, 225–237.

Olsen, R. W. (1988) Barbiturates. *Int. Anesth. Clin.* **26**, 254–261.

Olsen, R. W., Fischer, J. B., and Dunwiddie, T. V. (1986) Barbiturate enhancement of γ-aminobutyric acid receptor binding and function as a mechanism of anesthesia, in *Molecular and Cellular Mechanisms of Anesthetics* (Roth, S. H. and Miller K. W. eds.), Plenum Press, New York, pp. 165–177.

Olsen, R. W. and Sapp, D. W. (1995) Neuroactive steroid modulation of GABA$_A$ receptors, in *GABA$_A$ Receptors and Anxiety from Neurobiology to Treatment: Advances in Biochemical Psychopharmacology*, vol. 48. (Biggio, G., Sanna, E., Serra, M., and Costa, E., ed.), Raven, New York, pp. 57–74.

Orser, B. A., Wang, L.-Y., Pennefather, P. S., and Macdonald, J. F. (1994) Propofol modulates activation and desensitization of GABA$_A$ receptors in cultured murine hippocampal neurons. *J. Neurosci.* **14**, 7747–7760.

Peters, J. A., Kirkness, E. F., Callachan, H., Lambert J. J., and Turner, A. J. (1988) Modulation of the GABA$_A$ receptor by depressant barbiturates and pregnane steroids. Br. J. Pharmacol. **94**, 1257–1269.

Peters, J. A., Lambert, J. J., and Cottrell, G. A. (1989) An electrophysiological investigation of the characteristics and functions of GABA$_A$ receptors on bovine adrenomedullary chromaffin cells. Pflügers Arch. **415**, 95–103.

Phillipps, G. H. (1975) Structure-activity relationships in steroid anaesthetics. J. Steroid Biochem. **6**, 607–613.

Pistis, M., Belelli, D., Peters, J. A., and Lambert, J. J. (1996) Modulation of recombinant glycine and GABA$_A$ receptors by general anaesthetics: a comparative study. Soc. Neurosci. Abs. **22**, (in press).

Prince, R. J. and Simmonds, M. A. (1993) Differential antagonism by epipregnanolone of alphaxalone and prenanolone potentiation of [^{3}H]flunitrazepem binding suggests more than one class of binding site for steroids at GABA$_A$ receptors. Neuropharmacology **32**, 59–63.

Pritchett, D. B., Sontheimer, H., Gorman, C. M., Kettenman, H., Seeburg, P. H., and Scholfield, P. R. (1988) Transient expression shows ligand-gating and allosteric potentiation of GABA$_A$ receptor subunits. Science **242**, 1306–1308.

Proctor, W. R., Mynlieff, M., and Dunwiddie, T. V. (1986) Facilitatory action of etomidate and pentobarbital on recurrent inhibition in rat hippocampal pyramidal neurons. J. Neurosci. **6**, 3161–3168.

Puia, G., Costa, E., and Vicini, S. (1994) Functional diversity of GABA-activated Cl$^-$ currents in Purkinje versus granule neurons in rat cerebellar slices. Neuron **12**, 117–126.

Puia, G., Ducic, I., Vicini, S., and Costa, E. (1993) Does neurosteroid modulatory efficacy depend on GABA$_A$ receptor subunit composition? Receptors Channels **1**, 135–142.

Puia, G., Santi, M. R., Vicini, S. Pritchett, D. B., Purdy, R. H., Paul, S. M., Seeburg, P. H., and Costa, E. (1990) Neurosteroids act on recombinant human GABA$_A$ receptors. Neuron **4**, 759–765.

Robertson, B. (1989) Actions of anaesthetics and avermectin on GABA$_A$ chloride channels in mammalian dorsal root ganglion neurones. Br. J. Pharmacol. **98**, 167–176.

Rogers, C. J., Twyman, R. E., and Macdonald, R. L. (1994) Benzodiazepine and β-carboline regulation of single GABA$_A$ receptor channels of mouse spinal neurones in culture. J. Physiol. **475.1**, 69–82.

Sanna, E., Garau, F., and Harris, R. A. (1995a) Novel properties of homomeric (β_1 γ-aminobutyric acid type A receptors: actions of the anaesthetics propofol and pentobarbital. Mol. Pharmacol. **47**, 213–217.

Sanna, E., Mascia, M. P., Klein, R. L., Whiting, P. Biggio, G., and Harris, R. A. (1995b) Actions of the general anesthetic propofol on recombinant human GABA$_A$ receptors: influence of receptor subunits. J. Pharmacol. Exp. Ther. **274**, 353–360.

Saxena, N. C., and Macdonald, R. L. (1994) Assembly of GABA$_A$ receptor subunits: role of the δ subunit. J. Neurosci. **14**, 7077–7086.

Schulz, D. W., and Macdonald, R. L. (1981) Barbiturate enhancement of GABA-mediated inhibition and activation of chloride ion conductance: correlation with anticonvulsant and anesthetic actions. Brain Res. **209**, 177–188.

Scholfield, C. M. (1980) Potentiation of inhibition by general anaesthetics in neurones of the olfactory cortex in vitro. Pflügers Arch. **383**, 249–255.

Segal, M. and Barker, J. L. (1984) Rat hippocampal neurones in culture: voltage-clamp analysis of inhibitory synaptic connections. J. Neurophysiol. **52**, 469–487

Selye, H. (1941) Anesthetic effect of steroid hormones. *Proc. Soc. Exp. Biol. Med.* **46,** 116–121.

Shingai, R., Sutherland, M. L., and Barnard, E. A. (1991) Effects of subunit types of the cloned GABA$_A$ receptor on the response to a neurosteroid. *Eur. J. Pharmacol.* **206,** 77–80.

Sieghart, W. (1995) Structure and pharmacology of γ-aminobutyric acid$_A$ receptor subtypes. *Pharmacol. Rev.* **47,** 182–234.

Sigel, E., Baur, R., Malherbe, P., and Möhler, H. (1989) The rat β1-subunit of the GABA$_A$ receptor forms a picrotoxin-sensitive anion channel open in the absence of GABA. *FEBS Lett.* **257,** 377–379.

Sigel, E., Baur, R., Trube, G., Möhler, H., and Malherbe, P. (1990) The effect of subunit composition of rat brain GABA$_A$ receptors on channel function. *Neuron* **5,** 703–711.

Smith, G. B., and Olsen, R. W. (1995) Functional domains of GABA$_A$ receptors. *Trends Pharmacol. Sci.* **16,** 162–168.

Stevenson, A., Wingrove, P. B., Whiting, P. J., and Wafford, K. A. (1995) β-carboline γ-aminobutyric acid$_A$ receptor inverse agonists modulate γ-aminobutyric acid via the loreclezole binding site as well as the benzodiazepine site. *Mol. Pharmacol.* **48,** 965–969.

Study, R. E. and Barker, J. L. (1981) Diazepam and (–) pentobarbital: fluctuation analysis reveals different mechanisms for potentiation of γ-aminobutyric acid responses in cultured central neurones. *Proc. Natl. Acad. Sci. USA* **78,** 7180–7184.

Tanelian, D. L., Kosek, P., Mody, I., and MacIver, B. (1993) The role of the GABA$_A$ receptor/choride channel complex in anesthesia. *Anesthesiology* **78,** 757–776.

Thompson, S. A., Whiting, P. J., and Wafford, K. A. (1996) Barbiturate interactions at the human GABA$_A$ receptor: dependence on receptor subunit composition. *Br. J. Pharmacol.* **117,** 521–527.

Thyagarajan, R., Ramanjaneyulu, R., and Ticku, M. K. (1983) Enhancement of diazepam and γ-aminobutyric acid binding by (+) etomidate and pentobarbital. *J. Neurochem.* **41,** 578–585.

Ticku, R. K. and Rastogi, S. K. (1986) Barbiturate-sensitive sites in the benzodiazepine-GABA receptor-ionophore complex, in *Molecular and Cellular Mechanisms of Anaesthetics* (Roth, S. H., and Miller K. W., eds.), Plenum Press, New York, pp. 179–188.

Turner, D. M., Ransom, R. W., Yang, J. S.-J., and Olsen, R. W. (1989) Steroid anesthetics and naturally occurring analogues modulate the γ-aminobutyric acid receptor complex at a site distinct from barbiturates. *J. Pharmacol. Exp. Ther.* **248,** 960–966.

Twyman, R. E. and Macdonald, R. L. (1992) Neurosteroid regulation of GABA$_A$ receptor single-channel kinetic properties of mouse spinal cord neurons in culture. *J. Physiol.* **456,** 215–245.

Tyndale, R. F., Olsen, R. W., and Tobin, A. J. (1995) GABA$_A$ receptors, in *Ligand- and Voltage-gated Ion Channels. Handbook of Receptors and Channels* (North, R. A., ed.), CRC, Boca Raton, FL, pp. 265–290.

Uchida, I., Cestari, I. N., and Yang, J. (1996) The differential bicuculline and SR95531 antagonism of chloride current directly induced by pentobarbital in cultured postnatal hippocampal neurons. *Eur. J. Pharmacol.* in press.

Uchida, I., Katamachi, G., Burt, D., and Yang, J. (1995) Etomidate potentiation of GABA$_A$ receptor gated current depends on subunit composition. *Neurosci. Letts.* **185,** 203–206.

Valeyev, A. Y., Barker, J. L., Cruciani, R. A., Lange, G. D., Smallwood, V. V., and Mahan, L. C. (1993) Characterization of the γ-aminbutyric acid A receptor channel complex composed of α1β2 and α1β3 subunits from rat brain. *J. Pharmacol. Exp. Ther.* **265,** 985–991.

Vicini, S., Mienville, J.-M., and Costa, E. (1987) Actions of benzodiazepine and β-carboline derivatives on γ-aminobutyric acid-activated Cl⁻ channels recorded from membrane patches of neonatal rat cortical neurons in culture. *J. Pharmacol. Exp. Ther.* **243,** 1195–1201.

Wafford, K. A., Thompson, S. A., Thomas, D., Sikela, J., Wilcox, A. S., and Whiting, P. J. (1996) Functional characterization of human $GABA_A$ receptors containing the α4 subunit. Manuscript submitted for publication.

Wingrove, P. B., Wafford, K. A., Bain, C., and Whiting, P. J. (1994) The modulatory action of loreclezole at the γ-aminobutyric acid type A receptor is determined by a single amino acid in the β_2 and β_3 subunit. *Proc. Natl. Acad. Sci. USA* **91,** 4569–4573.

Whiting, P. J., McKernan, R. M., and Wafford, K. A. (1995) Structure and pharmacology of vertebrate $GABA_A$ receptor subtypes. *Int. Rev. Neurobiol.* **38,** 95–138.

Woodward, R. M., Polenzani, L., and Miledi, R. (1992) Effects of steroids on γ-aminobutyric acid receptors expressed in *Xenopus* oocytes by poly (A)+ RNA from mammalian brain and retina. *Mol. Pharmacol.* **41,** 89–103.

Yang, J. and Uchida, I. (1996) Mechanisms of etomidate potentiation of $GABA_A$ receptor-gated currents in cultured post-natal hippocampal neurons. *Neuroscience* (in press).

Zimmermann S. A., Jones M. V., and Harrison N. L. (1994) Potentiation of γ-aminobutyric $acid_A$ Cl⁻ current correlates with in vivo anesthetic potency. *J. Pharmacol. Exp. Ther.* **270,** 987–991.

CHAPTER 6

Electrophysiology of GABA$_B$ Receptors

Rudolf A. Deisz

1. Introduction

The last decade has seen a tremendous increase in the understanding of the cellular and molecular mechanisms of synaptic transmission. This gain in knowledge is also reflected in the number of excellent reviews concerning synaptic transmission in general (Mayer and Westbrook, 1987; Siggins and Gruol, 1986; Nicoll et al., 1990), and on specific aspects of synaptic functioning. Synaptic inhibition in the visual cortex was reviewed by Connors (1992) and the ionic mechanisms of inhibition received an in-depth treatment by Kaila (1995). Thompson (1994) presented a complete survey of the modulation of synaptic inhibition in the hippocampus. The modulation of calcium channels by neurotransmitters (reviewed by Anwyl [1991] and Dolphin [1991]) is of particular interest in the present context. Most relevant to the issue addressed here are previous reviews covering the physiology and pharmacology of GABA$_B$ receptors by Bowery (1993), Mott and Lewis (1994), and Misgeld et al. (1995).

2. Synaptic Transmission in the Central Nervous System

Numerous molecular, neurochemical, and electrophysiological studies have firmly established the current concepts of synaptic transmission as the basis for the integrative properties of the central nervous system (CNS). In essence, the action potential arriving in terminal regions releases transmitter molecules through a cascade of cellular events. Upon binding to specific recognition sites on postsynaptic neurons, transmitters induce diverse cellular reactions, depending upon the transmitter and neuron involved, and even on the cellular history of the neuron.

The GABA Receptors Eds.: S. J. Enna and N. G. Bowery
Humana Press Inc., Totowa, NJ

The details of this chain of events are far from being fully understood. The cellular cascades involved in the liberation of transmitter (for review, *see* Südhof et al., 1993) are still a matter of debate (*see* Neher and Penner, 1994). Once released, a given transmitter exerts postsynaptic responses, which can be distinguished into two principal categories: the flux of ions through transmitter-gated channels and the induction of intracellular changes of second messenger systems through metabotropic receptors. But the molecular and functional diversity of receptors, for both excitatory (*see* Seeburg, 1993) and inhibitory amino acids, precludes the precise prediction of a synaptic response in a given area. The diversity of synaptic responses determined by the families of receptors is further multiplied by the interaction with intrinsic currents and use-dependent changes of synaptic transmission, which finally govern neuronal information processing.

Regarding receptors for GABA, the main inhibitory transmitters in the CNS, two types of receptors have been demonstrated. The classical GABA receptor, now termed $GABA_A$ receptor, has been purified and cloned. The $GABA_A$ receptor is probably a pentamer arrangement of subunits, with homologies in primary sequence and membrane topology (Schofield et al., 1987). The subunit composition of the receptor governs the biophysical properties (Verdoorn et al., 1990) and the mRNAs encoding distinct subunits display a specific pattern in both the adult brain (Wisden et al., 1992) and during development (Laurie et al., 1992). The $GABA_A$ receptors are the target for several centrally active drugs, including barbiturates and benzodiazepines (*see* Chapter 2 of this volume).

The second class of GABA receptors, the $GABA_B$ receptors, are operationally defined by their selective activation by baclofen and their lack of sensitivity towards bicuculline (Bowery et al., 1980; for review, *see* Bowery, 1993). Although earlier work had demonstrated distinct actions of baclofen on synaptic transmission in the spinal cord (Pierau and Zimmermann, 1973) and the excitability of cortical neurons (Curtis et al., 1974; Davies and Watkins, 1974), the work by Bowery et al., 1980) firmly established that baclofen interacts with a distinct receptor. During the past few years, an impressive amount of work was devoted to the mechanisms of $GABA_B$ action in the CNS. A major factor spurring the advance in the understanding of $GABA_B$ receptor function was the availability of antagonists. The development of potent $GABA_B$ antagonists (Olpe et al., 1990; Froestl et al., 1992) greatly facilitated the investigations on the various facets of $GABA_B$ receptors, but the physiological functions of $GABA_B$ receptors are just beginning to emerge.

The focus of this review will be the electrophysiological characterization of $GABA_B$ receptor-mediated effects, although some data obtained with other methods will also be included. Considering the exhaustive recent reviews by Mott and Lewis (1994) and Misgeld et al. (1995), the key features of $GABA_B$ receptor function will be discussed. Evidence will be evaluated for a diversity of $GABA_B$ receptors and for a distinct inhibitory system utilizing the same transmitter as the $GABA_A$ inhibition, but a separate receptor and a discrete population of interneurons. In addition, the discrete differences will be delineated in $GABA_B$ receptor effector systems at pre- and postsynaptic sites in several structures.

3. Structure of the $GABA_B$ Receptors

$GABA_B$ receptors were solubilized from a crude synaptosomal fraction of bovine cerebral cortex. The isolation and purification of the $GABA_B$ receptor revealed that these receptors are a homogeneous population of proteins of about 80 kDa (Kuriyama and Ohmori, 1990). This differs markedly from the size of $GABA_A$ receptor subunits, indicating that $GABA_B$ receptors are entirely different from the $GABA_A$ receptors. The loss of $GABA_B$ receptor coupling to G proteins after solubilization, similar to the dopamine D2 receptor, was taken as evidence for similar transduction mechanisms (Kuriyama and Ohmori, 1990). The monoclonal antibody raised against the 80 kDa protein antagonized the binding of baclofen by more than 90%, indicating this protein constitutes the sole baclofen binding capacity (Kuriyama et al., 1992; *see also* Chapter 9 of this volume). However, some splice variants, differing in size below the resolution of the protein separation, cannot be excluded. Until the $GABA_B$ receptor has been cloned, the question of subtypes of the $GABA_B$ receptor as molecular entities is unsolved. Regarding the molecular properties and transmembrane topology of the $GABA_B$ receptors, some evidence indicates $GABA_B$ receptors are related to the family of the seven membrane-spanning proteins. A specific antisense oligonucleotide to mRNA encoding these proteins decreased the $GABA_B$ receptors in cerebellar granule cells (Holopainen and Wojcik, 1993).

4. Postsynaptic Effects of Baclofen

4.1. Action of Agonists

4.1.1. Postsynaptic Potential Changes by Baclofen

The cellular actions of baclofen, the prototypic agonist for the $GABA_B$ receptor, have been extensively studied in many areas of the CNS. The first intracellular examination of the actions of baclofen in hippocampal CA3 neurons and granule cells in the dentate gyrus yielded a multitude of effects on membrane potential and excitatory and inhibitory postsynaptic potentials (Klee et al., 1981; Misgeld et al., 1982). Together with a series of subsequent investigations (Newberry and Nicoll, 1984, 1985; Andrade et al., 1986), these data established the basic properties of baclofen-induced conductance in hippocampal neurons. The baclofen-induced hyperpolarization and increase in membrane conductance is, unlike the bicuculline-sensitive GABA response, insensitive to changes in intracellular or extracellular chloride. The reversal potential of the baclofen responses shifted by 48 mV in response to a tenfold change in extracellular potassium, consistent with a potassium conductance increase (Newberry and Nicoll, 1985). The persistence of the baclofen response, after blockade of synaptic transmission by cadmium or tetrodotoxin (TTX), ascertained that the response is postsynaptically mediated and not related to a calcium activated potassium current (Newberry and Nicoll, 1985). The effects of baclofen are similar to GABA responses in the presence of bicuculline and to a late inhibitory postsynaptic potential (Newberry and Nicoll, 1985).

Early extracellular recordings in the neocortex in vivo indicate that baclofen causes a pronounced depression of excitability (Curtis et al., 1974; Davies and Watkins, 1974). Subsequent work in the neocortical slice revealed that baclofen hyperpolarizes the majority of neurons, increases membrane conductance (Howe et al., 1987a; Connors et al., 1988; Deisz and Prince, 1989), and produces outward currents when the neurons are recorded in the voltage clamp mode (Howe et al., 1987a). The hyperpolarizations are fairly small and are associated with a small decrease in resistance of 15–30% (Howe et al., 1987a). The baclofen-induced conductance was estimated to be about 12 nS (Connors et al., 1988). The reversal potential of the baclofen response corresponded to the potassium equilibrium potential (Howe et al., 1987a; Connors et al., 1988), indicating that baclofen activates a potassium conductance increase, similar to findings in hippocampal neurons. A baclofen-induced hyperpolarization and conductance increase has since been described in many areas of the CNS, including suprachiasmatic nucleus (Jiang et al., 1995), nucleus accumbens (Uchimura and North, 1991), lateral parabrachial neurons (Christie and North, 1988), dorsal lateral geniculate nucleus (Soltesz et al., 1988), and substantia nigra (Lacey et al., 1988; Häusser and Yung, 1994). It is interesting to note that astrocytes are also endowed with $GABA_B$ receptors inducing a hyperpolarization (Hösli et al., 1990), although little is known about the physiological function of these receptors. The reduction of the baclofen or bicuculline-insensitive GABA response by phaclofen, or any of the more recent antagonists of the CGP family (CGP 35348 or CGP 55845A; for details, *see* Olpe et al., 1990; *see also* Chapter 10 of this volume), has often been employed to verify the involvement of $GABA_B$ receptors (Dutar and Nicoll, 1988b; Soltesz et al., 1988).

However, some notable exceptions exist. For instance, several authors (Calabresi et al., 1991; Seabrook et al., 1991; Nisenbaum et al., 1993) have consistently reported no detectable postsynaptic effects in the neostriatum, despite clear evidence for the presence of GABA$_B$ receptors on inhibitory and excitatory terminals (Calabresi et al., 1991; Nisenbaum et al., 1993). Also in the hippocampus a marked difference in the baclofen responsiveness exists between area CA3 and dentate gyrus. Granule cells respond only with a marginal hyperpolarization and conductance increase, compared to CA3 neurons, indicating a lower density of receptors (Misgeld et al., 1984), or a different state of the GABA$_B$-mediated signaling cascade.

Comparison of the baclofen responsiveness revealed comparable half-maximal concentrations of 1.5 μM in substantia nigra (Lacey et al., 1988) and 1 μM in the lateral parabrachial neurons (Christie and North, 1988) and neocortex (Howe et al., 1987a) (determined as the change of threshold for action potential generation). The difference between this electrophysiologically determined effectiveness of baclofen and the K_d determined in binding studies, ranging typically between 30–80 nM (Bowery et al., 1983), is unclear. Nevertheless, both methods reveal a stereoselective effect of baclofen, the (–)-baclofen isomer is consistently reported to be more potent in electrophysiological experiments (Newberry and Nicoll, 1985; Howe et al., 1987a) and in binding studies (Bowery et al., 1983). The baclofen induced postsynaptic conductance is attenuated by GABA$_B$ receptor antagonists, phaclofen (Dutar and Nicoll, 1988a,b), and the more recent antagonists.

4.1.2. Second Messengers Involved in the Action of Baclofen

4.1.2.1. G Protein Involvement

Several lines of evidence indicate that the postsynaptic conductance increase by baclofen is mediated through G proteins. Early binding experiments demonstrated that guanyl nucleotides inhibit GABA$_B$ receptor binding (Hill et al., 1984; Asano et al., 1985). The diminished binding affinity corresponds to the abolition of postsynaptic baclofen responses in hippocampal CA1 neurons after treatment with pertussis toxin (Andrade et al., 1986), which inactivates the α subunit of some, but not all G proteins. In addition, the GDP analog GDPβS greatly attenuates the response to baclofen, and the GTP analog GTPγS mimics the effect of baclofen application (Andrade et al., 1986). Dutar and Nicoll (1988b) confirmed and extended these data. Pertussis toxin pretreatment (intracerebroventricular injection 3 d before the slices were obtained) not only abolishes the postsynaptic baclofen response, but also the late inhibitory postsynaptic potential (IPSP). These findings have also been confirmed in the CA3 area of hippocampal slices maintained in organotypic culture (Thompson and Gähwiler, 1992). Following an incubation of the cultures with pertussis toxin (500 ng/mL for 48 h), postsynaptic potential and conductance changes induced by baclofen are abolished.

The pertussis toxin sensitivity of G protein-mediated conductance of substantia nigra neurons, however, appears controversial; both pertussis toxin sensitivity of dopamine responses (Innis and Aghajanian, 1987a) and insensitivity of baclofen and dopamine responses have been reported (Lacey et al., 1988). Intracerebroventricular injection of pertussis toxin was ineffective in antagonizing the baclofen-induced conductance (Lacey et al., 1988), yet the intracellular application of guanosine 5'0-(3-thiophosphate) (GTPγS) enhances the action of baclofen (and of dopamine). This indicates that both baclofen and dopamine responses are mediated by G proteins (Lacey et al., 1988). The lack of effect of pertussis toxin may suggest that pertussis toxin-insensitive G proteins are involved in the coupling of $GABA_B$ receptors to potassium conductance. The alternative explanation is that diffusional limitations prevented an access of pertussis toxin to the substantia nigra (Lacey et al., 1988). In fact, when pertussis toxin is applied more locally in the anterior substantia nigra, baclofen and dopamine responses are antagonized (Innis and Aghajanian, 1987a). Local pertussis toxin application caused a much greater depression of baclofen responses compared to intracerebroventricular injection (Innis et al., 1988). Biochemical data demonstrates that the sensitivities to serotonin and baclofen correlated with the concentration of the remaining non-ADP ribosylated G proteins (Innis et al., 1988). These data provide evidence that pertussis toxin-sensitive G proteins are crucial for the coupling of $GABA_B$ receptors to the potassium conductance.

4.1.2.2. THE ROLE OF ADENYLATE CYCLASE

The prominent biochemical effect of baclofen is the inhibition of basal adenylate cyclase activity (Wojcik and Neff, 1984). The subunit of G proteins inhibiting adenylate cyclase was shown to be the $G_{i\alpha}$ (Taussig et al., 1993). Despite the detailed knowledge about the cellular cascades involved in the modulation of adenylate cyclase, the electrophysiological consequences of these changes remained obscure until recently. Evidence now indicates that adenylate cyclase plays a crucial role in the slow afterhyperpolarization mediated by a calcium-dependent potassium conductance (Gerber and Gähwiler, 1994). Both baclofen and adenosine enhance (after a transient depression, attributed to technical limitations) the I_{AHP} of hippocampal CA3 neurons. Conversely, isoproterenol, which stimulates adenylate cyclase through β-adrenergic receptors, caused a pronounced depression of I_{AHP}, indicating that the activity of the adenylate cyclase plays a crucial role in the magnitude of the slow afterhyperpolarization. The crucial experiment of this series was the observation that inhibition of cyclic AMP-dependent kinase prevented the baclofen-induced enhancement of I_{AHP} (Gerber and Gähwiler, 1994). Considering previous evidence that the usual $GABA_B$-induced potassium conductance is not related to I_{AHP} (Newberry and Nicoll, 1984, 1985), these data indicate that activation of $GABA_B$ receptors has a dual and independent effect on neuronal excitability, through at least two signaling pathways and distinct types of potassium currents. A further control mechanism of neuronal excitability by baclofen may be through the phosphatidylinositol pathway (Ohmori and Kuriyama, 1989).

4.1.3. Single Channel Currents Induced by Baclofen

Despite the wealth of evidence of macroscopic currents induced by baclofen, a scan of the literature reveals only a few reports investigating the properties of single channels activated by baclofen. This may be a result of technical difficulties involved in the recording of G protein mediated single channel activity, because the G proteins might be diluted if either inside-out or outside-out patches were used for single channel current measurements. An elegant way of circumventing these problems was used by Premkumar et al. (1990), who recorded single-channel activity in the cell-attached mode, following application of GABA or baclofen outside of the patched area of membrane. This procedure preserves the internal milieu of the neurons, but requires a diffusible messenger between the receptor and the channel, located outside and inside of the membrane patch in the orifice of the electrode, respectively. GABA or baclofen induced single channel currents of 4.2–4.7 pA, when the patch was polarized by –40 mV, i.e., the transmembrane gradient was reduced by 40 mV. From these measurements, a single-channel conductance of 64–73 pS was estimated (Premkumar et al., 1990). The single channel currents were insensitive to bicuculline and blocked by high concentrations of saclofen (Premkumar et al., 1990). These channels were mediated by a G protein messenger system, because neurons pretreated for 20–40 h with pertussis toxin never exhibited channel events. Between the application of the agonist and the onset of single-channel activity, 30–90 s elapsed. This was taken as evidence for exaggerated diffusional delays between agonist binding and channel opening, under conditions of spatial separation of channel and receptor. The reversal potential (rather, the zero-current potential under these experimental conditions) was 25 mV more negative at extracellular 5 mM potassium, and shifted by 19 mV when channels were recorded with electrodes containing 15 mM potassium. Both values are close to those expected for a potassium selective ion channel. A puzzling finding is the progressive increase in current amplitudes during prolonged exposure to the agonist. It has been tentatively attributed to recruitment of cooperative elementary channels, perhaps related to the slow increase in second messenger concentration (Premkumar et al., 1990). It remains to be seen whether a similar effect can be detected in macroscopic currents during prolonged exposure to baclofen, so far a pronounced sensitization of the response to baclofen during a continuous application, has not been observed. The slow development of single channel current amplitudes may relate to a delayed I_{AHP} conductance through adenylate cyclase inhibition (Gerber and Gähwiler, 1994), adding to conventional $GABA_B$ potassium conductance.

4.1.4. The Properties of the Late IPSP

Originally established by the pioneering work in the hippocampus (Alger, 1984; Newberry and Nicoll, 1984, 1985), a comparatively slow synaptic inhibition has since been found in several areas of the CNS. This early work presented evidence toward a novel type of synaptic response activating a potassium conductance, rather than an indirect effect, such as a calcium-activated potassium conductance through the preceding excitatory postsynaptic potential (EPSP). Experimental conditions interfering with calcium-dependent potassium conductance increase, e.g., by injecting ethylene-bis(oxyethylene-nitrilo)tetraacetic acid (EGTA), thereby increasing the intracellular buffering power, had little effect on the late IPSP (Lancaster and Wheal, 1984; Newberry and Nicoll, 1984). The similarity between the late IPSP and the baclofen-induced responses, in terms of the magnitude of the conductance change and the reversal potential, was the main argument for the involvement of $GABA_B$ receptors in the late IPSP in the early work (Howe et al., 1987b). The reduction of the late IPSP by the $GABA_B$ receptor antagonist, phaclofen, concomitant to the depression of the baclofen-induced hyperpolarization and conductance increase (Dutar and Nicoll, 1988a), provided some evidence for the involvement of $GABA_B$ receptors in the late IPSP.

A late IPSP (Fig. 1) has also been described in neocortical neurons of many species, such as rat, cat (Connors et al., 1988), guinea pig (Deisz and Prince, 1989), and man (McCormick, 1989). The late IPSP of neocortical neurons is also mediated by a conductance increase for potassium ions. The reversal potential is close to the expected equilibrium potential for potassium (Howe et al., 1987a,b), and changes in extracellular potassium concentration shift the reversal potential of the $IPSP_B$ in the expected direction for a Nernst potential toward potassium ions (Howe et al., 1987b; Thompson et al., 1988, Fig. 2). The late IPSP is only slightly reduced by 500 μM phaclofen (Fig. 3), but the more potent antagonists (2-OH-saclofen and CGP 35348) cause more marked depressions of the late IPSP.

This type of synaptic response has been observed in many parts of the CNS. A similar late IPSP is elicited in projection cells of the cat dorsal lateral geniculate nucleus by optic tract stimulation. The evoked late IPSP is, as in the neocortex, preceded by an EPSP and an early bicuculline-sensitive $IPSP_A$, and depends upon a potassium conductance increase (Soltesz et al.,

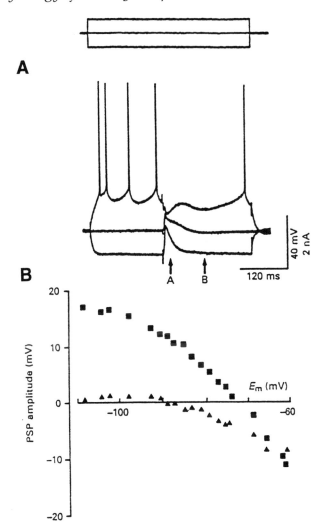

Fig. 1. Properties of early and late IPSPs of cortical neurons of guinea pig. (A) Changes in membrane potential and evoked synaptic responses (bottom traces) by current injection (top traces). The amplitudes of the early and late IPSP were determined at the time indicated by arrow A and B, respectively. (B) The amplitudes of both components were plotted vs the membrane potential measured before the stimulus artifact (reprinted with permission from Deisz and Prince, 1989).

1989b). However, in ventral lateral geniculate of the rat, optic tract stimulation fails to elicit a late IPSP, despite the presence of GABA$_B$ receptors on these neurons (Soltesz et al., 1989a). The late IPSP was indeed reduced by phaclofen (Soltesz et al., 1988). A late IPSP, blocked by CGP 35348, was

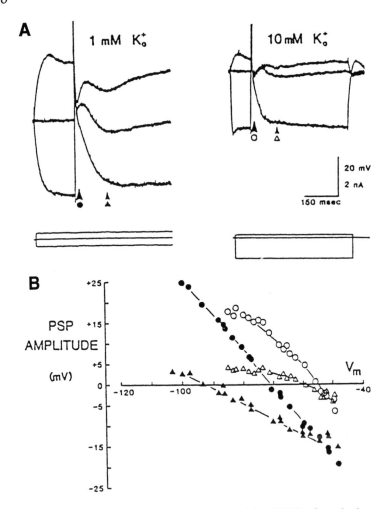

Fig. 2. Potassium dependence of the early and late IPSP of cortical neurons of guinea pig. **(A)** The amplitudes of early (circles) and late IPSPs (triangles) were determined at various membrane potentials obtained by current injection (bottom traces) in the presence of 1 mM and 10 mM extracellular potassium. **(B)** The amplitudes of both responses were plotted vs the membrane potential; the filled and open symbols denote 1 and 10 mM potassium, respectively. The shift in reversal potential of the late IPSP by about 35 mV is consistent with an increase in potassium conductance during the late IPSP (reprinted with permission from Thompson et al., 1988).

also demonstrated in dopamine neurones of the substantia nigra (Häusser and Yung, 1994).

Detailed measurements of the properties of the late inhibitory postsynaptic currents (IPSC) in hippocampal CA3 area revealed a conductance of

control

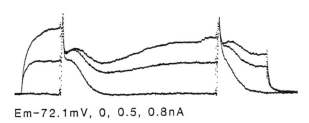

Em−72.1mV, 0, 0.5, 0.8nA

500µM Phaclofen

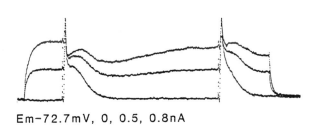

Em−72.7mV, 0, 0.5, 0.8nA

Fig. 3. Effects of phaclofen on the late IPSP of neocortical neurons. The traces show intracellular recordings before and during the bath application of 500 µ*M* phaclofen. The neuron was depolarized from resting membrane potential by current injection (as indicated). Note the slight depression of the late IPSP without detectable effect on the paired pulse depression (Deisz et al., 1996).

about 12 nS (Hablitz and Thalmann, 1987). The currents exhibited a strong dependence on the extracellular potassium concentration, consistent with the view of being caused by a potassium conductance increase. This current reached its peak between 120–150 ms and decayed in a single exponential manner with a time constant of 185 ms. Hablitz and Thalmann (1987) also provided evidence that this synaptic potential is not mediated by a calcium-activated potassium conductance. Both intracellular injection of EGTA or forskolin application virtually abolished the slow afterhyperpolarization following a train of action potentials, but the synaptic response persisted.

Also, the properties of isolated $GABA_B$ receptor-mediated IPSPs of granule cells in the dentate gyrus are characterized in detail (Otis et al., 1993). These IPSPs were isolated by the application of (CNQX) and (D-APV) to eliminate excitatory transmission, and picrotoxin to abolish the fast inhibitory transmission. These currents displayed the appropriate behavior for an increased potassium conductance. A fourfold increase of potassium concentration (from 1.5 mM to 6.8 mM) shifted the reversal potential of the current from 97.9 to 73.2 mV. The pharmacology of these responses also was in line with $GABA_B$-mediated events. These synaptic potentials were reduced in a dose-dependent fashion by CGP 35348 and abolished by intracellular QX 314, or by replacing potassium with cesium (Otis et al., 1993). These isolated IPSPs exhibited an average activation time constant of 45 ms and two inactivation time constants of 110 and 512 ms. The activation and inactivation time constants were not dependent on the voltage between –45 and –95 mV. The mean slope conductance (in 2.5 mM extracellular potassium) was 1.5 nS. Both CGP 35348 (between 200 and 800 µM) and a 2-hydroxy-saclofen (0.5–1.0 mM) antagonized the isolated current (Otis et al., 1993). Similar measurements have also been carried out on hippocampal CA neurons (Ling and Benardo, 1994). A slow inhibitory component was isolated by the application of the N-methyl-D-aspartate (NMDA), non-NMDA, and $GABA_A$ receptor antagonists CPP, CNQX, and picrotoxin, respectively. The rising phase was best fitted with an activation time constant of 73 ms. The decay was fitted by a double exponential with inactivation time constants of 46 and 247 ms. This synaptic component was blocked by saclofen (500 µM), indicating the involvement of $GABA_B$ receptors (Ling and Benardo, 1994). The question remains whether the improvements in techniques (single electrode clamp with sharp microelectrodes vs patch-clamp recordings) or the different morphology of these two types of hippocampal neurons (CA vs granule cells of the dentate gyrus) account for the differences in behavior of these currents.

Ample evidence from hippocampal neurons, both in the acute slice in area CA1 (Dutar and Nicoll, 1988b) and area CA3 (Thalmann, 1988), as well as from the CA3 area in organotypic culture (Thompson and Gähwiler, 1992), have shown that pertussis toxin treatment effectively antagonizes the $IPSP_B$. These data indicate that synaptically released GABA activates postsynaptic $GABA_B$ receptors and the subsequent activation of a potassium current through G proteins would generate the $IPSP_B$. However, comparison of giant IPSPs, bicuculline-insensitive GABA responses and baclofen responses, have revealed marked differences in these apparently similar responses (Jarolimek et al., 1994). Both the 4-AP-induced giant $IPSP_B$, caused by a hyperexcitability of hilar neurons (Müller and Misgeld, 1990), and the baclofen response were potassium-mediated events and blocked by

2-OH-saclofen (500 μM), CGP 35348 (100 μM), intracellular TEA, or extracellular barium ions (Jarolimek et al., 1994), indicating that both responses are mediated by increases in GABA$_B$ receptor-induced potassium conductance. However, the two responses differed markedly in their sensitivity towards intracellular and extracellular cesium ions (Jarolimek et al., 1994), suggesting functionally different types of potassium effector systems. This adds to previous evidence that the two responses involve separate pathways, the response to exogenous baclofen being sensitive, the response to endogenous GABA being insensitive to carbachol (an agonist for muscarinic receptors; Müller and Misgeld, 1989). These differences were tentatively attributed to a spatial separation of the receptors, so that the exogenous GABA$_B$ agonist would activate only one receptor effector system (Jarolimek et al., 1994). It remains to be established to what extent the adenylate cyclase-dependent potassium conductance is involved in these different responses (Gerber and Gähwiler, 1994).

4.1.5. Physiological Implications of the GABA$_B$ Conductance

In the neocortex, the magnitude of baclofen-induced potential and conductance changes are comparatively small, yet these effects are sufficient to alter neuronal excitability. Although baclofen had no effect on the threshold voltage for action potential generation or action potential parameters of rat neocortical neurons, the amplitude of depolarizing current necessary to evoke action potentials was increased (Howe et al., 1987a). Similar findings were also obtained in guinea pig neocortical neurons. Threshold depolarizations that normally were sufficient to elicit just a few action potentials failed to do so during the application of baclofen. However, depolarizations with slightly increased current pulses indicated essentially unaltered excitability (Deisz and Prince, 1989). This notion is also supported by the effects of baclofen on plots of the firing frequency vs current intensity (F/I). Such F/I curves exhibit two components, a very steep initial range for the first interspike interval (primary slope), which flattens abruptly to a much smaller secondary slope. Baclofen shifted the onset of the primary slope by about 0.3 nA to the right, i.e., to higher current intensities, but the steepness of the primary slope was increased (Connors et al., 1988). The secondary slope of the F/I relationship, however, was not significantly different from control. Regarding the transfer function represented by the primary slope, the baclofen-induced conductance has a dual effect, an increase in threshold and an increase in sensitivity (or gain). This action of baclofen, and perhaps also the late IPSP, would tend to reduce the noise level of background activity, thereby improving the signal-to-noise ratio and the dynamic response behavior.

4.2. Cellular Effects of GABA$_B$ Antagonists

4.2.1. Effects of GABA$_B$ Antagonists on Neuronal Excitability

Only a few reports investigated possible effects of GABA$_B$ receptor antagonists on neuronal properties. The application of GABA$_B$ antagonists may provide some clues about the contribution of a tonic GABA$_B$ receptor activation to the control of neuronal excitability. In the hippocampus, neither phaclofen nor CGP 35348 exhibited significant effects on the neuronal input resistance determined by hyperpolarizing current steps (Olpe et al., 1990). The excitability in the hippocampus was unaffected by phaclofen (Karlsson and Olpe, 1989). This finding was corroborated and extended in the neocortex, where the application of the GABA$_B$ antagonists phaclofen (500 μM), 2-OH-saclofen (200 μM), and CGP 35348 (up to 1 mM), caused no detectable change in neuronal properties. Neither resting membrane potential, nor neuronal input resistance, nor direct excitability were consistently affected (Deisz et al., 1993, 1996). The lack of effect of GABA$_B$ receptor antagonists on membrane properties suggests that a tonic activation of GABA$_B$ receptors is unlikely. Since either mechanism, the conventional potassium conductance increase or the enhancement of I$_{AHP}$, depend on elevated GABA activity, the lack of effect of GABA$_B$ antagonists therefore suggests that the GABA concentration in the vicinity of the receptors is too low, perhaps because of the quiescent interneurons contacting GABA$_B$ receptors (Otis and Mody, 1992).

4.2.2. Effects of GABA$_B$ Antagonists on the Late IPSP

Since the first demonstration of a depression of the late IPSP by GABA$_B$ receptor antagonists (Dutar and Nicoll, 1988a), numerous studies confirmed a reduction of the amplitude of the late IPSP by GABA$_B$ antagonists. A late IPSP was depressed in the lateral geniculate nucleus (Soltesz et al., 1988), neocortex (Karlsson et al., 1988; Deisz et al., 1993, 1996), and hippocampus (Otis et al., 1993). This depression by GABA$_B$ antagonists certainly indicates a participation of GABA$_B$ receptors, but does not rule out the contribution of other transmitters to the late IPSP, e.g., other transmitters activating the same conductance (Andrade et al., 1986). Only a quantitative evaluation of the effects of GABA$_B$ antagonists would reveal to what extent the late IPSP is caused by the activation of GABA$_B$ receptors. In the neocortex, for instance, application of phaclofen (500 μM), 2-OH-saclofen (200 μM) and CGP 35348 (100 μM) reduced the IPSP by 23, 52, and 70%, respectively. The component remaining in high concentrations of CGP 35348 (up to 1 mM) was attributed to the tail of the preceding IPSP$_A$, because concomitant to the reduction of the IPSP$_B$, the predominating ion species is changing from a potassium to an anion conductance (Deisz et al., 1996).

In addition to a depression by selective receptor antagonists, the IPSP$_B$ of cortical neurons is also reduced or eliminated by conditions interfering with GABA$_B$ receptor-mediated increases in potassium conductance, e.g., barium ions (Gähwiler and Brown, 1985; Newberry and Nicoll, 1985). Barium ions virtually eliminate the IPSP$_B$ (Deisz et al., 1992, 1996, Fig. 4). These barium experiments also provide an estimate for the participation of potassium conductances activated by receptors other than GABA$_B$ to the IPSP$_B$. Barium should antagonize not only GABA$_B$, but also other G protein-dependent potassium conductances (Lacey et al., 1988). Since the residual conductance was of the same magnitude (about 30%) in the presence of CGP 35348 and barium (Deisz et al., 1996), the residual component is not a result of another transmitter converging onto potassium channels (Andrade et al., 1986); rather, it is because of the residual conductance from the preceding IPSP$_A$ (Deisz et al., 1996).

Also, lidocaine derivatives are known to abolish G protein-mediated potassium conductances, as first reported for QX 572 and 5HT responses (Segal, 1988). Indeed, intracellular QX 314 application virtually eliminates the late synaptic current (Fig. 5). The intracellular elimination of GABA$_B$ responses by QX 314 is particularly useful for isolating the IPSP$_A$ and for studying presynaptic GABA$_B$ effects (e.g., Deisz et al., 1996). Taken together, these data indicate that an isolated late IPSP would be exclusively generated by GABA$_B$ receptors activating a G protein-mediated potassium conductance. Hence it seems justified to name the late IPSP, IPSP$_B$, at least in the neocortex.

4.3. Modulation of Calcium Conductances by Baclofen

4.3.1. Subtypes of Calcium Currents

A variety of neurotransmitters were shown to modulate calcium currents in various preparations (for review, *see* Anwyl, 1991). Before discussing the modulation of calcium currents by GABA$_B$ receptors, however, it seems appropriate to briefly reiterate the present classification of calcium currents. On the basis of single-channel kinetics and conductances, voltage dependence, and pharmacological properties, neuronal calcium channels can be separated into at least six major classes. The low voltage-activated calcium channel originally described by Llinás and co-workers in the inferior olive (Llinás and Yarom, 1981a,b) and thalamic neurons (Jahnsen and Llinás, 1984a,b) is now usually referred to as T-current, because of its transient nature (Nowycky et al., 1985; Fox et al., 1987). The T-current, also demonstrated in other central and peripheral neurons (Carbone and Lux, 1984; Sutor and Zieglgänsberger, 1987), is characterized by a low activation threshold (about −70 mV) and complete inactivation at membrane potentials above

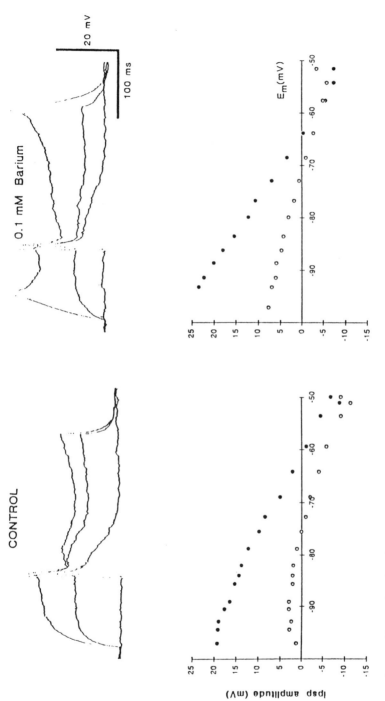

Fig. 4. Effects of barium ions on the early and late IPSP of neocortical neurons. (Top) Intracellular recordings in the absence and presence of 0.1 mM barium ions, as indicated. To evoke comparable changes in membrane potential, despite the changes in membrane input resistance, the amplitude of injected current was decreased. (Bottom) Plot of the amplitudes of the early (filled symbols) and late IPSP (open symbols) vs membrane potential. Both the monotonic decay of the IPSP$_A$ and the shift in reversal potential at the peak time of the previous late IPSP indicates the absence of any significant late conductance other than the IPSP$_A$ (Deisz et al., 1996, unpublished).

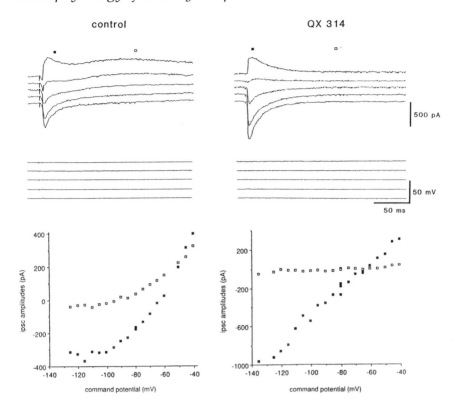

Fig. 5. Effects of QX 314 on synaptic currents of rat neocortical neurons. **(Top)** Synaptic currents (Top traces) following orthodromic stimulation at various command potential (Bottom traces) in control conditions and in the presence of intracellular QX 314 (holding potential −80 mV, switched voltage clamp, switching frequency 20 kHz). The traces from a control neuron (potassium acetate filled microelectrode) are shown at the left; the traces in the left panel show records from a neuron recorded with a microelectrode containing 100 mM QX 314 in the normal filling solution. The amplitudes of the early and late IPSC were measured at the times indicated by filled and open symbols respectively. **(Bottom)** Plots of the amplitudes of the synaptic currents vs the command potential. The filled and open symbols denote the early and late IPSP, respectively. Comparison of the traces, and the corresponding plots shown below, reveals a complete elimination of the late IPSP. The nonlinear behavior of the IPSP$_A$, a result of shunting by the hyperpolarization activated cation conductance, was eliminated by QX 314 (Deisz, unpublished observations).

−60 mV. The high-threshold calcium currents, both sensitive to ω CgTX VIA, can be distinguished by their activation, inactivation and sensitivity to dihydropyridine into L-type channels (for long-lasting, dihydropyridine-sensitive, threshold near 0 mV, little inactivation) and N-type channels (for neither, dihydropyridine-sensitive, intermediate threshold about –40 mV, pronounced inactivation) (Fox et al., 1987). P-type channels, originally described by Llinás et al. (1989), do not respond to the dihydropyridine or ω conotoxin-type blockers, and have an activation threshold between the T-type and N-type currents, (for review, *see* Llinás et al., 1992). The family of calcium currents grew further by distinguishing Q-type and R-type channels from P-type channels (Randall and Tsien, 1995). Recent evidence indicates that several calcium current subtypes participate in the liberation of transmitter in the hippocampus (Wheeler et al., 1994). The different properties in threshold and kinetics of individual calcium currents, as well as the specific modulation by neurotransmitters, may provide a means for subtle changes in the kinetics of presynaptic calcium entry.

4.3.2. Modulation of Calcium Channels by Baclofen

The original observations by Dunlap (1981) of shortened calcium-dependent action potentials by baclofen might, at first sight, readily explain the reduced transmitter release. The established role of calcium in transmitter release (e.g., Llinás et al., 1981) makes the modulation of calcium currents by neurotransmitters an interesting hypothesis for presynaptic inhibition (Dunlap and Fischbach, 1981). However, the shortening of calcium action potentials by baclofen was removed by injection of cesium (Désarmenien et al., 1984), indicating that the shortening of calcium action potentials may have been caused by a baclofen-activated potassium conductance, rather than a decreased calcium current *per se*. Patch-clamp measurements revealed that both T and L or N calcium currents of cultured avian dorsal root ganglion neurons were reduced by both baclofen and GABA in a bicuculline-insensitive manner (Deisz and Lux, 1985). The measurements were carried out with symmetrical cesium chloride across the membrane, a condition which should eliminate all other contaminating conductances; these data provided evidence that net calcium current had been reduced (Deisz and Lux, 1985). Reduction of calcium currents by baclofen has been confirmed in dorsal root ganglion neurons of several species (Dolphin and Scott, 1986; Robertson and Taylor, 1986), and central neurons (Scholz and Miller, 1991; Guyon and Leresche, 1995). The depression of calcium currents by baclofen has also been confirmed by direct measurements of intracellular calcium activity in synaptosomes (Bowery and Williams, 1986) and bovine chromaffin cells (Doroshenko and Neher, 1991). More recently, a decrease in presynaptic calcium entry by baclofen was directly demonstrated in area CA1 (Wu and Saggau, 1995).

Moreover, it was shown that the modulation of calcium currents by baclofen was reduced by pertussis toxin or intracellular application of guanyl nucleotide analogs (Holz et al., 1986; Scott and Dolphin, 1986), conditions interfering with the G protein transduction mechanism. The intracellular elevation of cyclic AMP precludes the depression of T and N/L type calcium currents (Deisz and Lux, 1986), perhaps relating to the protein kinase C-dependent phosphorylation implicated in the noradrenaline depression of calcium currents (Rane and Dunlap, 1986). This pathway may be a peculiarity of avian and bullfrog DRG cells, because it is not involved in baclofen modulation of calcium currents of rat DRG cells (Dolphin et al., 1989). GABA$_B$ receptor activation causes a depression of both high- and low-threshold calcium currents in the lamprey spinal cord (Matsushima et al., 1993), indicating that a modulation of calcium currents by GABA$_B$ receptors is a comparatively old phylogenetical mechanism. At any rate, the G protein-linked modulation of calcium currents is in mammalian neurons, like the postsynaptic potassium conductance increase by baclofen, shared by several transmitters and neuromodulators, including opioid peptides (Hescheler et al., 1987) and noradrenaline (Bean, 1989).

Despite the differences in pharmacology of the subtypes of calcium currents mentioned above, a common feature of all calcium currents described so far seems to be the modulation by baclofen. The modulation of N- and L-type currents by baclofen is well-established (e.g., Scholz and Miller, 1991); in addition, P-type channels were shown to be sensitive to a modulation by baclofen in a G protein-dependent fashion (Mintz and Bean, 1993). Recently, a modulation of R-type channels by baclofen was reported in thalamocortical cells (Guyon and Leresche, 1995).

The modulation of calcium currents by baclofen does not occur in all cells, rather, distinct differences exist between different neurons and even in a given type of neuron under different experimental conditions. In thalamocortical cells, both R- and N-currents were depressed by baclofen, while neither L- nor T-currents were affected (Guyon and Leresche, 1995). However, in dorsal root ganglion cells, T-currents are markedly reduced by baclofen (Deisz and Lux, 1985; Scott et al., 1990). This difference in sensitivity of T-currents may partly be the result of intracellular factors. For instance, the presence of 10 µM intracellular ATP attenuated the modulation of the T-current by 50 µM baclofen from a 46 to a 22% depression, without significant effects on the baclofen-induced depression of the L- (or N-) current (Deisz and Lux, 1985, 1986). In experiments using low intracellular ATP (2 mM) (Scott et al., 1990), or ATP-free (Deisz and Lux, 1985), an effect of baclofen on T-current can be observed; with higher ATP levels (4 mM) (Guyon and Leresche, 1995), an effect is absent. The T-current also presents an interesting feature from the general depression of calcium currents by baclofen. At low concentrations of baclofen (2 µM), the T-current in rat dorsal root ganglion cells was enhanced; only at higher concentrations (10 μM) is the usual depression observed (Scott et al., 1990).

These data indicate that different calcium currents exhibit distinct sensitivities to $GABA_B$ agonists; in addition, recent evidence suggests that the $GABA_B$ modulation of calcium currents displays a distinct difference toward $GABA_B$ antagonists. In thalamocortical cells, both R- and N-type calcium currents are depressed by baclofen (Guyon and Leresche, 1995). However, the baclofen-induced depression differs markedly in its sensitivity toward $GABA_B$ antagonists (Guyon and Leresche, 1995). The baclofen-induced depression of N-type calcium currents is antagonized by CGP 35348, the depression of R-type calcium current, however, is not antagonized by a reasonable concentration of CGP 35348 (100 μM), and is only blocked by the most potent antagonist CGP 55845 (Guyon and Leresche, 1995).

Unlike the G protein-linked potassium channels, where a convergence of various neurotransmitters has been repeatedly demonstrated, a small amount of data available indicate a convergence of different neurotransmitters onto the same calcium current. Some evidence for convergence through different biochemical pathways was provided by Diversé-Pierluissi and Dunlap (1995). Both norepinephrine and GABA reduce calcium currents of avian dorsal root ganglion cells, the norepinephrine effect is eliminated by an intracellular proteinkinase C pseudosubstrate (PKC 19-31, blocking the effect of proteinkinase C), but GABA modulation of the calcium current persisted. This provides some evidence for independent, transmitter-activated pathways to calcium currents, but may involve separate calcium currents, because the current was not irrefutably isolated. It remains to be seen whether a given calcium current is modulated by different neurotransmitters when stringent criteria for the isolation are applied.

5. Evidence for $GABA_B$ Interneurons

5.1. Electrophysiological Findings

The first evidence of distinct types of interneurons mediating the $GABA_A$ and $GABA_B$ IPSPs was probably the observation of 4-aminopyridine 4-AP-enhanced slow IPSP, indicating that only the interneurons releasing GABA onto $GABA_B$ receptors exhibited a 4-AP-sensitive alteration in excitability (Segal, 1990). This conclusion is supported by several lines of evidence indicating that $GABA_A$- and $GABA_B$-mediated synaptic potentials are activated by different interneurons. In the amygdala and the ventral tegmental area, the $IPSP_A$ is depressed by muscarine, but the 2-OH-saclofen sensitive $IPSP_B$ is unaffected by muscarine (Sugita et al., 1992). Conversely, the $IPSP_A$ is unaffected by 5HT, and the $IPSP_B$ is strongly reduced by 5HT. These differences in the responsiveness of presynaptic terminals were taken as evidence for two types of GABA-ergic interneurons mediating the two synaptic responses (Sugita et al., 1992). Also, two types of inhibitory interneurons in the striatum have been proposed, based on the sensitivity to baclofen (Seabrook et al., 1991).

Further support for the presence of separate interneurons stems from observations in the dentate gyrus (Otis and Mody, 1992). Spontaneous release activates only postsynaptic $GABA_A$ receptors, stimulation of the molecular layer elicits both fast $GABA_A$- and slow $GABA_B$-mediated synaptic components. Several possibilities may account for this effect: The two postsynaptic responses may be mediated by separate interneurons differing in their spontaneous activity; interneurons releasing GABA in the vicinity of postsynaptic $GABA_A$ receptors exhibiting a high spontaneous activity; and those interneurons releasing GABA onto postsynaptic $GABA_B$ receptors being quiescent (Otis and Mody, 1992). These authors also considered several other possibilities. For instance, a spatial separation of $GABA_A$ and $GABA_B$ receptors may preclude the activation of post-synaptic $GABA_B$ receptors under conditions of small amounts of released GABA; and only under high-release conditions, such as a spill-over of GABA, impaired GABA uptake, and the like, may GABA reach $GABA_B$ sites (Isaacson et al., 1993). Otis and Mody (1992) also considered the possibility that the $GABA_B$-mediated event is brought about by another transmitter, perhaps coreleased with GABA under certain stimulus conditions, as originally envisaged by Müller and Misgeld (1990). Such a coreleased transmitter appears unlikely to contribute to the $IPSP_B$ of neocortical neurons (Deisz et al., 1996).

5.2. Anatomical Evidence

Different classes of interneurons have also been demonstrated by histochemical methods in the neocortex of old world monkeys. In virtually all GABA-ergic interneurons, an immunoreactivity for the two types of calcium-binding proteins, parvalbumin and calbindin-28, is detectable. However, the majority of neurons, except a few cells in layer IV displaying immunoreactivity for both calcium-binding proteins, exhibit immunoreactivity for only one of the calcium-binding proteins. The basket neurons are characterized by immunoreactivity for parvalbumin, calbindin immunoreactivity is almost exclusively found in double bouquet neurons (Hendry et al., 1989). These immunohistochemical data indicate that the separate classes of interneurons may also differ in terms of calcium homeostasis and calcium currents present. The selective pattern of synapses formed by basket cells, contacting predominantly somata and proximal dendrites (Somogyi, 1990), might indicate that the two populations of interneurons serve different functions in the neocortex. Yet, a discrete association with postsynaptic responses, as suggested in hippocampus, has not been firmly established in the neocortex.

The concept of distinct groups of interneurons is further supported by the selectivity of the input. Double anterograde tracing from the septum and the median raphe nucleus, together with immunostaining of interneurons (containing calbindin, parvalbumin, or cholecystokinin), was used to evaluate whether the two pathways converge onto distinct types of interneurons. The septal afferents innervated the parvalbumin-containing interneurons, but raphe axons avoided the parvalbumin-containing interneurons. This selectivity was taken as evidence that the different subcortical nuclei modulate different types of inhibitory circuits in the hippocampus (Miettinen and Freund, 1992).

Taken together, the electrophysiological and anatomical data lend support for the hypothesis that the GABA$_B$ IPSP is not simply an effect of GABA dumped into the extracellular space and escaping its proper location; rather, it seems to be a distinct inhibitory pathway with separate afferents onto distinct sets of interneurons synapsing onto specific regions.

6. Modulation of Synaptic Transmission by GABA$_B$ Agonists

6.1. Excitatory Transmission

Since the original observation of EPSPs reduced by baclofen in the spinal cord (Pierau and Zimmermann, 1973), a wealth of evidence has accumulated that indicates a pronounced effect of baclofen on synaptic transmission. In many neurons of the CNS, a depressant effect of baclofen on excitatory synaptic transmission was demonstrated. However, a general depressant action of baclofen cannot be inferred, rather the net effect of baclofen is markedly different in different structures. Misgeld et al. (1984) compared the effects of baclofen on excitatory and inhibitory transmission onto pyramidal neurons of the CA3 area and granule cells in the dentate gyrus. Low concentrations of baclofen (10–25 μ*M*) caused small hyperpolarization of about 5 mV and decreased the IPSP of granule cells. The decrease in the IPSP was so pronounced that the EPSP evoked by perforant-path stimulation was enhanced. The effects of baclofen resembled those of bicuculline, giving rise to repetitive firing. In the CA3 area, however, baclofen at the same concentrations caused a marked increase in membrane conductance and potential by about 15 mV. The synaptic responses evoked by mossy fiber stimulation were decreased (Misgeld et al., 1984). These early findings have been reiterated because they demonstrate that the net effect of baclofen may depend upon the site investigated.

Baclofen-induced depression of EPSPs are also demonstrated in neocortical neurons. The half-maximal concentration of the racemic mixture ($\pm$)-baclofen was about 1 μM, similar to the half-maximal concentration for the postsynaptic effect (Howe et al., 1987a). However, these effects were not observed under conditions of more localized application. Small doses of baclofen applied in the vicinity of the recorded neurons failed to antagonize the EPSPs (Connors et al., 1988), perhaps because the localized action did not reach the excitatory input at more distal parts of the dendrite. In any case, the EC$_{50}$ for the depression of the EPSP in the neocortex is about 1 μM for ($\pm$)-baclofen (Howe et al., 1987a) and, in the neostriatum, 800 nM for ($-$)-baclofen (Calabresi et al., 1991). Considering the much higher potency of ($-$)-baclofen over the racemate, the fairly high concentration required in the neostriatum may reflect differences in sensitivity between different areas.

6.1.1. Pertussis Toxin Sensitivity of Presynaptic Responses

Numerous studies have investigated the effects of baclofen on the excitatory synaptic transmission in the hippocampus. From these, only a few were selected because of limitations of space. The original observations by Dutar and Nicoll (1988b) revealed that the baclofen-induced depression of EPSPs persisted in slices from animals pretreated with pertussis toxin. In these neurons, the baclofen-induced postsynaptic effects and the IPSP$_B$ were abolished, indicating that pertussis toxin had effectively interrupted the G protein cascade (Dutar and Nicoll, 1988b). This eliminates the possibility that pertussis toxin may not have reached the area investigated (Innis et al., 1988). Phaclofen, the only available antagonist at the time, failed to reverse the depression of glutamatergic transmission by baclofen, despite an effective antagonistic effect at postsynaptic sites. This difference was used as an argument to propose different types of GABA$_B$ receptors (Dutar and Nicoll, 1988b). Subsequent work has shown that part of the problem to antagonize the presynaptic action may have been caused by the poor efficacy of phaclofen (Yoon and Rothman, 1991). Nevertheless, a pertussis toxin-insensitive depression of EPSP is confirmed in area CA1 (Colmers and Pittman, 1989), although the insensitivity to pertussis toxin of the presynaptic baclofen effect may have been the result of an insufficient concentration (Stratton et al., 1989). The basic concept was also confirmed in the CA3 area of organotypic slice culture, where baclofen caused a marked depression of isolated non-NMDA EPSP by 87% (Thompson and Gähwiler, 1992). Following pertussis toxin pretreatment, the postsynaptic potential and conductance change induced by baclofen are abolished, yet the presynaptic action of baclofen on glutamatergic terminals persists (Thompson and Gähwiler, 1992;

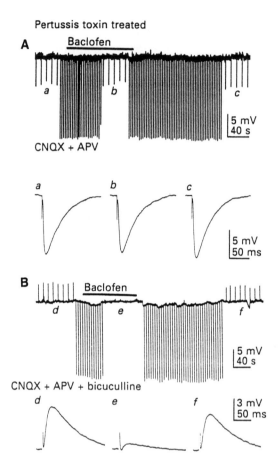

Fig. 6. Effects of pertusis toxin treatment on pre- and postsynaptic baclofen responses in area CA3; **(A)** upper trace chart recording of a CA3 neuron treated for 48 h with 500 ng/mL pertussis toxin. Baclofen fails to evoke a significant hyperpolarization and conductance increase (determined with hyperpolarizing current steps 0.2 nA). The monosynaptic IPSPs (in the presence of CNQX and D-APV, 20 μ*M* each), evoked before (a), during (b), and after (c) application of baclofen, were averaged and displayed at different scales in panels a–c. The pretreatment with pertussis toxin prevents both the postsynaptic effect and the presynaptic attenuation of the IPSP by baclofen. **(B)** Upper trace, chart recording of a CA3 cell after pertusis toxin treatment. EPSPs were evoked in the presence of CNQX and D-APV (20 μ*M* each), and bicuculline (4 μ*M*) before (d), during (e), and after (f) the application of baclofen. The averaged EPSPs are displayed in d–f at an enlarged scale. Note the persistence of presynaptic baclofen effect in the absence of detectable postsynaptic effects (reprinted with permission from Thompson and Gähwiler, 1992).

see Fig. 6). In cultured hippocampal neurons, however, pertussis toxin prevents the depression of EPSPs by baclofen (Scholz and Miler, 1991). These data indicate that the cellular cascades associated with presynaptic GABA$_B$ receptors at excitatory terminals not only differ from postsynaptic ones and from those at inhibitory terminals, but also may vary between excitatory terminals of different regions.

Some similarities between different regions may be inferred, however. The cellular cascades involved in the baclofen-induced depression of EPSP at spiny striatal neurons (Nisenbaum et al., 1993) have not yet been determined directly. Nevertheless, binding data (Knott et al., 1993) provide some clues toward the pertussis toxin sensitivity of presynaptic terminals. These authors find no effect of pertussis toxin on GABA binding to GABA$_B$ sites in the striatum (Knott et al., 1993). This implies that all GABA$_B$ binding in the striatum are pertussis toxin-insensitive. The lack of pertussis toxin effects may indicate that the presynaptic GABA$_B$ receptors of the neostriatum are pertussis toxin insensitive, like some of the hippocampus glutamatergic terminals.

6.1.2. Antagonist Sensitivity
of Presynaptic GABA$_B$ Receptors on Excitatory Terminals

If the presynaptic receptors involved in the modulation of glutamate release were of the B type, an antagonism by the established GABA$_B$ receptors might be anticipated. Several reports confirmed the view that antagonists of GABA$_B$ receptors antagonize, or at least attenuate, the GABA or baclofen-induced depression of EPSP/Cs. In a dissociated culture of hippocampal neurons, GABA (5 μM, in the presence of bicuculline) depressed EPSPs by 64% in control, and in the presence of 100 μM 2-OH-saclofen, the depression was reduced to 9.8% (Yoon and Rothman, 1991). This clearly indicates that 2-OH-saclofen antagonizes a presynaptic GABA$_B$ receptor effect on excitatory terminals. This effect was, however, much weaker at higher concentrations of GABA$_B$ agonists (Yoon and Rothman, 1991). At higher concentrations, 2-OH-saclofen (200 μM) antagonized the baclofen-induced depression in a similar system (Scholz and Miller, 1991). Also, CGP 35348 effectively abolished the baclofen-induced depression of EPSP/Cs in organotypic hippocampal cultures in the CA3 area (Thompson and Gähwiler, 1992). However, barium ions, which block the postsynaptic potassium conductance increase (Gähwiler and Brown, 1985; Newberry and Nicoll, 1985), fail to antagonize the presynaptic effects of baclofen (Fig. 7), indicating a presumably pertussis toxin-insensitive coupling of GABA$_B$ receptors to calcium channels (Thompson and Gähwiler, 1992).

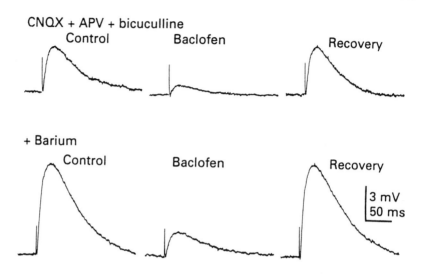

Fig. 7. Effects of barium on presynaptic baclofen action at excitatory terminals in area CA3. Isolated EPSPs, elicited in the presence of CNQX and D-APV (20 µ*M* each) and bicuculline (4 µ*M*), are shown before, during, and after the bath application of 10 µ*M* baclofen. In control conditions, baclofen caused a 78% decrease in EPSP amplitude and a 7 mV hyperpolarization. After bath application of 1 m*M* barium, baclofen caused a 72% decrease in EPSP amplitude, without significant effects on membrane potential (reprinted with permission from Thompson and Gähwiler, 1992).

6.2. Inhibitory Transmission

Following the demonstration of a GABA$_B$ receptor-mediated depression of inhibition in the neocortex, many laboratories corroborated and extended this finding. Presynaptic GABA$_B$ receptors have since been demonstrated on inhibitory terminals in the hippocampus, neocortex, neostriatum, nucleus accumbens, and lateral geniculate. Compared to the detailed knowledge in the hippocampus, the data from other structures are fragmentary. The presynaptic GABA$_B$ receptors appear similar in terms of baclofen sensitivity. A half-maximal effect of (−)-baclofen was obtained at 800 n*M* in the striatum (Calabresi et al., 1991), and in the neocortex, a half-maximal concentration, for (±)-baclofen of 1 µ*M* was obtained (Howe et al., 1987a).

Despite this similarity of presynaptic terminals toward baclofen, there is considerable evidence to underscore a diversity in presynaptic GABA$_B$ receptors of inhibitory terminals and the associated ionic mechanisms in different areas of the CNS, and even in a given structure. Concerning the pre-

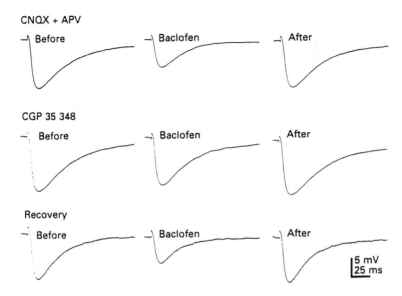

Fig. 8. Effects of CGP 35348 on presynaptic GABA_B receptors on inhibitory interneurons. Pharmacologically isolated IPSPs (by the presence of 20 μM CNQX and 20 μM D-APV) are evoked before, during, and after bath application of 1 μM baclofen. The 45% depression of the IPSP, obtained in control condition, is reduced to a 10% depression in the presence of CGP 35348 (reprinted with permission from Thompson and Gähwiler, 1992).

synaptic mechanisms involved in the baclofen depression, experiments with barium ions are particularly useful. As mentioned in Section 4.2.2., barium ions should abolish a GABA_B receptor-mediated potassium conductance increase, but they should spare GABA_B receptor-mediated calcium current modulation. Application of barium ions reduced both the baclofen-induced increase in membrane conductance and the depression of the IPSP. From this observation, it was proposed that both pre- and postsynaptic GABA_B receptors share the same conductance mechanism (Misgeld et al., 1989). Similar findings were made in the CA3 region using pharmacologically isolated IPSPs (Thompson and Gähwiler, 1992). The baclofen-induced depression of IPSPs is effectively antagonized by CGP 35348 (*see* Fig. 8) and by 1 mM barium (Thompson and Gähwiler, 1992; Fig. 9). Both responses to baclofen, the postsynaptic conductance increase and the baclofen-induced depression of the IPSP, are antagonized by pertussis toxin (Thompson and Gähwiler, 1992; *see* Fig. 5). These data indicate that presynaptic GABA_B receptors of GABA-ergic terminals in area CA3 are probably coupled, via pertussis

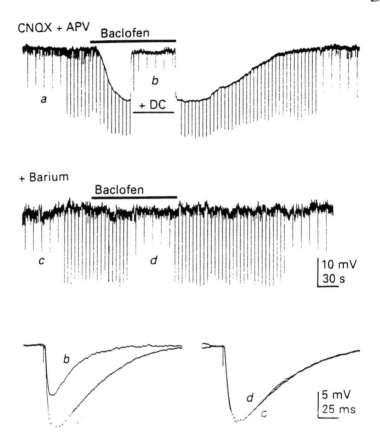

Fig. 9. Effects of barium on post synaptic baclofen responses and on presynaptic responses at inhibitory terminals in area CA3. **(Top)** Chart recordings of a CA3 neuron in the presence of CNQX and D-APV. Bath application of 10 µ*M* baclofen causes a hyperpolarization of 18 mV and a 40% depression of the monosynaptic IPSP. The increase in membrane conductance by baclofen is obvious from the decrease in the large downward excursions of membrane potential induced by repetitive current injection of 0.3 nA. **(Middle)** In the presence of barium, the baclofen-induced changes in membrane potential and conductance are abolished. **(Bottom)** The isolated IPSPs evoked under the different experimental conditions are displayed at enlarged scaling. Comparison of the IPSPs reveals that barium effectively antagonized the presynaptic depression of the IPSP by baclofen (reprinted with permission from Thompson and Gähwiler, 1992).

toxin-sensitive G proteins, to a similar conductance mechanism as those located postsynaptically.

These data differ markedly from those obtained in the CA1 area, where the baclofen-induced depression of IPSPs is not antagonized by barium

control

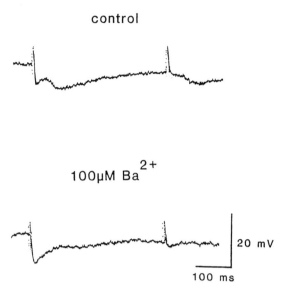

$100\mu M\ Ba^{2+}$

20 mV

100 ms

Fig. 10. Barium effects on paired-pulse depression of neocortical IPSPs. A pair of stimuli elicits a markedly smaller second IPSP, because of the negative feedback of GABA on its own release. Application of barium eliminates the $IPSP_B$ evoked by the first stimulus, but fails to alleviate paired-pulse depression (modified from Deisz et al., 1996).

ions (Lambert et al., 1991). Also, barium fails to antagonize the paired-pulse depression in the neocortex, used as an index for presynaptic $GABA_B$ receptor activation (Deisz et al., 1992, 1996; Fig. 10). The data concerning the barium sensitivity indicate that two types of presynaptic $GABA_B$ receptor effector systems exist in hippocampal CA1 and CA3, the former being similar to that of neocortical neurons.

Also the pertussis toxin-sensitivity of the $GABA_B$ effect on inhibitory terminals appears to differ between various parts of the CNS. As mentioned above, a presynaptic pertussis toxin-sensitivity of the $GABA_B$ responses is well-established at inhibitory terminals in the hippocampus CA3 area (Thompson and Gähwiler, 1992); however, indirect evidence suggests a pertussis toxin-resistant mechanism in the striatum. As mentioned in Section 6.1.1., pertussis toxin reduces GABA binding to $GABA_B$ sites in several brain areas, but not in the striatum (Knott et al., 1993). This lack of pertussis toxin on GABA binding to $GABA_B$ sites in the striatum also suggests that $GABA_B$ receptors on inhibitory terminals are pertussis toxin-insensitive. Therefore, the presynaptic depression of inhibition by $GABA_B$ receptors in the striatum (Nisenbaum et al., 1993) might be pertussis toxin-insensitive.

6.3. Frequency-Dependent Depression of Inhibition

Use-dependent depression of inhibition is well established in both hippocampal and neocortical neurons (McCarren and Alger, 1985; Deisz and Prince, 1989). A negative feedback of GABA on its own release was proposed to underlie the frequency-dependent depression of $IPSP_A$ and $IPSP_B$ in the neocortex (Deisz and Prince, 1986, 1989). A frequency-dependent depression of inhibition is firmly established using either repetitive or paired stimulation with short intervals (Pacelli et al., 1991; Thompson and Gähwiler, 1989; Lambert and Wilson, 1994; Davies et al., 1990; but *see* Häusser and Yung, 1994). Before discussing the evidence in favor of a presynaptic effect for the decrease in inhibition, the contribution of altered ionic gradients to the $IPSP_A$ depression must be briefly considered. A decrease in the reversal potential often contributes to the decline in inhibition (McCarren and Alger, 1985; Thompson and Gähwiler, 1989); others find little effect on the ionic gradient (Nathan and Lambert, 1991; Pacelli et al., 1991). More recently, a predominant change in the ionic gradient was proposed to underlie the depression of $GABA_A$ inhibition at higher frequencies (Ling and Benardo, 1995). These experiments were carried out at 27°C, perhaps impairing the temperature-dependent chloride transport system of central neurons (Thompson et al., 1988), which, in turn, would facilitate use-dependent deterioration of the chloride gradient. It is noteworthy that in the neocortex the shift in reversal potential was only apparent and not associated with a true change in reversal potential (Deisz and Prince, 1989). This smaller effect of repetitive stimulation on the chloride gradient in the neocortex, compared to the hippocampus, may be a result of the faster chloride extrusion. In the neocortex, a time constant on the order of 7 s was determined (Thompson et al., 1988); in hippocampal CA3 neurons, a half-time of about 20 s was obtained (Misgeld et al., 1986).

The elegant work by Davies et al. (1990) established the use of paired-pulse stimulation to investigate frequency-dependent depression of inhibition and the properties of presynaptic $GABA_B$ receptors. Since then it was often confirmed that use-dependent depression of inhibition is caused by presynaptic $GABA_B$ receptors (Thompson and Gähwiler, 1992; Davies and Collingridge, 1993; Lambert and Wilson, 1994; Pitler and Alger, 1994). A notable exception are small IPSPs of dopamine neurons in the substantia nigra, which exhibit no significant paired-pulse depression despite a marked reduction by baclofen (Hausser and Yung, 1994). Paired-pulse depression of IPSPs in the dentate gyrus can be antagonized by 2-OH saclofen (400 μM) (Mott and Lewis, 1991). Likewise the paired-pulse depression in area CA1 can be antagonized by high concentrations of phaclofen (0.4–2 mM), 2-OH saclofen (0.02–0.4 mM), or CGP 35348 (0.01–1.0 mM) (Davies and Collingridge, 1993). Comparison of the pre- and postsynaptic IC$_{50}$ values revealed that the postsynaptic GABA$_B$ receptors are 5–10 times more sensitive to the antagonists. This difference in sensitivity towards antagonists between pre- and postsynaptic GABA may also account for the failure to detect significant effects of GABA$_B$ antagonists on paired-pulse depression (Wilcox and Dichter, 1994). To discard the possibility of a presynaptic autoinhibition through GABA$_B$ receptors, on the basis of a persistence of paired-pulse depression in the presence of 100 μM CGP 35348 (Wilcox and Dichter, 1994), therefore seems premature.

This clearly illuminates the controversy about the pharmacology of presynaptic receptors modulating GABA release. In this context, the data of Yoon and Rothman (1991) are particularly relevant. At low baclofen concentrations (1 μM), 2-OH-saclofen antagonized the baclofen-induced depression of inhibition, yet it exerted no detectable effect on paired-pulse depression (Yoon and Rothman, 1991). These findings are in accordance with data from the neocortex, where 200 μM 2-OH-saclofen failed to antagonize paired-pulse depression (Deisz et al., 1992, 1993). But in the neocortex, paired-pulse depression was also resistant to concentrations of CGP 35348 up to 1 mM (Deisz et al., 1992, 1996). The graph in Fig. 11 compares the effects of 500 μM phaclofen, 200 μM 2-OH-saclofen, and 100 μM CGP 35348 on the conductance of the late IPSP and on paired-pulse depression, the former being progressively reduced, the latter being unaffected. In addition, CGP 35348 fails to antagonize the depressant effect of low baclofen concentrations (Deisz et al., 1996). This might suggest that other presynaptic mechanisms predominate the modulation of GABA release, e.g., co-release of other molecules affecting the release of GABA. However, recent experiments on isolated IPSPs in cortical neurons revealed that the more potent GABA$_B$ antagonist, CGP 55845A, reduces paired-pulse depression. The usual depression of a second IPSP by about 60% (at 500 ms interstimulus interval) was reduced to below 10% by CGP 55845A (Deisz, 1996). This indicates that GABA$_B$ receptors modulate presynaptic GABA release. The failure of CGP 35348 to antagonize presynaptic depression of release through GABA$_B$ receptors may relate to the distinct pharmacological differences of presynaptic calcium currents.

Like the GABA$_A$-mediated inhibition, the isolated GABA$_B$-mediated inhibition exhibits a pronounced paired-pulse depression (Otis et al., 1993). In area CA1, stimulation with 1 Hz decreases the isolated IPSP$_B$ to less than 20% of control amplitudes. This depression of the amplitude is not mediated by a change in the ionic gradient and the unchanged kinetics of the response indicate a presynaptic mechanism (Ling and Benardo, 1994). These data

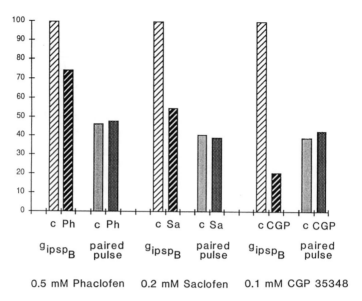

Fig. 11. Comparison of the effects of 0.5 m*M* phaclofen, 0.2 m*M* 2-OH-saclofen (denoted saclofen), and 0.1 m*M* CGP 35348 on the conductance of the late IPSP (left pair of columns in each group) and on paired-pulse depression (right pair of columns). The conductance of the late IPSP (gipsp$_B$) is progressively reduced, from left to right, corresponding to the increased potency of the antagonists. Paired-pulse depression is virtually unaffected (reprinted with permission from Deisz et al., 1996).

correspond to the frequency dependent depression of the IPSP$_B$ of neocortical neurones (Deisz and Prince, 1989). Comparison of the time course of the isolated postsynaptic IPSP$_B$ and the time course of presynaptic action revealed that the presynaptic effect lasts longer (Otis et al., 1993). A detailed analysis of the temporal properties of paired-pulse depression revealed further complications. In the hippocampal CA3 area, the ratio of the first to the second IPSP was on average 0.64, i.e., the second IPSP was maximally reduced by 36%, at an interstimulus interval of about 150 ms. Paired-pulse depression at interstimulus intervals up to 200 ms was reduced to about 10% in the presence of CGP 55845H, but at larger interstimulus intervals (1–2 s), a paired-pulse depression was virtually unaffected. The remaining paired-pulse depression was neither antagonized by the opioid antagonist naloxone (10 μ*M*), nor by the muscarinic antagonist atropine (10 μ*M*), indicating that neither of these receptors is involved (Lambert and Wilson, 1994). These authors attribute the CGP 55845-insensitive component to an altered release of

GABA because it is associated with an increase in the variability of amplitude and occurs at low intensity-evoked IPSPs.

The differences in the sensitivity of inhibitory transmission may relate to the different types of presynaptic calcium currents involved. At least two types of calcium currents were proposed to be involved in the release of GABA in the striatum (Pin and Bockaert, 1990), and other regions may utilize a different combination of presynaptic calcium currents. Baclofen depressed both N-type and R-type calcium currents, but the GABA_B antagonist CGP 35348 only antagonized the baclofen depression of N-type currents. CGP 55845, however, antagonized both the baclofen-induced depression of N-type and R-type calcium currents (Guyon and Leresche, 1995). If a comparable pharmacological profile of presynaptic calcium currents exists in the neocortex, R-type calcium currents may be responsible for release of GABA.

The presynaptic GABA_B receptors at inhibitory terminals may subserve the obvious function of conserving transmitter. When repetitive stimulation has liberated high amounts of GABA, an additional GABA release would exert no further effects and would be a waste of transmitter. In addition, a subtle disinhibition by presynaptic GABAB receptors enables, under normal conditions, long-term changes of excitatory transmission (*see* Section 8.1.). The function of GABA_B receptors at glutamatergic terminals, however, is less obvious when the spatial distribution of GABA is restricted to the vicinity of the terminal and selective activation were absent. The diffusional equilibration of GABA is controlled by a saturable GABA uptake at invertebrate synapses (Deisz et al., 1984) as well as in the hippocampus (Hablitz and Lebeda, 1985). Isaacson et al. (1993) nicely confirmed that blockade of GABA uptake facilitates the spread of GABA (by monitoring extracellular GABA activity with a patch electrode) and enhances paired-pulse depression, in line with previous evidence of augmented feedback depression of GABA release by nipecotic acid (Deisz and Prince, 1989). Impairment of uptake either by a selective blocker or saturation by brief repetitive stimulation, enabled GABA to spill over and reach glutamatergic terminals (Isaacson et al., 1993). Therefore, the GABA_B receptors on glutamatergic terminals add a highly nonlinear component to cortical inhibition which is governed by the spatio-temporal properties of inhibition through the efficacy of uptake.

7. Interaction of Other Transmitter Systems with GABA_B Function

7.1. Intracellular Convergence

A striking feature of G protein-mediated potassium conductance is the convergence of several neurotransmitter receptors onto the same potassium conductance mechanism, originally shown by Andrade et al. (1986). Application of either 5-HT or baclofen caused a comparable membrane hyperpolarization, the response to 5-HT could be antagonized by spiperone. This provided evidence for the independence of the two receptors. If the receptors and their associated effectors were separate entities, the combined application of both substances should yield a response close to the sum of the two individual responses. However, near-maximal responses to both 5-HT and baclofen were not additive when both were given in combination. This was taken as evidence that the two receptors converge onto a common potassium conductance (Andrade et al., 1986). Both responses were not mediated through an inhibition of adenylate cyclase, because 8-Br-cyclic AMP, a membrane-permeable analog of cyclic AMP, had no effect on the 5-HT or baclofen responses. The effectiveness of antagonizing the blockade of adenylate cyclase was verified by the abolition of the I_{AHP}. Conditions interfering with the G protein cascade (pertussin toxin, GTP-γS) blocked both responses. Similar observations have subsequently been reported in a variety of neurons and for several transmitters (Innis and Aghajanian, 1987b; Christie and North, 1988; Lacey et al., 1988). For instance, in lateral parabrachial neurons, M_2-muscarinic and μ-opioid peptide receptors utilize the same effector system as $GABA_B$ receptors (Christie and North, 1988). In the substantia nigra, the effects of dopamine were reduced by a preceding maximal application of baclofen (Lacey et al., 1988), indicating a convergence of different receptors onto the same potassium current effector system. However, the baclofen-induced conductance was about twice that of dopamine (Lacey et al., 1988), indicating that despite some convergence, different effector systems are present.

Some evidence toward differences in G protein-mediated potassium conductance is provided by single channel recordings. In cultured hippocampal neurons, 5HT and $GABA_B$ receptors activate separate channel entities (Premkumar and Gage, 1994). Several parameters usually considered hallmarks for classes of channels are remarkably different between the channels activated by 5HT and baclofen. The channels activated by baclofen had a much higher single channel conductance (67 pS), mean open time (2.86 ms), and burst length (21.27 ms), compared to the channels activated by serotonin (36 pS, 0.74 ms, 3.41 ms, respectively). In addition, the baclofen-activated channels exhibited a pronounced voltage dependence of their open probability, mean open time, and mean burst length; 5HT-activated channels were voltage invariant. Since some patches exhibited exclusively baclofen- or 5HT-activated channels, and other patches contained both types of channels, separate channels activated by the two receptors are proposed (Premkumar and Gage, 1994). To account for the above convergence, two explanations are given. If the two G protein pathways activated by 5HT and $GABA_B$ receptors utilize different G protein subtypes, the distinct differences in channel properties might be brought about by the two types of G proteins, imposing distinct biophysical differences on a given population of channels. Alternatively, if the channels activated by 5HT and GABA$_B$ were separate entities, the occlusion experiments still might work if some intermediate step (e.g., available G protein concentration) limits the maximal response of the two populations of channels.

In addition to the convergence, a given transmitter receptor may activate through different G protein's several effector systems. A likely substrate for a divergence of GABA$_B$ receptors are the different subtypes of G proteins. GABA$_B$ receptors, for instance, interact with a specific set of some, but not all, G proteins (Morishita et al., 1990). Certainly different structures utilize different GABA effector pathways, as mentioned above. In particular, the differences in barium sensitivity of baclofen responses between inhibitory neurons synapsing onto CA1 and CA3 suggest a divergence of presynaptic GABA$_B$ receptors onto separate effector systems. Some inhibitory interneurons are equipped with GABA$_B$ receptors associated with a potassium conductance increase (Misgeld et al., 1989); others, e.g., in area CA1, are endowed with GABA$_B$ receptors linked to calcium currents (Pitler and Alger, 1994). This may be taken as evidence that in different areas the presynaptic mechanisms associated with the GABA$_B$ receptor are different.

These experiments indicate that G protein-mediated cascades can both diverge from a similar receptor to several effectors and converge from various transmitter receptors onto at least closely related effectors. The convergence implies that the effect of a given transmitter would be modified by the concomitant action of another transmitter, utilizing the same effector system. The transmitter effect varies between a full effect in the absence of the other transmitter sharing the effector system, and a marginal effect if the competing transmitter were present. The convergence of different transmitter systems onto a certain effector system, together with the divergence of a given transmitter to diverse effector systems provides a novel dimension of synaptic integration.

7.2. Synaptic Interactions

The interaction between several transmitters by the convergence onto the same channels, or closely related channels, is only one type of interaction between GABA$_B$ receptors and other transmitters. During the past few years, an additional type of interaction has been found in several structures. In the amygdala, 5HT decreases the IPSP$_B$ by a presynaptic mechanism (Sugita et al., 1992). The isolated IPSP$_B$ in the dopamine neurons of the substantia nigra pars compacta or the ventral tegmental area was decreased by 5HT via presynaptic 5HT$_{1b}$ receptors (Johnson et al., 1992). In midbrain dopamine neurons, the isolated IPSP$_B$ was also reduced through activation of presynaptic adenosine receptors (Wu et al., 1995). The μ receptor-selective opioid peptide D-Ala^2,N-Me-Phe^4,Gly^5-ol enkephalin (DAMGO) reduces the amplitude of pharmacologically isolated GABA$_B$-mediated IPSPs (Pawelzik et al., 1996) and the IPSP$_B$ exhibits a pronounced frequency dependence through presynaptic GABA$_B$ receptors (Deisz and Prince, 1989). This indicates that inhibitory terminals in the neocortex are endowed with at least two types of receptors. These few examples indicate that GABA$_B$ receptor-mediated transmission can be modulated by several other transmitter receptors, 5HT$_{1b}$ and adenosine in the midbrain, and μ-opioid peptides and GABA$_B$ in the neocortex. The question arises whether the presynaptic effects of, for instance, μ-opioid peptide and GABA$_B$ receptors, are localized on separate interneurons or on the same interneuron and terminal. The next question would be whether, at a given interneuron, different receptors share a common transduction system or utilize different effector systems.

7.3. Interaction with Intrinsic Currents

Another interesting feature of the IPSP$_B$ is the interaction with intrinsic membrane currents in different preparations. In the thalamus, the slow GABA$_B$-mediated IPSP contributes to the deinactivation of the T-current and plays an important role in thalamic oscillations (for review, *see* Crunelli and Leresche, 1991). By comparison, in the neocortex, under normal conditions, very little rebound excitation is noted, although neocortical pyramidal neurons are equipped with T-currents (Sutor and Zieglgänsberger, 1987). Apart from obvious differences in the magnitude of the T-current and GABA$_B$ inhibition, further differences must be considered. A crucial factor for the generation of rebound excitation through the T-current may be the time-course of the IPSP$_B$. For instance, in the neocortex the decay of the IPSP$_B$ may be sufficiently slow to cause an inactivation of the T-current without significant activation. Thus, differences in the time-course of the IPSP$_B$ might contribute to the absence or presence of rebound excitation. But the time-course of the IPSP$_B$ is comparable in thalamic and neocortical neurons judging by published figures. The differences in rebound excitation may also be the result of baclofen sensitivity of the T-current. The T-currents of neocortical neurons may be sensitive to baclofen (similar to those of dorsal root ganglion cells), as opposed to the baclofen-insensitive T-current of thalamic neurons (Guyon and Leresche, 1995). The comparison indicates that GABA$_B$ inhibition could serve two opposite functions in different neurons, depending upon the relative magnitudes of GABA$_B$ inhibition and T-current and their interaction.

Another interesting feature in this context is the modulation of A-currents by baclofen. A-currents are transient voltage-activated potassium currents, which exhibit a pronounced steady-state inactivation at membrane potentials less negative than about -70 mV. Baclofen (200 μM) induces a shift of the half-maximal inactivation from about -85 to near -45 mV (Saint et al., 1990). The hypothesis of Saint et al. (1990), that this shift of the A-current inactivation may contribute to modulation of transmitter release from presynaptic terminals by accelerating action potential repolarization, is unlikely, however. About 10-fold lower concentrations of baclofen already decrease calcium currents, and at 100-fold lower concentrations, baclofen significantly depress the IPSP in the neocortex.

8. Physiological and Clinical Implications of GABA$_B$ Receptors

8.1. GABA$_B$ Receptors and the Induction of LTP

Long-term potentiation (LTP) represents an established model for plasticity in the CNS (for review, *see* Bliss and Collingridge, 1993). The interest in both LTP and *N*-methyl-D-aspartic acid (NMDA) receptor function increased tremendously following the demonstration of behavioral deficits and the depression of LTP by application of NMDA receptor antagonists (Morris et al., 1986). A key feature of the NMDA receptor is the voltage-dependent enhancement of the NMDA receptor-mediated response caused by removal of the Mg^{++} block (Nowak et al., 1984). This property constitutes an AND-gate, relevant for learning and memory.

Early experiments had shown that high frequency stimulation causes a dual effect: a depression of inhibition and an enhancement of NMDA components (Stelzer et al., 1987). These authors proposed that high frequency stimulation would enhance NMDA receptor-mediated EPSP, and the resulting calcium influx through NMDA channels (McDermott et al., 1986) would, in turn, decrease inhibition (Stelzer et al., 1987). The facilitation of NMDA receptor-mediated EPSP components by paired stimulation (Metherate and Ashe, 1994) seems compatible with the view of Stelzer et al. (1987). But Metherate and Ashe (1994) presented evidence that the increase of NMDA receptor-mediated excitation is caused by a decreased inhibition. The sequence of events is exactly opposite to that proposed previously (Stelzer et al., 1987), the initial step being the decrease of inhibition, unveiling the NMDA components, rather than the enhancement of NMDA components depressing the IPSP. However, considerable evidence indicates the presence of a long-term potentiation independent of NMDA receptors (e.g., in the visual cortex, Bear et al., 1992). The voltage dependent enhancement of the EPSP via recruitment of T currents (Deisz et al., 1991), also presents an AND-gate and provides localized calcium increases (Markram and Sakmann, 1994). In fact, LTP of visual cortex was attributed to a recruitment of T currents by the EPSP (Komatsu and Iwakiri, 1992). Like the NMDA receptor-dependent LTP, this LTP would benefit from a disinhibition, because inhibition prevents the recruitment of the T current (Deisz et al. 1991). From these considerations it appears likely that not only NMDA receptor-dependent LTP (Davies et al., 1991; Mott and Lewis, 1991) but also the NMDA-receptor-independent LTP requires disinhibition.

8.2. GABA$_B$ Function During Development and Aging

The data reviewed so far were mostly obtained from adult animals. Recent evidence indicates that GABA$_B$ function exhibits marked changes during development. Fukuda et al. (1993) demonstrated that the presynaptic expression of GABA$_B$ receptors precedes that of postsynaptic GABA$_B$ receptors. Only about 10% of the neurons at postnatal d 7–10 exhibited an IPSP$_B$; at postnatal d 22–24, 5 out of 12 neurons exhibited an IPSP$_B$. On the other hand, at postnatal d 7, the paired-pulse depression of the IPSP$_A$ is already present, with a similar time-course and magnitude as during later development (Fukuda et al., 1993).

Also, a marked developmental change of the GABA$_B$ systems in the hippocampal CA3 area was reported (Gaiarsa et al., 1995). Comparison of the currents induced by baclofen (30 µM) at different postnatal days revealed a marked increase in current amplitude from d 3 (78 pA) to postnatal d 30 (412 pA). Baclofen reduced the amplitude of calcium currents of CA3 pyramidal neurons at postnatal d 6, but not at d 3. By contrast, the baclofen-induced depression of GABA$_B$-mediated and glutamatergic synaptic potentials was already present at birth. GABA$_B$ receptor function also appears to change during aging. Comparison of young and aged rats revealed a significant decrease in the amplitude of the IPSP$_B$, without detectable changes in the IPSP$_A$. The postsynaptic responsiveness to baclofen is unaltered; in young animals, baclofen induced a conductance of 6.4 nS and in aged rats the maximal response decreased to 4.8 nS. This slight decline with age was statistically insignificant (Billard et al., 1995). Paired-pulse depression, employed as an index for presynaptic GABA$_B$ function, was also not significantly different between young and aged rats (Billard et al., 1995). The smaller IPSP$_B$ in the aged rats was attributed to a selective impairment of those interneurons responsible for GABA$_B$ inhibition (Billard et al., 1995).

The early presence of use-dependent depression of inhibition through GABA$_B$ receptors (Fukuda et al., 1993) may contribute to plasticity during critical phases of cortical development. This use-dependent disinhibition may unleash NMDA receptor-mediated components (Metherate and Ashe, 1994), facilitating the expression of long-term potentiation, similar to the adult hippocampus (Davies et al., 1991; Mott and Lewis, 1991). It remains to be seen whether the change in GABA$_B$ coupling to effector systems during postnatal development, as suggested by the data of Gaiarsa et al. (1995), is also present in other structures.

8.3. GABA$_B$ and Antidepressants

An interesting feature of the GABA$_B$ receptors is their modulation by antidepressant drugs (Lloyd et al., 1985). Administered acutely, antidepressant drugs are without significant effects on neurochemical measures of GABA function, including GABA synthesis, uptake, and the levels of GABA$_A$ and GABA$_B$ receptors (Lloyd, 1990). However, prolonged administration of several antidepressants (amitriptyline, desipramine, fluoxetine) caused a pronounced increase in GABA$_B$ binding in rat frontal cortex (Lloyd, 1990), although the neurochemical indices of GABA-ergic function remained unaltered. From the data presented above, it is obvious that without a physiological control, the increased GABA$_B$ binding is difficult to relate to a level of inhibition. If postsynaptically located, the increase in GABA$_B$ binding might cause enhancement of the IPSP$_B$; if presynaptically located it may even cause weaker inhibition through enhanced feedback. In any case, these findings have been confirmed, to some extent (Pratt and Bowery, 1993). Chronic treatment with desipramine increased GABA$_B$ receptor density in the outer laminar region of rat frontal cortex by about 50%, but amitriptyline was without effect. Others have failed to demonstrate an up-regulation of GABA$_B$ binding by antidepressants (Cross and Horton, 1987; McManus and Greenshaw, 1991). The discrete location of the GABA$_B$ receptor up-regulation (Pratt and Bowery, 1993) may have precluded the detection when larger tissue samples are pooled. Nevertheless, up-regulation exhibits interesting differences between GABA$_B$ receptor antagonists: The GABA$_B$ receptor binding was also increased by CGP 36742, but not by the more commonly used CGP 35348 (Pratt and Bowery, 1993).

This selectivity for certain antidepressants and GABA$_B$ antagonists points toward a fairly specific effect. It would be interesting to determine the cellular sites of this GABA$_B$ up-regulation, whether it is pre- or postsynaptically located, and, hence the functional consequences of this antidepressant-induced effect.

8.4. GABA$_B$ Receptors and Epilepsy

Compared to the ease of eliciting paroxysmal depolarization shifts following the application of GABA$_A$ antagonists (Gutnick et al., 1982), the application of GABA$_B$ antagonists exerts little effect on neuronal and synaptic excitability under normal conditions in the neocortex (Deisz et al., 1993,

1996) or hippocampus (Malouf et al., 1995). In the presence of convulsant drugs (bicuculline, penicillin) or magnesium, however, antagonists of $GABA_B$ receptors increase excitability in area CA3 in 50–75% of the slices; the main effect is an increase in the frequency of spontaneous epileptiform activity recorded extracellularly (Karlsson et al., 1992). The increase in frequency may be, in part, attributed to the appearance of repetitive after-discharges, following the application of $GABA_B$ antagonists in the presence of bicuculline (10 μM) (Malouf et al., 1995). In addition, intracellular recordings in area CA1 revealed a slight increase in the duration of bicuculline-induced paroxysmal depolarizations in the presence of CGP 35348 (Karlsson et al., 1992). These data suggest that postsynaptic $GABA_B$ receptors of hippocampal and neocortical neurons contribute little to the control of excitability under control conditions. On the other hand, activation of presynaptic $GABA_B$ receptors and the resulting decreased release of GABA has significant effects on excitability. This mechanism comes into play during use-dependent depression of inhibition (for review, *see* Prince et al., 1992), long known to induce epileptiform activity (Ben-Ari et al., 1979), and during focal baclofen application in the neocortex (van Rijn et al., 1987) and the hippocampus dentate gyrus (Misgeld et al., 1984).

In addition, $GABA_B$ receptors appear to play a major role in absence epilepsy. In an animal model of absence epilepsy (Vergnes et al., 1990), $GABA_B$ antagonists exert marked beneficial effects (Marescaux et al., 1992; Snead, 1992), indicating that $GABA_B$ inhibition is involved. The cellular mechanisms and changes in circuitry involved in the 3/s spike wave discharges are not fully understood, but thalamic circuitry appears to play a major role. The activation and deinactivation properties of T-type calcium current of thalamic neurons (Jahnsen and Llinás, 1984a,b) are well established to govern thalamic oscillations. Thalamic neurons of genetically absent epilepsy-prone rats from Strasbourg have larger amplitudes of T-currents (Tsakiridou et al., 1995). Considering that subtle modulations of the T-current are sufficient to control rhythmic activity in the thalamus (Huguenard and Prince, 1994), the larger T-currents *per se* may contribute to a generation of the spike wave discharge. The role of $GABA_B$ antagonists in such a monocausal thalamic model may be the attenuation of the $GABA_B$ IPSP, which, in turn, would reduce deinactivation of the T-current and abolish the oscillatory mode (Huguenard and Prince, 1994). On the other hand, a cortical contribution of thalamic oscillations is well established, and cortical stimulation evokes rhythmic discharges in ventrolateral thalamic relay cells (Steriade, 1984). In addition, cortical lesioning interrupts thalamic oscillations (Vergnes et al., 1990), which is difficult to equate with monocausal origin of spike wave discharges. In this context, frequency dependence of cortical inhibition may play a central role. At interstimulus intervals of about 300 ms, cortical inhibition is reduced to such an extent that no net inhibition remains. Further stimuli would reduce inhibition even more and unveils the concomitantly evoked EPSP, i.e., at about 3 Hz cortical activity inverts from inhibition to excitation (Deisz, 1996). Thus, the frequency-dependent depression of inhibition may gate a re-entry excitation of the thalamus, giving rise to reverberative activity of the thalamocortical corticothalamic loop near 3 Hz.

Acknowledgments

Some of the original work referred to was supported by the Deutsche Forschungsgemeinschaft (SFB 220). I am most grateful to J. Mullington, K. Bohr, and to U. Misgeld for reading the manuscript and to S. M. Thompson for the permission to reproduce some of his figures.

References

Alger, B. E. (1984) Characteristics of a slow hyperpolarizing synaptic potential in rat hippocampal pyramidal cells *in vitro. J. Neurophysiol.* **52**, 892–910.

Andrade, R., Malenka, R. C., and Nicoll, R. A. (1986) A G protein couples serotonin and GABA_B receptors to the same channels in hippocampus. *Science* **234**, 1261–1265.

Anwyl, R. (1991) Modulation of vertebrate neuronal calcium channels by transmitters. *Brain Res. Rev.* **16**, 265–281.

Asano, T., Ui, M., and Ogasawara, N. (1985) Prevention of the agonist binding to γ-aminobutyric acid B receptors by guanine nucleotides and islet-activating protein, pertussis toxin in bovine cerebral cortex. *J. Biol. Chem.* **260**, 12,653–12,658.

Bean, B. P. (1989) Neurotransmitter inhibition of neuronal calcium currents by changes in channel voltage dependence. *Nature* **340**, 153–156.

Bear, M. F., Press, W. A., and Connors, B. W. (1992) Long-term potentiation in slices of kitten visual cortex and the effects of NMDA receptor blockade. *J. Neurphysiol.* **67**, 841–851.

Ben-Ari, Y., Kmjevic, K., and Reinhardt, W. (1979) Hippocampal seizures and failure of inhibition. *Can. J. Physiol. Pharmacol.* **57**, 1462–1466.

Billard, J. M., Lamour, Y., and Dutar, P. (1995) Decreased monosynaptic GABA_B-mediated inhibitory postsynaptic potentials in hippocampal CA1 pyramidal cells in the aged rat: pharmacological characterization and possible mechanisms. *J. Neurophysiol.* **74**, 539–546.

Bliss, T. V. P. and Collingridge, G. L. (1993) A synaptic model of memory: long-term potentiation in the hippocampus. *Nature* **361**, 31–39.

Bowery, N. G. (1993) GABA_B receptor pharmacology. *Ann. Rev. Pharmacol. Toxicol.* **33**, 109–147.

Bowery, N. G., Hill, D. R., and Hudson, A. L. (1983) Characterisation of GABA_B receptor binding sites on rat whole brain synaptic membranes. *Br. J. Pharmacol.* **78**, 191–206.

Bowery, N. G., Hill, D. R., Hudson, A. L., Doble, A., Middlemiss, D. N., Shaw, J., and Turnbull, M. (1980) (–)Baclofen decreases neurotransmitter release in the mammalian CNS by an action at a novel GABA receptor. *Nature* **283**, 92–94.

Bowery, N. G. and Williams, L. C. (1986) GABA$_B$ receptor activation inhibits the increase in nerve terminal Ca^{++} induced by depolarization. *Br. J. Pharmacol.* **86,** 37P.

Calabresi, P., Mercuri, N. B., DeMurtas, M., and Bernardi, G. (1991) Involvement of GABA systems in feedback regulation of glutamate-and GABA-mediated synaptic potentials in rat neostriatum. *J. Physiol.* **440,** 581–599.

Carbone, E. and Lux, H. D. (1984) A low voltage-activated fully inactivating Ca channel in vertebrate sensory neurones. *Nature* **310,** 501,502.

Christie, M. J. and North, R. A. (1988) Agonists at µ-opioid, M$_2$-muscarinic and GABA$_B$-receptors increase the same potassium conductance in rat lateral parabrachial neurones. *Br. J. Pharmacol.* **95,** 896–902.

Colmers, W. F. and Pittman, Q. J. (1989) Presynaptic inhibition by neuropeptide Y and baclofen in hippocampus: insensitivity to pertussis toxin treatment. *Brain Res.* **498,** 99–104.

Connors, B. W. (1992) GABA$_A$-and GABA$_B$-mediated processes in visual cortex, in *Progress in Brain Research*, vol. 90 (Mize, R. R., Marc, R. E., and Sillito, A. M., eds.), Elsevier Science, pp. 335–348.

Connors, B. W., Malenka, R. C., and Silva, L. R. (1988) Two inhibitory postsynaptic potentials and GABA$_A$ and GABA$_B$ receptor-mediated responses in neocortex of rat and cat. *J. Physiol.* **406,** 443–468.

Cross, J. A. and Horton, R. W. (1987) Are increases in GABA$_B$ receptors consistent findings following chronic antidepressant administration? *Eur. J. Pharmacol.* **141,** 159–162.

Crunelli, V. and Leresche, N. (1991) A role for GABA$_B$ receptors in excitation and inhibition of thalamocortical cells. *Trends Neurosci.* 14, 16–21.

Curtis, D. R., Game, C. J. A., Johnston, G. A. R., and McCulloch, R. M. (1974) Central effects of β-(ρ-chlorophenyl)-γ-aminobutyric acid. *Brain Res.* **70,** 493–499.

Davies, C. H. and Collingridge, G. L. (1993) The physiological regulation of synaptic inhibition by GABA$_B$ autoreceptors in rat hippocampus. *J. Physiol.* **472,** 245–265.

Davies, C. H., Davies, S. N., and Collingridge, G. L. (1990) Paired-pulse depression of monosynaptic GABA-mediated inhibitory postsynaptic responses in rat hippocampus. *J. Physiol.* **424,** 513–531.

Davies, C. H., Starkey, S. J., Pozza, M. F., and Collingridge, G. L. (1991) GABA$_B$ autoreceptors regulate the induction of LTP. *Nature* **349,** 609–611.

Davies, J. and Watkins, J. C. (1974) The action of β-phenyl-GABA derivatives on neurones of the cat cerebral cortex. *Brain Res.* **70,** 501–505.

Deisz, R. A. (1996) GABA$_B$ receptors of inhibitory interneurons mediate the frequency-dependent depression inhibition of rat neocortex in vitro. *J. Physiol.* **491,** 139,140.

Deisz, R. A., Billard, J. M., and Zieglgänsberger, W. (1992) Evidence for two types of GABA$_B$ receptors located pre- and postsynaptically in the neocortical slice in vitro. *J. Physiol.* **446,** 514P.

Deisz, R. A., Billard, J. M., and Zieglgänsberger, W. (1993) Pre-and postsynaptic GABA$_B$ receptors of rat neocortical neurons differ in their pharmacological properties. *Neurosci. Lett.* **154,** 209–212.

Deisz, R. A., Billard, J. M., and Zieglgänsberger, W. (1996) Presynaptic and postsynaptic GABA$_B$ receptors of neocortical neurones of the rat *in vitro*: differences in pharmacology and ionic mechanisms. *Synapse* (in press).

Deisz, R. A., Dose, M., and Lux, H. D. (1984) The time course of GABA action on the crayfish stretch receptor: evidence for a saturable GABA uptake. *Neurosci. Lett.* **47,** 245–250.

Deisz, R. A., Fortin, G., and Zieglgänsberger, W. (1991) Voltage dependence of excitatory postsynaptic potentials of rat neocortical. neurons. *J. Neurophysiol.* **65**, 371–382.

Deisz, R. A. and Lux, H. D. (1985) γ-Aminobutyric acid-induced depression of calcium currents of chick sensory neurons. *Neurosci. Lett.* **56**, 205–210.

Deisz, R. A. and Lux, H. D. (1986) Depression of calcium currents of chick sensory neurons by gamma-aminobutyric acid persists after elimination of other net currents, in *Calcium Electrogenesis and Neuronal Functioning* (Heinemann, U., Klee, M., Neher, E. and Singer, W., eds.), Springer-Verlag, Berlin, pp. 229–235.

Deisz, R. A. and Prince, D. A. (1986) Presynaptic GABA feedback causes frequency-dependent depression of IPSPs in neocortical neurons. *Soc. Neurosci.* **12**, 19.

Deisz, R. A. and Prince, D. A. (1989) Frequency-dependent depression of inhibition in guinea-pig neocortex *in vitro* by GABA$_B$ receptor feedback on GABA release. *J. Physiol.* **412**, 513–541.

Deisz, R. A. and Zieglgänsberger, W. (1992) Distinguishing pre- and postsynaptic GABA$_B$ receptors in the neocortical slice *in vitro*. *Pharmacol. Commun.* **2**, 38–40.

Désarmenien, M., Feltz, P., Occhipinti, G., Santangelo, F., and Schlichter, R. (1984) Coexistence of GABA$_A$ and GABA$_B$ receptors on Aδ and C primary afferents. *Br. J. Pharmacol.* **81**, 327–333.

Diversé-Pierluissi, M. and Dunlap, K. (1995) Interaction of convergent pathways that inhibit N-type calcium currents in sensory neurons. *Neuroscience* **65**, 477–483.

Dolphin, A. C. (1991) Regulation of calcium channel activity by GTP binding proteins and second messengers. *Biochem. Biophys. Acta* **1091**, 68–80.

Dolphin, A. C., McGuirk, S. M., and Scott, R. H. (1989) An investigation into the mechanisms of inhibition of calcium channel currents in cultured sensory neurones of the rat by guanine nucleotide analogues and (–)baclofen. *Br. J. Pharmacol.* **97**, 263–273.

Dolphin, A. C. and Scott, R. H. (1986) Inhibition of calcium currents in cultured rat dorsal root ganglion neurones by (–)baclofen. *Br. J. Pharmacol.* **88**, 213–220.

Doroshenko, P. and Neher, E. (1991) Pertussis-toxin sensitive inhibition by (–)baclofen of Ca signals in bovine chromaffin cells. *Pflügers Archiv.* **419**, 444–449.

Dunlap, K. (1981) Two types of γ-aminobutyric acid receptor on embryonic sensory neurones. *Br. J. Pharmacol.* **74**, 579–585.

Dunlap, K. and Fischbach, G. D. (1981) Neurotransmitters decrease the calcium conductance activated by depolarization of embryonic chick sensory neurones. *J. Physiol.* **317**, 519–535.

Dutar, P. and Nicoll, R. A. (1988a) A physiological role for GABA$_B$ receptors in the central nervous system. *Nature* **332**, 156–158.

Dutar, P. and Nicoll, R. A. (1988b) Pre- and postsynaptic GABA$_B$ receptors in the hippocampus have different pharmacological properties. *Neuron* **1**, 585–591.

Fox, A. P., Nowycky, M. C., and Tsien, R. W. (1987) Kinetic and pharmacological properties distinguishing three types of calcium currents in chick sensory neurones. *J. Physiol.* **394**, 149–172.

Froestl, W., Mickel, S. J., von Sprecher, G., Bittiger, H., and Olpe, H.-R. (1992) Chemistry of new GABA$_B$ antagonists. *Pharmacol. Comm.* **2**, 52–56.

Fukuda, A., Mody, I., and Prince, D. A. (1993) Differential ontogenesis of presynaptic and postsynaptic GABA$_B$ inhibition in rat somatosensory cortex. *J. Neurophysiol.* **70**, 448–452.

Gähwiler, B. H. and Brown, D. A. (1985) GABA$_B$-receptor-activated K$^+$ current in voltage-clamped CA3 pyramidal cells in hippocampal cultures. *Proc. Natl. Acad. Sci. USA* **82**, 1558–1562.

Gaiarsa, J.-L., Tseeb, V., and Ben-Ari, Y. (1995) Postnatal development of pre-and postsynaptic GABA$_B$-mediated inhibition in the CA3 hippocampal region of the rat. *J. Neurophysiol.* **73,** 246–255.

Gerber, U. and Gähwiler, B. H. (1994) GABA$_B$ and adenosine receptors mediate enhancement of the K$^+$ current, I$_{AHP}$, by reducing adenylyl cyclase activity in rat CA3 hippocampal neurons. *J. Neurophysiol.* **72,** 2360–2367.

Gutnick, M. J., Connors, B. W., and Prince, D. A. (1982) Mechanism of neocortical epileptogenesis *in vitro. J. Neurophysiol.* **48,** 1321–1335.

Guyon, A. and Leresche, N. (1995) Modulation by different GABA$_B$ receptor types of voltage activated calcium currents in rat thalamocortical neurones. *J. Physiol.* **485,** 29–42.

Hablitz, J. J. and Lebeda, F. J. (1985) Role of uptake in γ-aminobutyric acid (GABA)-mediated responses in guinea pig hippocampal neurons. *Cell. Mol. Neurobiol.* **5,** 353–371.

Hablitz, J. J. and Thalmann, R. H. (1987) Conductance changes underlying a late synaptic hyperpolarization in hippocampal CA3 neurons. *J. Neurophysiol.* **58,** 160–179.

Häusser, M. A. and Yung, W. H. (1994) Inhibitory synaptic potentials in guinea-pig substantia nigra dopamine neurones *in vitro. J. Physiol.* **479,** 401–422.

Hendry, S. H. C., Jones, E. G., Emson, P. C., Lawson, D. E. M., Heizmann, C. W., and Streit, P. (1989) Two classes of cortical GABA neurons defined by differential calcium binding protein immunoreactivities. *Exp. Brain Res.* **76,** 467–472.

Hescheler, J., Rosenthal, W., Trautwein, W., and Schultz, G. (1987) The GTP-binding protein, G$_o$, regulates neuronal calcium channels. *Nature* **325,** 445–447.

Hill, D. R., Bowery, N. G., and Hudson, A. L. (1984) Inhibition of GABA$_B$ receptor binding by guanyl nucleotides. *J. Neurochem.* **42,** 652–657.

Holopainen, I. and Wojcik, W. J. (1993) A specific antisense oligodeoxynucleotide to mRNAs encoding receptors with seven transmembrane spanning regions decreases muscarinic m2 and γ-aminobutyric acid B receptors in rat cerebellar granule cells. *J. Pharmacol. Exp. Ther.* **264,** 423–430.

Holz, G. G., Rane, S. G., and Dunlap, K. (1986) GTP-binding proteins mediate transmitter inhibition of voltage-dependent calcium channels. *Nature* **319,** 670–672.

Hösli, L., Hösli, E., Redle, S., Rojas, J., and Schramek, H. (1990) Action of baclofen, GABA and antagonists on the membrane potential of cultures astrocytes of rat spinal cord. *Neurosci. Lett.* **117,** 307–312.

Howe, J. R., Sutor, B., and Zieglgänsberger, W. (1987a) Baclofen reduces post-synaptic potentials of rat cortical neurones by an action other than its hyperpolarizing action. *J. Physiol.* **384,** 539–569.

Howe, J. R., Sutor, B., and Zieglgänsberger, W. (1987b) Characteristics of long-duration inhibitory postsynaptic potentials in rat neocortical neurones *in vitro. Cell. Mol. Neurobiol.* **7,** 1–18.

Huguenard, J. R. and Prince, D. A. (1994) Intrathalamic rhythmicity studied *in vitro*: nominal T-current modulation causes robust antioscillatory effects. *J. Neurosci.* **14,** 5485–5502.

Innis, R. B. and Aghajanian, G. K. (1987a) Pertussis toxin blocks autoreceptor-mediated inhibition of dopaminergic neurons in rat substantia nigra. *Brain Res.* **411,** 139–143.

Innis, R. B. and Aghajanian, G. K. (1987b) Pertussis toxin blocks 5-HT$_{1A}$ and GABA$_B$ receptor-mediated inhibition of serotonergic neurons. *Eur. J. Pharmacol.* **143,** 195–204.

Innis, R. B., Nestler, E. J., and Aghajanian, G. K. (1988) Evidence for G protein mediation of serotonin-and GABA$_B$-induced hyperpolarization of rat dorsal raphe neurons. *Brain Res.* **459,** 27–36.

Isaacson, J. S., Solis, J. M., and Nicoll, R. A. (1993) Local and diffuse synaptic actions of GABA in the hippocampus. *Neuron* **10**, 165–175.

Jahnsen, H. and Llinás, R. (1984a) Electrophysiological properties of guinea-pig thalamic neurones: an *in vitro* study. *J. Physiol.* **349**, 205–226.

Jahnsen, H. and Llinás, R. (1984b) Ionic basis for the electroresponsiveness and oscillatory properties of guinea-pig thalamic neurones *in vitro*. *J. Physiol.* **349**, 227–247.

Jarolimek, W., Bijak, M., and Misgeld, U. (1994) Differences in the Cs block of baclofen and 4-aminopyridine induced potassium currents of guinea pig CA3 neurons *in vitro*. *Synapse* **18**, 169–177.

Jiang, Z.-G., Allen, C. N., and North, R. A. (1995) Presynaptic inhibition by baclofen of retino-hypothalamic excitatory synaptic transmission in rat suprachiasmatic nucleus. *Neuroscience* **64**, 813–819.

Johnson, S. W., Mercuri, N. B., and North, R. A. (1992) 5-Hydroxytryptamine$_{1B}$ receptors block the GABA$_B$ synaptic potential in rat dopamine neurons. *J. Neurosci.* **12**, 2000–2006.

Kaila, K. (1995) Ionic basis for GABA$_A$ receptor channel function in the nervous system. *Prog. Neurobiol.* **42**, 489–537.

Kaila, K., Voipio, J., Paalasmaa, P., Pasternack, M. and Deisz, R. A. (1993) The role of bicarbonate in GABA$_A$ receptor-mediated IPSPs of rat neocortical neurones. *J. Physiol.* **464**, 273–289.

Karlsson, G., Kolb, C., Hausdorf, A., Portet, C., Schmutz, M., and Olpe, H.-R. (1992) GABA$_B$ receptors in various *in vitro* and *in vivo* models of epilepsy: a study with the GABA$_B$ receptor blocker CGP 35348. *Neuroscience* **47**, 63–68.

Karlsson, G. and Olpe, H.-R. (1989) Inhibitory processes in normal and epileptic-like rat hippocampal slices: the role of GABA$_B$ receptors. *Eur. J. Pharmacol.* **163**, 285–290.

Karlsson, G., Pozza, M., and Olpe, H.-R. (1988) Phaclofen: a GABA$_B$ blocker reduces long-duration inhibition in the neocortex. *Eur. J. Pharmacol.* **148**, 485–486.

Klee, M. R., Misgeld, U., and Zeise, M. L. (1981) Pharmacological differences between CA3 and dentate granule cells in hippocampal slices, in *Cellular Analogues of Conditioning and Neural Plasticity.* (Feher, O. and Joo, F., eds.), Pergamon and Akadémiai Kiadó, Budapest, pp. 145–154.

Knott, C., Maguire, J. J., Moratalla, R., and Bowery, N. G. (1993) Regional effects of pertussis toxin *in vivo* and *in vitro* on GABA$_B$ receptor binding in rat brain. *Neuroscience* **52**, 73–81.

Komatsu, Y. and Iwakiri, M. (1992) Low-threshold Ca^{2+} channels mediate induction of long-term potentiation in kitten visual cortex. *J. Neurophysiol.* **67**, 401–410.

Kuriyama, K., Nakayasu, H., Mizutani, H., Hanai, K., and Kimura, H. (1992) Structure and function of GABA$_B$ receptor in bovine cerebral cortex: analysis using the purified receptor and monoclonal antibody. *Pharmacol. Comm.* **2**, 15–19.

Kuriyama, K. and Ohmori, Y. (1990) Solubilization and partial purification of cerebral GABA$_B$ receptors, in *GABA$_B$ Receptors in Mammalian Function* (Bowery, N. G., Bittiger, H., and Olpe, H.-R., eds.), Wiley, Chichester, UK, pp. 183–193.

Lacey, M. G., Mercuri, N. B., and North, R. A. (1988) On the potassium conductance increase activated by GABA$_B$ and dopamine D2 receptors in rat substantia nigra neurones. *J. Physiol.* **401**, 437–453.

Lambert, N. A., Harrison, N. L., and Teyler, T. J. (1991) Baclofen-induced disinhibition in area CA1 of rat hippocampus is resistant to extracellular Ba^{2+}. *Brain Res.* **547**, 349–352.

Lambert, N. A. and Wilson, W. A. (1994) Temporally distinct mechanisms of use-dependent depression at inhibitory synapses in the rat hippocampus in vitro. *J. Neurophysiol.* **72,** 121–130.

Lancaster, B. and Wheal, H. V. (1984) The synaptically evoked late hyperpolarisation in CA1 pyramidal cells is resistant to intracellular EGTA. *Neuroscience* **12,** 267–276.

Laurie, D. J., Wisden, W., and Seeburg, P. H. (1992) The distribution of thirteen $GABA_A$ receptor subunit mRNAs in the rat brain. III. Embryonic and postnatal development. *J. Neurosci.* **12,** 4151–4172.

Ling, D. S. F. and Benardo, L. S. (1994) Properties of isolated $GABA_B$-mediated inhibitory postsynaptic currents in hippocampal pyramidal cells. *Neuroscience* **63,** 937–944.

Ling, D. S. F. and Benardo, L. S. (1995) Activity-dependent depression of monosynaptic fast IPSCs in hippocampus: contributions from reductions in chloride driving force and conductance. *Brain Res.* **670,** 142–146.

Llinás, R., Steinberg, I. Z., and Walton, K. (1981) Relationship between presynaptic calcium current and postsynaptic potential in squid giant synapse. *Biophys. J.* **33,** 323–352.

Llinás, R., Sugimori, M., Lin, J.-W., and Cherksey, B. (1989) Blocking and isolation of a calcium channel from neurons in mammals and cephalopods utilizing a toxin fraction (FTX) from funnel-web spider poison. *Proc. Natl. Acad. Sci. USA* **86,** 1689–1693.

Llinás, R., Sugimori, M., Hillman, D. E., and Cherksey, B. (1992) Distribution and functional significance of the P-type, voltage-dependent Ca^{2+} channels in the mammalian central nervous system. *Trends Neurosci.* **9,** 351–355.

Llinás, R. and Yarom, Y. (1981a) Properties and distribution of ionic conductances generating electroresponsiveness of mammalian inferior olivary neurones *in vitro*. *J. Physiol.* **315,** 569–584.

Llinás, R. and Yarom, Y. (1981b) Electrophysiology of mammalian inferior olivary neurones *in vitro*. Different types of voltage-dependent ionic conductances. *J. Physiol.* **315,** 549–567.

Lloyd, K. G. (1990) Antidepressants and $GABA_B$ site upregulation, in *$GABA_B$ Receptors in Mammalian Function* (Bowery, N. G., Bittiger, H., and Olpe, H.-R., eds.), John Wiley, Chichester, UK, pp. 297–307.

Lloyd, K. G., Thuret, F., and Pilc, A. (1985) Upregulation of γ-aminobutyric acid ($GABA_B$) binding sites in rat frontal cortex: a common action of repeated administration of different classes of antidepressants and electroshock. *J. Pharmacol. Exp. Ther.* **235,** 191–199.

Malouf, A. T., Robbins, C. A., and Schwartzkroin, P. A. (1990) Phaclofen inhibition of the slow inhibitory postsynaptic potential in hippocampal slice cultures: a possible role for the $GABA_B$-mediated inhibitory postsynaptic potential. *Neuroscience* **35,** 53–61.

Marescaux, C., Liu, Z., Bernasconi, R., and Vergnes, M. (1992) $GABA_B$ receptors are involved in the occurrence of absence seizures in rats. *Pharmacol. Commun.* **2,** 57–62.

Markram, H. and Sakmann, B. (1994) Calcium transients in dendrites of neocortical neurons evoked by single subthreshold excitatory postsynaptic potentials via low-voltage activated calcium channels. *Proc. Natl. Acad. Sci. USA* **91,** 5207–5211.

Matsushima, T., Tegner, J., Hill, R. H., and Grillner, S. (1993) $GABA_B$ receptor activation causes a depression of low and high-voltage activated Ca^{2+} current, postinhibitory rebound, and postspike afterhyperpolarization in lamprey neurons. *J. Neurophysiol.* **70,** 2606–2619.

Mayer, M. L. and Westbrook, G. L. (1987) The physiology of excitatory amino acids in the vertebrate central nervous system. *Prog. Neurobiol.* **28,** 197–276.

McCarren, M. and Alger, B. E. (1985) Use-dependent depression of IPSPs in rat hippocampal pyramidal cells in vitro. *J. Neurophysiol.* **53**, 557–571.

McCormick, D. A. (1989) GABA as an inhibitory transmitter in human cerebral cortex. *J. Neurophysiol.* **62**, 1018–1027.

McDermott, A. B., Mayer, M. L., Westbrook, G. L., Smith, S. J., and Barker, J. L. (1986) NMDA-receptor activation increases cytoplasmic calcium concentration in cultured spinal cord neurons. *Nature* **321**, 519–522.

McManus, D. J. and Greenshaw, A. J. (1991) Differential effects of antidepressants on GABA$_B$ and β-adrenergic receptors in rat cerebral cortex. *Biochem. Pharmacol.* **42**, 1525–1528.

Metherate, R. and Ashe, J. H. (1994) Facilitation of an NMDA receptor-mediated EPSP by paired-pulse stimulation in rat neocortex via depression of GABAergic IPSPs. *J. Physiol.* **481**, 331–348.

Miettinen, R. and Freund, T. F. (1992) Convergence and segregation of septal and median raphe inputs onto different subsets of hippocampal inhibitory interneurons. *Brain Res.* **594**, 263–272.

Mintz, I. M. and Bean, B. P. (1993) GABA$_B$ receptor inhibition of P-type channels in central neurons. *Neuron* **10**, 889–898.

Misgeld, U., Bijak, M., and Jarolimek, W. (1995) A physiological role of GABA$_B$ receptors and the effects of baclofen in the mammalian central nervous system. *Prog. Neurobiol.* **46**, 423–462.

Misgeld, U., Deisz, R. A., Dodt, H. U., and Lux, H. D. (1986) The role of chloride transport in postsynaptic inhibition of hippocampal neurons. *Science* **232**, 1413–1415.

Misgeld, U., Klee, M. R., and Zeise, M. L. (1982) Differences in burst characteristics and drug sensitivity between CA3 neurons and granule cells, in *Physiology and Pharmacology of Epileptogenic Phenomena* (Klee, M. R., Lux, H. D., and Speckmann, E. J., eds.), Raven, New York, pp. 131–139.

Misgeld, U., Klee, M. R., and Zeise, M. L. (1984) Differences in baclofen-sensitivity between CA3 neurons and granule cells of the guinea pig hippocampus in vitro. *Neurosci. Lett.* **47**, 307–311.

Misgeld, U., Müller, W., and Brunner, H. (1989) Effects of (–)baclofen on inhibitory neurons in the guinea pig hippocampal slice. *Pflügers Archiv.* **414**, 139–144.

Morishita, R., Kato, K., and Asano, T. (1990) GABA$_B$ receptors couple to G proteins G$_o$, G$_o$* and G$_{i1}$ but not to G$_{i2}$. *FEBS Lett.* **271**, 231–235.

Morris, R. G. M., Anderson, E., Lynch, G. S., and Baudry, M. (1986) Selective impairment of learning and blockade of long-term potentiation by an N-methyl-D-aspartate receptor antagonist, AP5. *Nature* **319**, 774–776.

Mott, D. D. and Lewis, D. V. (1991) Facilitation of the induction of long-term potentiation by GABA$_B$ receptors. *Science* **252**, 1718–1720.

Mott, D. D. and Lewis, D. V. (1994) The pharmacology and function of central GABA$_B$ receptors, in *International Review of Neurobiology*, vol 36 (Bradley, R. J. and Harris, R. A., eds.), Academic, New York, pp. 97–223.

Müller, W. and Misgeld, U. (1989) Carbachol reduces I$_{K, Baclofen}$, but not I$_{K, GABA}$ in guinea pig hippocampal slices. *Neurosci. Lett.* **102**, 229–234.

Müller, W. and Misgeld, U. (1990) Inhibitory role of dentate hilus neurons in guinea pig hippocampal slice. *J. Neurophysiol.* **64**, 46–56.

Nathan, T. and Lambert, J. D. C. (1991) Depression of the fast IPSP underlies paired-pulse facilitation in area CA1 of the rat hippocampus. *J. Neurophysiol.* **66**, 1704–1715.

Neher, E. and Penner, R. (1994) Mice sans synaptotagmin. *Nature* **372**, 316,317.

Newberry, N. R. and Nicoll, R. A. (1984) A bicuculline-resistant inhibitory post-synaptic potential in rat hippocampal pyramidal cells *in vitro. J. Physiol.* **348**, 239–254.

Newberry, N. R. and Nicoll, R. A. (1985) Comparison of the action of baclofen with gamma-aminobutyric acid on rat hippocampal pyramidal cells *in vitro. J. Physiol.* **360**, 161–185.

Nicoll, R. A., Malenka, R. C., and Kauer, J. A. (1990) Functional comparison of neurotransmitter receptor subtypes in mammalian central nervous system. *Physiol. Rev.* **70**, 513–565.

Nisenbaum, E. S., Berger, T. W., and Grace, A. A. (1993) Depression of glutamatergic and GABAergic synaptic responses in striatal spiny neurons by stimulation of presynaptic $GABA_B$ receptors. *Synapse* **14**, 221–242.

Nowak, L., Bregestovski, P., Ascher, P., Herbert, A., and Prochiantz, A. (1984) Magnesium gates glutamate-activated channels in mouse central neurones. *Nature* **307**, 462–465.

Nowycky, M. C., Fox, A. P., and Tsien, R. W. (1985) Three types of neuronal calcium channel with different calcium agonist sensitivity. *Nature* **316**, 440–443.

Ohmori, Y. and Kuriyama, K. (1989) Negative coupling of γ-aminobutyric acid ($GABA_B$) receptor with phosphatidylinositol turnover in the brain. *Neurochem. Int.* **15**, 359–363.

Olpe, H.-R., Karlsson, G., Pozza, M. F., Brugger, F., Steinmann, M., Van Riezen, H., Fagg, G., Hall, R. G., Froestl, and Bittiger, H. (1990) CGP 35348: a centrally active blocker of $GABA_B$ receptors. *Eur. J. Pharmacol.* **187**, 27–38.

Otis, T. S., DeKoninck, Y., and Mody, I. (1993) Characterization of synaptically elicited $GABA_B$ responses using patch-clamp recordings in rat hippocampal slices. *J. Physiol.* **463**, 391–407.

Otis, T. S. and Mody, I. (1992) Differential activation of $GABA_A$ and $GABA_B$ receptors by spontaneously released transmitter. *J. Neurophysiol.* **67**, 227–235.

Pacelli, G. J., Su, W., and Kelso, S. R. (1991) Activity-induced decrease in early and late inhibitory synaptic conductances in hippocampus. *Synapse* **7**, 1–13.

Pawelzik, H., Martin, G., Deisz, R. A., and Zieglgänsberger, W. (1996) The μ-opioid agonist DAMGO differentially modulates NMDA and non-NDMA-mediated synaptic transmission in rat neocortical neurons *in vitro* (in preparation).

Pierau, F.-K. and Zimmermann, P. (1973) Action of a GABA-derivative on postsynaptic potentials and membrane properties of cats' spinal motoneurones. *Brain Res.* **54**, 376–380.

Pin, J.-P. and Bockaert, J. (1990) ω Conotoxin GVIA and dihydropyridines discriminate two types of Ca2+ channels involved in GABA release from striatal neurons in culture. *Eur. J. Pharmacol.* **188**, 81–84.

Pitler, T. A. and Alger, B. E. (1994) Differences between presynaptic and postsynaptic $GABA_B$ mechanisms in rat hippocampal pyramidal cells. *J. Neurophysiol.* **72**, 2317–2327.

Pratt, G. D. and Bowery, N. G. (1993) Repeated administration of desipramine and a $GABA_B$ receptor antagonist, CGP 36742, discretely up-regulates $GABA_B$ receptor binding in rat frontal cortex. *Br. J. Pharmacol.* **110**, 724–735.

Premkumar, L. S., Chung, S.-H., and Gage, P. W. (1990) GABA-induced potassium channels in cultured neurons. *Proc. Royal Soc. Lond. B* **241**, 153–158.

Premkumar, L. S. and Gage, P. W. (1994) Potassium channels activated by $GABA_B$ agonists and serotonin in cultured hippocampal neurons. *J. Neurophysiol.* **71**, 2570–2575.

Prince, D. A., Deisz, R. A., Thompson, S. M., and Chagnac-Amitai, Y. (1992) Functional alterations in GABAergic inhibition during activity. *Epilepsy Res.* **8**, 31–38.

Randall, A. and Tsien, R. W. (1995) Pharmacological dissection of multiple types of Ca^{2+} channel currents in rat cerebellar granule neurons. *J. Neurosci.* **15,** 2995–3012.

Rane, S. G. and Dunlap, K. (1986) Kinase C activator 1,2-oleoylacetylglycerol attenuates voltage-dependent calcium currents in sensory neurons. *Proc. Natl. Acad. Sci. USA* **83,** 184–188.

Robertson, B. and Taylor, W. R. (1986) Effects of γ-aminobutyric acid and (–)-baclofen on calcium and potassium currents in cat dorsal root ganglion neurones in vitro. *Br. J. Pharmacol.* **89,** 661–672.

Saint, D. A., Thomas, T., and Gage, P. W. (1990) GABA$_B$ agonists modulate a transient potassium current in cultured mammalian hippocampal neurons. *Neurosci. Lett.* **118,** 9–13.

Schofield, P. R., Darlison, M. G., Fujita, N., Burt, D. R., Stephenson, F. A., Rodriguez, H., Rhee, L. M., Ramachandran, J., Reale, V., Glencorse, T. A., Seeburg, P. H., and Barnard, E. A. (1987) Sequence and functional expression of the GABA$_A$ receptor shows a ligand-gated receptor super-family. *Nature* **328,** 221–227.

Scholz, K. P. and Miller, R. J. (1991) GABA$_B$ receptor-mediated inhibition of Ca^{2+} currents and synaptic transmission in cultured rat hippocampal neurones. *J. Physiol.* **444,** 669–686.

Scott, R. H. and Dolphin, A. C. (1986) Regulation of calcium currents by a GTP analogue: potentiation of (–)-baclofen-mediated inhibition. *Neurosci. Lett.* **69,** 59–64.

Scott, R. H., Wootton, J. F., and Dolphin, A. C. (1990) Modulation of neuronal T-type calcium channel currents by photoactivation of intracellular guanosine 5'-0(3-Thio)triphosphate. *Neuroscience* **38,** 285–294.

Seabrook, G. R., Howson, W., and Lacey, M. G. (1991) Subpopulations of GABA-mediated synaptic potentials in slices of rat dorsal striatum are differentially modulated by presynaptic GABA$_B$ receptors. *Brain Res.* **562,** 332–334.

Seeburg, P. H. (1993) The molecular biology of mammalian glutamate receptor channels. *Trends Neurosci.* **16,** 359–365.

Segal, M. (1988) Effects of a lidocaine derivative QX-572 on CA1 neuronal responses to electrical and chemical stimuli in a hippocampal slice. *Neuroscience* **27,** 905–909.

Segal, M. (1990) A subset of local interneurons generate slow inhibitory postsynaptic potentials in hippocampal neurons. *Brain Res.* **511,** 163–164.

Siggins, G. R. and Gruol, D. L. (1986) Mechanisms of transmitter action in the vertebrate central nervous system, in *Handbook of Physiology—The Nervous System IV,* American Physiological Society, Bethesda, MD, pp. 1–114.

Snead, O. C. (1992) GABA$_B$ receptor mediated mechanisms in experimental absence seizures in rat. *Pharmacol. Commun.* **2,** 63–69.

Soltesz, I., Haby, M., Leresche, N., and Crunelli, V. (1988) The GABA$_B$ antagonist phaclofen inhibits the late K$^+$-dependent IPSP in cat and rat thalamic and hippocampal neurones. *Brain Res.* **448,** 351–354.

Soltesz, I., Lightowler, S., Leresche, N., and Crunelli, V. (1989a) Optic tract stimulation evokes GABA$_A$ but not GABA$_B$ IPSPs in the rat ventral lateral geniculate nucleus. *Brain Res.* **479,** 49–55.

Soltesz, I., Lightowler, S., Leresche, N., and Crunelli, V. (1989b) On the properties and origin of the GABA$_B$ inhibitory postsynaptic potential recorded in morphologically identified projection cells of the cat dorsal lateral geniculate nucleus. *Neuroscience* **33,** 23–33.

Somogyi, P. (1990) Synaptic organization of GABAergic neurons and GABA$_A$ receptors in the lateral geniculate nucleus and visual cortex, in *Neural Mechanisms of Visual Perception* (Lam, D. M. and Gilbert, C. D., eds.), Gulf, Houston, pp. 35–62.

Stelzer, A., Slater, N. T., and ten Bruggencate, G. (1987) Activation of NMDA receptors blocks GABAergic inhibition in an *in vitro* model of epilepsy. *Nature* **326**, 698–701.

Steriade, M. (1984) The excitatory-inhibitory response sequence in thalamic and neocortical cells: state-related changes and regulatory systems, in *Dynamic Aspects of Neocortical Function* (Edelmann, G. M., Gall, W. E., and Cowan, W. M., eds.), Wiley, New York, pp. 107–157.

Stratton, K. R., Cole, A. J., Pritchett, J., Eccles, C. U., Worley, P. F., and Baraban, J. M. (1989) Intrahippocampal injection of pertussis toxin blocks adenosine suppression of synaptic responses. *Brain Res.* **494**, 359–364.

Südhof, T. C., Petrenko, A. G., Whittaker, V. P., and Jahn, R. (1993) Molecular approaches to synaptic vesicle exocytosis. *Prog. Brain Res.* **98**, 235–240.

Sugita, S., Johnson, S. W., and North, R. A. (1992) Synaptic inputs to $GABA_A$ and $GABA_B$ receptors originate from discrete afferent neurons. *Neurosci. Lett.* **134**, 207–211.

Sutor, B. and Zieglgänsberger, W. (1987) A low-voltage activated, transient calcium current is responsible for the time-dependent depolarizing inward rectification of rat neocortical neurons in vitro. *Pflügers Archiv.* **410**, 102–111.

Taussig, R., Iñiguez-Lluhi, J. A., and Gilman, A. G. (1993) Inhibition of adenylyl cyclase by $G_{i\alpha}$. *Science* **261**, 218–221.

Thalmann, R. H. (1988) Evidence that guanosine triphosphate (GTP)-binding proteins control a synaptic response in brain: effect of pertussis toxin and GTPγS on the late inhibitory postsynaptic potential of hippocampal CA3 neurons. *J. Neurosci.* **8**, 4589–4602.

Thompson, S. M. (1994) Modulation of inhibitory synaptic transmission in the hippocampus. *Prog. Neurobiol.* **42**, 575–609.

Thompson, S. M., Deisz, R. A., and Prince, D. A. (1988) Relative contributions of passive equilibrium and active transport to the distribution of chloride in mammalian cortical neurons. *J. Neurophysiol.* **60**, 105–124.

Thompson, S. M. and Gähwiler, B. H. (1989) Activity-dependent disinhibition. I. Repetitive stimulation reduces IPSP driving force and conductance in hippocampus in vitro. *J. Neurophysiol.* **61**, 501–511.

Thompson, S. M. and Gähwiler, B. H. (1992) Comparison of the actions of baclofen at pre- and postsynaptic receptors in the rat hippocampus *in vitro. J. Physiol.* **451**, 329–345.

Tsakiridou, E., Bertollini, L., deCurtis, M., Avanzini, G., and Pape, H. C. (1995) Selective increase in T-type calcium conductance of reticular thalamic neurons in a rat model of absence epilepsy. *J. Neurosci.* **15**, 3110–3117.

Uchimura, N. and North, R. A. (1991) Baclofen and adenosine inhibit synaptic potentials mediated by γ-aminobutyric acid and glutamate release in rat nucleus accumbens. *J. Pharmacol. Exp. Ther.* **258**, 663–668.

Van Rijn, C. M., Van Berlo, M. J., Feenstra, M. G. P., Schoofs, M. L. F., and Hommes, O. R. (1987) R(−)-Baclofen: focal epilepsy after intracortical administration in the rat. *Epilepsy Res.* **1**, 321–327.

Verdoorn, T. A., Draguhn, A., Ymer, S., Seeburg, P. H., and Sakmann, B. (1990) Functional properties of recombinant rat $GABA_A$ receptors depend upon subunit composition. *Neuron* **4**, 919–928.

Vergnes, M., Marescaux, C., De Paulis, A., Micheletti, G., and Warter, J.-M. (1990) Spontaneous spike-and-wave discharges in Wistar rats: a model of genetic generalized nonconvulsive epilepsy, in *Generalized Epilepsy: Neurobiological Approaches* (Avoli, M., Gloor, P., Kostopoulos, G., and Naquet, R., eds.), Birkhäuser, Boston, pp. 238–253.

Wheeler, D. B., Randall, A., and Tsien, R. W. (1994) Roles of N-type and Q-type Ca^{2+} channels in supporting hippocampal synaptic transmission. *Science* **264**, 107–111.

Wilcox, K. S. and Dichter, M. A. (1994) Paired pulse depression in cultured hippocampal neurons is due to a presynaptic mechanism independent of GABA$_B$ autoreceptor activation. *J. Neurosci.* **14**, 1775–1788.

Wisden, W., Laurie, D. J., Monyer, H., and Seeburg, P. H. (1992) The distribution of 13 GABA$_A$ receptor subunit mRNAs in the rat brain. I. Telencephalon, diencephalon, mesencephalon. *J. Neurosci.* **12**, 1040–1062.

Wojcik, W. J. and Neff, N. H. (1984) γ-Aminobutyric acid B receptors are negatively coupled to adenylate cyclase in brain and in the cerebellum; these receptors may be associated with granule cells. *Mol. Pharmacol.* **25**, 24–28.

Wu, L.-G. and Saggau, P. (1995) GABA$_B$ receptor mediated presynaptic inhibition in guinea pig hippocampus is caused by reduction of presynaptic Ca^{2+} influx. *J. Physiol.* **485**, 649–657.

Wu, Y.-N., Mercuri, N. B., and Johnson, S. W. (1995) Presynaptic inhibition of γ-aminobutyric acid$_B$-mediated synaptic current by adenosine recorded *in vitro* in midbrain dopamine neurons. *J. Pharmacol. Exp. Ther.* **273**, 576–581.

Yoon, K.-W. and Rothman, S. M. (1991) The modulation of rat hippocampal synaptic conductances by baclofen and γ-aminobutyric acid. *J. Physiol.* **442**, 377–390.

CHAPTER 7

Pharmacology
of Mammalian GABA$_B$ Receptors

Norman G. Bowery

1. Introduction

At the time of publication of the first edition of *The GABA Receptors* in 1983, the concept of GABA receptor subtypes had only just emerged. Designation of the terms GABA$_A$ and GABA$_B$ to describe bicuculline-sensitive Cl$^-$-dependent and novel bicuculline-insensitive Cl$^-$-independent receptors, respectively, was introduced less than two years earlier (Hill and Bowery, 1981). There was no evidence for a physiological role for the novel GABA$_B$ site at that time and the molecular structure of fast channel-linked GABA$_A$ receptors was unknown. We now know that GABA$_B$ receptors have not only a physiological role in synaptic transmission (Dutar and Nicoll, 1988a), but may also be important in pathological conditions associated with pain and epilepsy. In addition, we now have information for the structural sequences of the GABA$_A$ receptor (*see* Chapter 2 of this volume), with evidence for marked heterogeneity (e.g., Olsen and Tobin, 1990). Evidence is also accruing for a potential subclassification of GABA$_B$ receptors based on pharmacological characteristics *(see* Section 3.4.)*. Thus, in little more than a decade we have gone from a single GABA receptor to a multiplicity of GABA sites, with at least two distinct classes of receptors namely GABA$_A$ and GABA$_B$. A third class GABA$_C$, associated with fast Cl$^-$ channels, has also been suggested (Johnston, 1995; *see also* Chapter 11 of this volume). This chapter summarizes the pharmacological properties of the GABA$_B$ receptor(s), making reference to its potential significance as a therapeutic target.

The background to GABA$_B$ receptors is unusual, because the selective agonist for the receptor was already in therapeutic use before its discovery. Baclofen (Lioresal CIBA-Geigy) had been in clinical medicine as a centrally-

The GABA Receptors Eds.: S. J. Enna and N. G. Bowery
Humana Press Inc., Totowa, NJ

active muscle relaxant drug for at least seven years before discovery of the novel GABA$_B$ receptor and obtaining of the apparent site of action for this compound (Bowery et al., 1980). Its selectivity for this receptor and lack of effect on the classical bicuculline-sensitive GABA$_A$ receptor not only provided a basis for the mechanism of action of baclofen, but also a selective ligand for pursuing basic research studies. Baclofen had originally been designed as a GABA-mimetic that would penetrate the blood-brain barrier (Keberle and Faigle, 1972; Bein, 1972) and, although it was shown to be a potent centrally active muscle relaxant, its link with the action of GABA was never established until its efficacy at the metabotropic GABA$_B$ receptor was demonstrated (Bowery et al., 1980). It was known that baclofen could suppress the evoked release of neurotransmitter glutamate from cerebral cortex (Potashner, 1978) and presynaptic events of the monosynaptic reflex in spinal cord (Fox et al., 1978). These effects could not be attributed to a GABA-mimetic action at the time; in retrospect, it seems likely that GABA$_B$ receptors were implicated in the observed effects.

2. GABA$_B$ Receptor Distribution and Ontogeny

GABA$_B$ receptors were first demonstrated on nerve terminals of the peripheral autonomic nervous system (Bowery et al., 1981), where they mediate a decrease in evoked neurotransmitter release. Both acetylcholine and noradrenaline release can be inhibited by GABA$_B$ receptor agonists, which decrease the contractile response to transmural stimulation of smooth muscle preparations, e.g., ileum and anococcygeus muscle (Bowery et al., 1981; Muhyaddin et al., 1982; Giotti et al., 1983a; Ong and Kerr, 1983; 1990), and a measurable reduction in the release of acetylcholine and noradrenaline (Bowery et al., 1981; Kleinrok and Kilbinger, 1983; Shirakawa et al., 1987).

There exists very little evidence for any physiological function for GABA$_B$ mechanisms in peripheral organs (for review, see Erdö and Bowery, 1986) with the possible exception of the enteric nervous system, where GABA-ergic neurons appear to modulate the output from cholinergic nerve terminals to influence the tone and motility of the intestine (Jessen et al., 1979; Jessen, 1990; Ong and Kerr, 1983; 1987; Parkman et al., 1993; Giotti et al., 1985). The receptors appear to be confined to nerve tissue within the periphery, although GABA$_B$ sites have been reported in rabbit oviduct and uterus, which may be of nonneural origin (Erdö, 1986).

In the central nervous system (CNS) GABA$_B$ binding sites are distributed in a heterogeneous manner with high densities in certain brain regions, such as the thalamus, the molecular layer of the cerebellar cortex, the interpeduncular nucleus, and the dorsal horn of the spinal cord (Bowery et al.,

1987; Chu et al., 1990; Turgeon and Albin, 1993). The pattern of binding differs from that of $GABA_A$ sites, although in many brain regions $GABA_B$ and $GABA_A$ sites appear to coexist (Bowery et al., 1987). This is perhaps not surprising, in light of the frequent and dual occurrence of $GABA_A$ and $GABA_B$ synaptic events in many brain regions (Thalman, 1988; Crunelli and Leresche, 1991; Karlsson et al., 1988; Lambert et al., 1989; Dutar and Nicoll, 1988a), indicating the presence of both GABA receptor types, even though the origin of the transmitter GABA may be from different inhibitory neurons for each receptor type (Benardo, 1994).

$GABA_B$ binding sites appear to be present in rodent brain at an early stage of life (Turgeon and Albin, 1993; Knott et al., 1993), and appear to increase in density in different regions 3–21 d postnatal before decreasing to the level detected in adult animals. In general, the characteristics of the receptors and their G protein-coupling in young animals appear to be similar to those in adults, although some indication of a distinct pharmacological profile has been suggested (Turgeon and Albin, 1993).

In adult mammalian brain, the wide distribution of $GABA_B$ receptor sites, as determined by receptor autoradiography (Bowery et al., 1987; Chu et al., 1990), is consistent with the presence of functional $GABA_B$ receptors on many neurons throughout the CNS, as demonstrated by electrophysiological techniques (*see* Mott and Lewis, 1994). Data from electrophysiological studies indicate that $GABA_B$ receptors are present on presynaptic terminals and at postsynaptic sites (Harrison, 1990; Harrison et al., 1988; Dutar and Nicoll, 1988b; Thompson and Gähwiler, 1992; Alford and Grillner, 1991). At presynaptic sites, $GABA_B$ receptor activation suppresses evoked release of neurotransmitter, whereas at the postsynaptic sites a long-lasting neuronal hyperpolarization occurs (Newberry and Nicoll, 1984; Crunelli and Leresche, 1991; Thalman, 1987; Colmers and Williams, 1988; Seabrook et al., 1990; Deisz et al., 1992).

Undoubtedly, the $GABA_B$ sites detected by ligand binding experiments reflect both post- and presynaptic sites, but there is no evidence at present that any of the binding sites are postsynaptic in origin. However, there is good evidence for the presence of presynaptic binding sites in, for example, the interpeduncular nucleus (Price et al., 1984) and dorsal horn of the spinal cord (Price et al., 1987).

The functional role of $GABA_B$ receptors on nerve terminals that are not GABA-ergic might be questionable since outside the spinal cord there is little or no evidence for any axo-axonic synapses. However, Isaacson et al. (1993) have provided good evidence that GABA released from an adjacent synapse can diffuse to a $GABA_B$ heteroceptor in sufficient concentrations to activate it in a manner consistent with a paracrine-like action. Presynaptic $GABA_B$

heteroreceptors may well have a functional physiological role modulating the release of many neurotransmitters.

The presence of GABA$_B$ receptors on nerve terminals as heteroreceptors has been noted on a variety of presumed nerve terminals within the CNS (Table 1). These include glutamate, noradrenaline, dopamine, acetylcholine, 5HT, cholecystokinin, and somatostatin in higher centers (Bowery et al., 1980; Schlicker et al., 1984; Reimann et al., 1982; Gray and Green, 1987; Bonanno and Raiteri, 1993; Raiteri, 1992) and substance P, glutamate, and CGRP in the spinal cord (Malcangio and Bowery, 1993b; Teoh et al., 1996a; Malcangio and Bowery, 1996; Kangra et al., 1991). In all cases, the activation of GABA$_B$ receptors suppresses the evoked release of neurotransmitter.

Neurons are not the only cell type within the brain that possess GABA$_B$ receptors. Astrocytes have also been shown to express GABA$_B$ receptors (*see* Fraser et al., 1994; Hosli et al., 1990) on their cell surface, but their role, if any, has not been established, even though cellular hyperpolarization is produced on receptor activation (Hosli et al., 1990).

3. GABA$_B$ Receptor Ligands

3.1. Agonists

Relatively few selective agonists for GABA$_B$ receptors have been reported. Of course, (±)-baclofen was the first selective agonist to be described, providing the basis for the pharmacological separation of GABA$_B$ from GABA$_A$ receptors (Hill and Bowery, 1981), with the (–)-isomer providing the active enantiomeric form. Subsequently, 3-aminopropyl phosphinic acid (APPA) emerged from the laboratory of Froestl et al. (1995a) soon followed by the methyl derivative, (3-aminopropyl) methyl phosphinic acid (AMPPA), by Howson et al. (1993). These compounds exhibited three- to sevenfold greater potency at GABA$_B$ receptors than (–)-baclofen, while retaining considerable selectivity for GABA$_B$ over GABA$_A$ receptors. (3-Amino-2 (S)-hydroxypropyl) methyl phosphinic acid also proved to be a selective GABA$_B$ agonist, with potency comparable to AMPPA, particularly as an inhibitor of monosynaptic reflexes in rat spinal cord (Froestl et al., 1995a). Moreover, the duration of action of AMPPA far exceeded baclofen as a muscle relaxant, and fewer side effects were noted. As a consequence, this GABA$_B$ agonist has been selected as a development candidate for the treatment of spasticity (Froestl et al., 1995a). The phosphonic derivative of APPA has mixed agonist/antagonist actions, the expression of which depends on the location of the GABA$_B$ receptor inside or outside the brain (Kerr et al., 1990). This may reflect partial agonist characteristics, which are certainly evident in the compound (3-aminopropyl) (difluromethyl) phosphinic acid. This compound acts

Table 1
Inhibition of Evoked Mediator Release
by GABA$_B$ Receptor Activation

Mediator	Region[a]			Ref.[b]
Amino Acids				
Glutamate	B	S		1,2,3,4,5
GABA	B	S		2,4,5,6,7
Aspartate	B	S		3,5
Amines				
Dopamine	B			8,9
Noradrenaline/Adrenaline	B		P	10,11
5HT	B			9,12,19
Peptides				
Substance P		S	P	13,14
CGRP		S	P	15,10
Somatostatin	B	S	P	2,16,17
Cholecystokinin	B	S		2,18
Acetylcholine	B		P	20,21

[a]GABA$_B$ receptor activation depresses evoked release of substances in higher centers of brain (B), spinal cord (S), and peripheral organs (P) in mammalian preparations. In peripheral organs the released substance derives from the neural input.

[b]1. Potashner, 1979; 2. Bonanno and Raiteri, 1983; 3. Teoh et al., 1996b; 4. Waldemeier et al., 1994; 5. Teoh et al., 1996a; 6. Pittaluga et al., 1987; 7. Kangra et al., 1991; 8. Reimann et al., 1982; 9. Bowery et al., 1980; 10. Bowery, 1993; 11. Rosensteinetal, 1990; 12. Gray and Green, 1987; 13. Malcangio and Bowery, 1993; 14. Ray et al., 1991; 15. Malcangio and Bowery, 1996; 16. Kawai and Unger, 1983; 17. Vasko and Harris, 1990; 18. Benoliel et al., 1992; 19. Schlicker et al., 1984; 20. Arenas et al., 1990; 21. Parkman et al., 1993.

as a full agonist at GABA$_B$ sites on somatostatin-releasing neurons, but as an antagonist at GABA$_B$ autoreceptors (Gemignani et al., 1994).

Structure-activity studies have failed to yield other more active agonists, although certain close analogs of GABA do exhibit activity at GABA$_B$ receptors. For example, 2-hydroxy GABA is a stereospecifically active agonist that has recently been resolved into 2 enantiomers (*see* Frydenvang et al., 1996). However, any structure so closely related to GABA, and so flexible, will almost certainly activate GABA$_A$ receptors, as well as making them nonselective. The two isomers of 2-hydroxy GABA exert opposite selectively for GABA$_A$ and GABA$_B$ receptors, but the distinction is only marginal and the level of affinity for either site is relatively low. Nevertheless, the information obtained from this study has provided a basis for agonist design.

Other compounds recently reported to be possible $GABA_B$ agonists include DN 2327 (Wada and Fukuda, 1991), ginsenoside (Kimura et al., 1994), and γ-hydroxybutyric acid (GHB) (Xie and Smart, 1992; Williams et al., 1995). In all cases, the potency of these compounds is very low and definite evidence to support their association with $GABA_B$ sites is lacking. The weak agonist activity of GHB (Bernasconi et al., 1992; Engberg and Wissbrandt, 1993) could explain the ability of this compound to produce an absence epilepsy-like syndrome in rats (Snead, 1991), where $GABA_B$ receptor mechanisms appear to play a crucial role *(see* Section 6.3.*)*.

3.2. Antagonists

The design and production of $GABA_B$ receptor antagonists has been much more fruitful than the search for agonists *(see* Chapter 10 of this volume). In brief, we have seen the introduction of compounds with increasing potency, affinity, and selectivity for the $GABA_B$ site, during the past 10 years. The initial breakthrough came with the discovery by Kerr et al. (1986; 1987) that the phosphonic acid derivative of baclofen, phaclofen, was a very weak but selective and competitive $GABA_B$ receptor antagonist at central and peripheral sites. This was shortly followed by the introduction of 2-hydroxysaclofen, the sulphonic acid derivative of baclofen by the same group (Curtis et al., 1988; Lambert et al., 1989). This derived from the observation by Giotti et al. (1983b) that 3-aminopropanesulphonic acid, the $GABA_A$-receptor agonist, was also a $GABA_B$ antagonist. 2-Hydroxy- saclofen was a major improvement over phaclofen with a 10-fold increase in affinity for the $GABA_B$ site (Ki 12 μM cf phaclofen 100 μM). However, neither of these antagonists cross the blood-brain barrier (Table 2).

The introduction of CGP35348 by Olpe et al. (1990) provided the next major advance, with an antagonist capable of crossing the blood-brain barrier. A further improvement occurred with the advent of CGP 36742, which gains access to the brain after oral administration (Olpe et al., 1993). Both of these compounds have affinities for the $GABA_B$ receptor that are comparable to that of 2-hydroxysaclofen (12 μM).

More recently has been the introduction of antagonists with much greater affinities (1000-fold) than either CGP 35348 or CGP 36742. Compounds such as CGP 55845 and CGP 54626 are examples of antagonists with nanomolar affinity. This has been an exciting breakthrough, providing ligands with such high affinity. This should facilitate the characterization of $GABA_B$ receptors. More details about these ligands are provided in Chapter 10. The most recently reported antagonist to have emerged comes from the Schering Plough laboratories, who have introduced the compound SCH 50911, (+)-5, 5-dimethyl-2-morpholineacetic acid hydrochloride. This

Table 2
Characteristics of Certain GABA_B Receptor Antagonists

Antagonist	Affinity	Brain penetrating	Active in CNS after oral administration	Reported selectivity	Ref.[a]
δ-aminovaleric acid		X	X	GABA_A agonist	1
3-aminopropane sulphonic acid	Low (>50 μM)	X	X	GABA_A agonist	2
Phaclofen		X	X	Inactive at pre-synaptic GABA_B sites	3,4 but see 5
2-hydroxy saclofen		X	X	Partial agonist?	6
CGP 35348	Moderate (4–40 μM)	√	X		
CGP 36742		√	√		
CGP 46381		√	√		
SCH 50911		√	√		
CGP 55845	High (2–10 nM)	√			
CGP 54626		√			
CGP 56999		√	√		
CGP 52432		√		Inactive on glutamate terminals in spinal cord	7
				Selective for GABA_B autoreceptors	8

√ = yes; X = no.

[a]1. Dickenson et al., 1988; 2. Giotti et al., 1983b; 3. Harrison, 1990; 4. Dutar and Nicoll, 1988b; 5. Raiteri et al., 1990; 6. Stuart and Redman, 1992; 7. Teoh et al., 1996a; 8. Lanza et al., 1993.

stereoselective antagonist readily gains access to the brain and is reported to be 3–20 times more potent than CGP 35348 in a variety of in vivo assays, and is orally active (Bolser et al., 1995)

All of the selective antagonists reported thus far appear to produce a surmountable antagonism of the $GABA_B$ receptor, with little or no evidence for any modulatory influences. However, Ong and Kerr (1994) have recently suggested that amiloride can allosterically modulate $GABA_B$ receptors in the mammalian cerebral cortex. Whether this is an effect restricted to a single substance remains to be seen, but allosteric modulation could have important consequences.

3.3. Structure of the GABA_B Receptor(s)

The $GABA_B$ receptor is possibly the only established G protein-coupled receptor which has yet to be identified. Attempts to express the receptor in *Xenopus* oocytes from crude mRNA prepared from rat brain cerebral cortex and cerebellum have proven to be only partially successful. Coupling to unexpected channel mechanisms (Sekiguchi et al., 1990), or a very low expression rate with only about 5–10% of injected oocytes showing any evidence of the receptor (Taniyama et al., 1991a,b), has inhibited progress. The limited responses observed have been attributed by one group to changes in pH (Woodward and Miledi, 1992).

Nakayasu et al. (1993) have described the generation of a monoclonal (Ig*M*) antibody from purified receptor protein. The protein was obtained by affinity chromatography, using baclofen attached to a sephadex column. The purified material suggested a molecular weight for the receptor of about 80 kDa. However, despite the fact that the monoclonal antibody has been used to detect receptor protein in peripheral tissues, further information about the receptor has still to emerge. It might be expected that a high degree of structural homology exists between the $GABA_B$ receptor and somatostatin and adenosine receptors, in view of the similar pharmacological responses obtained on activation.

3.4. Receptor Heterogeneity

One advantage of knowing the receptor structure is the possibility of obtaining numerous subtype sequences. It seems unlikely that the $GABA_B$ receptor exists in only a single form. The receptor is probably heterogeneous with different forms, for instance, at pre- and postsynaptic sites. Early indications of receptor subtyping arose from the differential effects of $GABA_B$ agonists, e.g., baclofen on the activity of adenylate cyclase stimulated by beta-adrenoceptor agonists or forskolin in brain slices (Hill et al., 1984; Karbon et al., 1984; Hill, 1985; Scherer et al., 1985; Cunningham and Enna,

Chapter 8 of this volume). The effects observed in this instance seemed comparable to those obtained with adenosine and mediated separately by A_1 and A_2 receptors. Little evidence has subsequently accrued to support the participation of distinct receptor subtypes in these effects.

Subsequent electrophysiological studies examining the activity of pre-and postsynaptic $GABA_B$ receptors suggested that there may well be a distinction between the receptors at these locations. This was based on the apparent insensitivity of presynaptic $GABA_B$ receptors to pertussis toxin and the weak $GABA_B$ antagonist, phaclofen (Dutar and Nicoll, 1988b; Alger and Nicoll, 1982; Harrison, 1990). The postsynaptic response to $GABA_B$ receptor stimulation of hippocampal neurons could be prevented by prior treatment with pertussis toxin or phaclofen, but the presynaptic effect, depression in excitatory transmission, could not. Deisz et al. (1993) have also indicated the existence of separate receptor types at pre- and postsynaptic sites in the rat neocortex; this is referred to in Chapter 6 of this volume. The types of potassium channels to which $GABA_B$ receptors are coupled at pre- and postsynaptic sites probably differ (Lambert and Wilson, 1993), but this does not necessarily implicate separate receptor types.

Data obtained from CA3 neurons in culture by Thompson and Gähwiler (1992) suggest that there is no difference between the receptors at pre- and postsynaptic sites and similarly, Seabrook and colleagues (1990) could obtain no distinction between presynaptic receptors in caudate putamen and postsynaptic receptors in the substantia nigra.

The differential effects obtained with pertussis toxin could have been the result of poor penetration to presynaptic sites, but this possibility has been negated by the observations of Potier and Dutar (1993), who have shown that presynaptic $GABA_B$ autoreceptor inhibitory mechanisms can be suppressed by pertussis toxin, while depression of excitatory transmission is unaffected. Santos et al. (1995) have obtained similar data in GABA-release experiments, using rat cerebrocortical synaptosomes. Does this indicate that $GABA_B$ receptors on GABA terminals differ from those on glutamate terminals, and how far do they both differ from postsynaptic receptors which may also be heterogeneous?

Possible distinctions within the presynaptic receptor family have been proposed by Bonnano and Raiteri (1993) and Gemignani et al. (1994), who have suggested that at least four types of $GABA_B$ receptor exist on glutamate, GABA, somatostatin, and choleocystokinin in releasing synaptosomes. Moreover, a baclofen-insensitive site exists on terminals within the spinal cord. These conclusions are based on the differential abilities of antagonists to reduce the $GABA_B$-mediated inhibition of K^+-evoked transmitter release from synaptosomes isolated from mammalian, including human, brain. These are very interesting and potentially important observations, but they have yet to be confirmed in other biochemical-release or electrophysiological-recording studies. Waldmeier and colleagues (1994), using an electrically-evoked release system in mammalian brain slices, have failed to find any evidence for receptor heterogeneity.

We have also failed to show any major pharmacological differences between $GABA_B$ receptor mechanisms controlling endogenous glutamate, GABA, and substance P release from rat spinal cord (Teoh et al., 1996a). Only one antagonist tested so far, CGP 56999, showed any selectivity for these release mechanisms. This compound blocked the inhibitory effect of baclofen on the evoked release of GABA and substance P, but was completely inactive over a wide concentration range against baclofen on glutamate release. We conclude that the receptor on glutamate terminals may differ from those on other terminals in the cord. However, this is based on data from a single antagonist. No other compound tested showed any separation (Teoh et al., 1996a).

Potential separation of postsynaptic sites in the cerebral cortex has been noted by Jarolimek et al. (1992), but this interesting observation also requires further studies to establish its pharmacological significance.

Evidence is mounting in favor of $GABA_B$ receptor heterogeneity, but there still remains much debate about the extent and significance of any separation. The recent advent of high-affinity antagonists may help resolve these questions, but, of course, when the receptor structure is elucidated, everything should become much clearer.

4. Second Messenger Events

4.1. Biochemical

$GABA_B$ receptors are coupled via G proteins to membrane K^+ and Ca^{++} channels as well as to adenylate, and possibly guanylate, and cyclase although the nature of the link to this latter enzyme has yet to be determined. Details of the G protein-coupled events are covered in Chapter 8 of this volume. At present, the reported influence of $GABA_B$ receptors on guanylate cyclase is limited to in vivo studies in the rat cerebellum (Bernasconi et al., 1994), and may well be an indirect action via a change in glutamate release.

4.2. Channels

Although the neuronal channel events that occur on activation of $GABA_B$ receptors are also mediated via G proteins, the changes are not dependent on alterations in cyclic AMP. Both appear to occur independently. A broad outline of events is presented here, with a fuller account in the Chapter 8.

The predominant response to $GABA_B$ receptor activation is an increase in K^+ conductance, producing neuronal hyperpolarization. This occurs throughout the brain (e.g., Newberry and Nicoll, 1984; Gähwiler and Brown,

1985; Robertson and Taylor, 1986; Gallagher et al., 1984; Lacey et al., 1988; Crunelli and Leresche, 1991). This mechanism manifests as a slow inhibitory postsynaptic potential following afferent fiber stimulation.

GABA$_B$ receptors are associated with more than one type of K$^+$ channel (Wagner and Dekin, 1993) and the K$^+$ channel associated with GABA$_B$ appears to be different from that opened by 5HT receptor activation (Premkumar and Gage, 1994), even though both receptor systems have been previously reported to be inactivated by pertussis toxin treatment (Andrade et al., 1986).

K$^+$ channel-associated GABA$_B$ receptors are not confined to postsynaptic sites, but are also present on presynaptic terminals; these could be responsible for modifying transmitter release, in addition to effects on Ca^{++} conductance mechanisms. It has been suggested that an A (K$^+$) current may be coupled to the GABA$_B$ receptor on presynaptic terminals (Saint et al., 1990), particularly since the current is pertussis toxin insensitive. However, despite this evidence for K$^+$ involvement, the hypothesis is not without criticism (*see* Harrison, 1990; Otis et al., 1993). Inhibition of terminal Ca^{++} conductance, first described by Dunlap (1981) and Desarmenien et al. (1984), seems to have a greater acceptance as a presynaptic mechanism for GABA$_B$-mediated suppression of transmitter release. Conversely, postsynaptic GABA$_B$-controlled Ca^{++} conductances have less significance than K$^+$-mediated events. The detection of GABA$_B$ Ca^{++} currents in dorsal root ganglion cells reflects the receptor-mediated events on primary afferent terminals in the spinal cord. GABA$_B$ receptors on these C and A neurons appear to be connected directly via G proteins to N and P, but not L, Ca^{++} channels (Dolphin, 1990). This appears to be the case elsewhere in the brain (Pfrieger et al., 1994; Tareilus et al., 1994; Wall and Dale, 1994), but low-threshold Ca^{++} T-currents, which are inactivated at normal resting membrane potentials, may also be involved in the response to GABA$_B$ receptor activation (Scott et al., 1990), particularly within the thalamus in relation to the generation of Ca^{++} spikes in the production of spontaneous spike and wave discharges associated with generalized epilepsy *(see* Section 6.3.*)*.

5. Physiological Role of GABA$_B$ Receptors

GABA$_B$ receptors have been implicated in a variety of physiological, as well as pharmacological, actions in mammals (Table 3). Both central and peripheral actions have been attributed to GABA$_B$ receptor mechanisms, and include the central control of hormone release, the cardiovascular system, and respiration (*see* Bowery, 1993; Lalley, 1983, Schmid et al., 1989; Amano and Kubo, 1993). The enteric nervous system of the intestine may be a particularly important focus of GABA$_B$ receptor control, possibly arising

Table 3
General Actions Produced by GABA$_B$ Receptor Activation In Vivo and In Vitro

Effect	Locus of action
Smooth muscle relaxation	Lung, bladder, intestine, urinary bladder
Smooth muscle contraction	Uterus, oviduct, gall bladder, some intestine
Antinociception	Spinal cord (higher centers may also be involved)
Neuronal hyperpolarization —long duration	CNS–numerous locations
Long-term potentiation —modulation	Hippocampus
Generation and exacerbation of absence epilepsy	Thalamic nuclei
Inhibition of cognitive function	Higher centers of CNS
Enhanced feeding	Higher centers
Vasopressor action	Nucleus tractus solitarius
Muscle relaxation	Spinal cord
Antitussive action	Cough centre in medulla
Respiratory depression	Brain stem
Insulin/glucagon release	Pancreas
Suppression of CRH and MSH release	Pituitary
Gastrin secretion altered	Vagal center
Inhibition of transmitter release	CNS and peripheral nerve terminals

from the presence of GABA-ergic neurons within the mammalian intestine (*see* Ong and Kerr, 1990). GABA$_B$ receptor activation suppresses intestinal activity although the overall effect depends on the intestinal region (Ong and Kerr, 1987). The lungs may be another locus for GABA$_B$ receptor activation although the evidence for any physiological function seems remote. Nevertheless, the ability of GABA$_B$ agonists to suppress bronchial hyperactivity, as well as to depress the release of acetylcholine and substance P, makes them potentially important as bronchiolar relaxants (Chapman et al., 1993).

Perhaps the most well-studied and documented physiological actions of GABA$_B$ systems within the brain are: first, generation of the late postsynaptic hyperpolarization event, which has been described in many regions, including the cerebral cortex (e.g., Karlsson et al., 1988), hippocampus (e.g., Dutar and Nicoll, 1988a) and thalamus (e.g., Soltesz et al., 1988), and second, the involvement of presynaptic GABA$_B$ autoreceptors in paired-pulse inhibition within the hippocampus (*see* Mott and Lewis, 1994, for a complete review of the electrophysiological events). Both of these events are synaptically mediated and appear to be responsible for modulating postsynaptic excitatory processing. The late hyperpolarization most frequently, if not always, accompanies a fast hyperpolarization produced by activation of $GABA_B$ receptors on the same neuron. $GABA_B$ autoreceptors, $GABA_B$ heteroreceptors on glutamate terminals, and postsynaptic $GABA_B$ sites all participate in determining the final postsynaptic response. Even heteroreceptors probably receive a paracrine-type input from adjacent GABA neurons (Isaacson et al., 1993) to contribute to the overall physiological response. However, until antagonists that truly differentiate between the receptor targets become available, the individual contribution of each component cannot be defined.

The influence of $GABA_B$ receptors on the generation of long term potentiation (LTP) in hippocampal neurons has been noted (Davies et al., 1990; Olpe and Karlsson, 1990; Mott and Lewis, 1991; Burgard and Sarvey, 1991). LTP can be produced in pyramidal neurons by activation of excitatory inputs (i.e., Schaffer collaterals), which mediate the long-term effects via the release of glutamate acting through N-methyl-D-aspartic acid (NMDA) receptors, at least in the initial phase. The release of excitatory amino acid transmitter appears to be modulated by the concomitant release of GABA from interneurons, which activates $GABA_B$, as well as $GABA_A$, receptors. Antagonism of $GABA_B$ autoreceptors alters this release to influence the generation of LTP. However, the nature of this modification appears to depend on the frequency of stimulation employed (Olpe and Karlsson, 1990; Mott and Lewis, 1991; and *see* Mott and Lewis, 1994, for review).

6. Pathological Role of $GABA_B$ Receptors

6.1. Cognition

The significant effects of baclofen and $GABA_B$ antagonists on the generation of LTP in the hippocampal slice might be expected to manifest in vivo as a modification in cognitive function. In fact, this has now been demonstrated in a variety of paradigms. Essentially, baclofen decreases cognitive function whilst $GABA_B$ antagonists not only reverse the deficit produced by baclofen, but can also enhance learning performance when administered alone in rodent and primate models (DeSousa et al., 1994; Stackmann and Walsh, 1994; Carletti et al., 1993; Swartzwelder et al., 1987; Mondadori et al., 1992; Castellano et al., 1989).

6.2. Nociception

Baclofen has antinociceptive activity in acute pain models, such as the tail flick and hot plate tests in rodents (Cutting and Jordan, 1975; Levy and Proudfit, 1977; Wilson and Yaksh, 1978; Aley and Kulkarni, 1991). This effect occurs at doses below the threshold for muscle relaxation, thus an impairment of locomotor activity can be excluded as a confounding reason for the effect.

By contrast, in chronic pain, baclofen fails to produce any antinociceptive activity, although it can be effective in certain cases of trigeminal neuralgia (Fromm et al., 1990; Fromm 1992; Fromm and Terence, 1987; Terence et al., 1985). The antinociceptive action of baclofen in acute pain probably stems from a reduction in the release of nociceptive transmitter from primary afferent fibers within the dorsal horn of the spinal cord (Henry, 1982). However, contribution from an action of baclofen within higher centers of the brain cannot be excluded (Sawynok, 1989).

We have recently shown that $GABA_B$ receptor activation in spinal cord slices prevents the release of substance P, glutamate, and CGRP evoked by electrical stimulation of the dorsal roots (Malcangio and Bowery, 1993b, 1996; Teoh et al., 1996). These three compounds have been associated with the transmission of nociceptive impulses in the spinal cord. Under normal conditions, $GABA_B$ receptor antagonists, administered alone to the preparation, produce little or no increase in transmitter release. However, during chronic inflammation produced by, e.g., complete Freunds adjuvant (monoarthritis), an increase in the concentration of GABA (up to 25% control) occurs in the dorsal horn (Castro-Lopes et al., 1992). This appears to facilitate the $GABA_B$ receptor control of substance P release. When a $GABA_B$ antagonist is now applied to the isolated spinal cord preparation, the evoked release of substance P is dramatically increased (Malcangio and Bowery, 1994). Moreover, when the antagonist is administered to monoarthritic rats, a striking increase in nociception occurs This contrasts markedly with the lack of effect in naive animals. These results suggest that an increase in $GABA_B$ innervation to primary afferent terminals occurs during chronic inflammation and this acts as a pathological antinociceptive process to decrease the enhanced sensory input. It would also provide an explanation for the lack of activity of baclofen in chronic pain caused by the existing maximal receptor activation by endogenous GABA.

6.3. Absence Epilepsy

Perhaps the most fascinating and recently recognized pathological role for $GABA_B$ receptor mechanisms is in the generation of absence epilepsy. Generalized nonconvulsive seizures (absence epilepsy) manifest in man as synchronous 3/s spike and wave discharges that can be detected on the surface of the cerebral cortex. These discharges appear to emanate from the thalamus and are conveyed by the thalamocortical pathway to the cortex. During the seizure periods, locomotor activity ceases, but the individuals do not convulse or lose consciousness. Similar changes can be noted in rodent models of the disorder (Vergnes et al., 1982; Liu et al., 1991; Snead, 1991,1995; Hosford et al., 1992). In these in vivo models, the administration of $GABA_B$ receptor antagonists completely suppresses the seizure discharges and behavioral symptoms (Hosford et al., 1992, 1995; Liu et al., 1992; Marescaux et al., 1992; Snead, 1995). The constancy of this effect has prompted Snead (1995) to include GABA$_B$ receptor antagonism as one of the criteria required for acceptance of a model as predictive of absence epilepsy in man.

The mechanism(s) underlying the production of seizures is still under investigation, but the involvement of the thalamic nuclei seems clear. Crunelli and Leresche (1991) have proposed a plausible explanation for the GABA$_B$ receptor involvement. Synaptic GABA$_B$-mediated late hypopolarizations can be detected in neurons in many brain regions, but only in the thalamus does the prolonged increase in membrane potential give rise to Ca^{++} spikes, presumably caused by deinactivation of Ca^{++} T-currents. Prevention of the hyperpolarization with a GABA$_B$ antagonist will indirectly prevent the Ca^{++} spiking and, presumably, the thalamocortically evoked discharges. Ca^{++} influx in isolated neuron preparations can be produced by GABA$_B$ agonists (Ito et al., 1995), in contrast to the GABA$_B$-mediated reduction in Ca^{++} conductance produced in dorsal root ganglion cells (Dunlap, 1981; Desarmenien et al., 1984). Administration of GABA$_B$ agonists in animal models of absence epilepsy exacerbates the seizure activity (Hosford et al., 1992; Liu et al., 1992), but only occurs if the agonist is administered systemically or by direct injection into the thalamus. Direct injection into other brain regions is without effect. It has been suggested that in the lethargic mouse model of absence, an increase in the number of GABA$_B$ receptors could account for the increase in seizure activity (Lin et al., 1993). However, no evidence for any increase in GABA$_B$ receptor binding sites could be obtained in genetically susceptible rat models, GAERS (Knight and Bowery, 1992), and WAG/Rj (Parry et al., 1996). An alternative possibility is that there is an abnormal increase in the endogenous extracellular GABA concentration, which, though modest, could be sufficient to produce an enhanced hyperpolarization (Richards et al., 1995). This might then provide an explanation for the action of γ-hydroxybutyric acid (GHB), which produces absence-like seizures in rodents (Snead, 1995). If GHB mimics the effect of the endogenous agonist GABA at GABA$_B$ receptors in the thalamus, then GABA$_B$ receptor antagonists would be expected to block the spike and wave discharges produced by GHB, which they do (Snead, 1992; Williams et al., 1995). It has been suggested that GHB is a weak GABA$_B$ receptor agonist under certain circumstances (Bernasconi et al., 1992; Xie and Smart, 1992; Engberg and Wissbrandt, 1993).

7. Therapeutic Significance of GABA$_B$ Ligands

The use of GABA$_B$ ligands in therapeutics is currently restricted to baclofen in the treatment of spasticity and, occasionally, trigeminal neuralgia. The antispastic effect of baclofen is believed to derive from the suppression of excitatory transmitter release to motoneurons in the spinal cord (Fox et al., 1978; Davies, 1981; Wullner et al., 1989), although contributions from postsynaptic effects within the spinal cord and higher centers have been considered (Stefanski et al., 1990; Turski et al., 1990; Azouvi et al., 1993). Nevertheless, it is clear that a spinal site of action is of paramount importance, since intrathecal administration of baclofen is reported to be an effective method for administration of the drug, reducing the incidence of side effects by limiting the level of baclofen outside the spinal cord (Penn et al., 1989; Albright et al., 1991; Penn and Mangieri, 1993).

Other potential uses for GABA$_B$ agonists may be in the treatment of asthma (Chapman et al., 1993), intractable hiccup (Fodstad and Nilsson, 1993; Krahn and Penner, 1994), intestinal disorders (Kerr and Ong, 1995), and alcohol-related disorders, including alcohol withdrawal symptoms (Humeniuk et al., 1993).

The potential therapeutic use of GABA$_B$ receptor antagonists was reviewed in 1993 (Bowery, 1993), when it was concluded that antiabsence epilepsy, cognitive enhancement, antidepressant, anxiolytic, and neuroprotective therapy were all feasible goals. Evidence in support of the first two categories has increased significantly since 1993; few studies have focused on the last three applications, although they are still viable possibilities.

8. Receptor Plasticity

One concern with the chronic use of GABA$_B$ ligands is the possibility of modifications occurring in receptor function. It has been recognized for many years that the response to baclofen, following prolonged treatment for spasticity, diminishes with time. We have examined this phenomenon in detail, using binding studies and functional assays to monitor the changes in GABA$_B$ receptor function following prolonged agonist or antagonis administration.

Within the spinal cord, after 21 d administration of (–)-baclofen (10 mg/kg/d), a marked reduction in the number of GABA$_B$ binding sites occurs; this is coupled with a concomitant reduction in the inhibitory response to (–)-baclofen on the evoked release of substance P and amino acids (Malcangio et al., 1993, 1994). Conversely, administration of a GABA$_B$ antagonist (CGP36742 or CGP46381, 100 mg/kg/d) produced a significant increase in the number of binding sites and the sensitivity to (–)-baclofen on the release of substance P and amino acids.

In the same rats, the evoked response of olfactory neurons to stimulation of the lateral olfactory tract was similarly depressed or enhanced, respectively, by agonist or antagonist administration (Malcangio et al., 1994) (Fig. 1). The

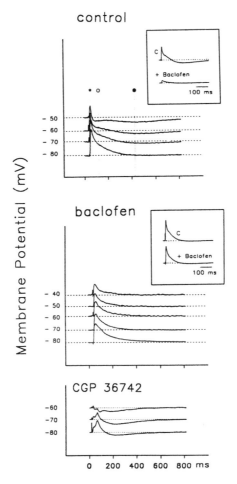

Fig. 1. Postsynaptic potentials recorded in three olfactory cortical neurons from control, (–)-baclofen and CGP 36742 pretreated rats. Rats were given a single daily ip injection of saline (0.1 mL control), (–)baclofen (10 mg/kg) or the $GABA_B$ antagonist, CGP 36742 (100 mg/kg) for 21 d. Twenty-four h after the last injection the rats were sacrificed and the brains removed and placed in Krebs solution (4°C). Intracellular recordings were made from the pyramidal cell layer of olfactory cortex slices (450 μm as described by Libri et al. [1994], *Neuroscience*, **59**, 331–347). Postsynaptic potentials obtained at membrane potentials indicated on the left, were evoked by high-intensity (15V 0.2ms) orthodromic stimulation of layer I. Three distinct peaks of the postsynaptic potential are labeled with an asterisk (EPSP), open circle (fast IPSP) and filled circle (slow IPSP). Insets show the inhibition of postsynaptic potentials by 10 μM (–)-baclofen. Note the absence of slow ipsps after baclofen pretreatment and the enhancement of IPSPs after CGP 36742. (Data kindly prepared by V. Libri.)

hyperpolarizing response to applied (–)-baclofen was similarly affected. We have also noted that prolonged treatment of rats with (–)-baclofen alters the response to neuronal stimulants, such as oxotremorine or metabotropic glutamate receptor agonists. Induction of an epileptiform response occurs that is dependent on the membrane potential (Libri et al., 1995).

Changes in $GABA_B$ receptor function with chronic ligand administration could be of major significance when long-term therapy is considered. Present experience with baclofen in long-term treatment indicates that many side effects can occur, often making the systemic administration of the drug unacceptable. Although these are mainly of acute origin, it is still possible that receptor plasticity may contribute. There is still much to do before we can understand the true significance of these long-term changes. Moreover, these changes may differ throughout the brain. We have recently examined the long-term response to baclofen in GAERS, in which baclofen administered ip produces a marked increase in seizure activity (*see* Section 6.3.). Chronic administration of baclofen (10 mg/kg/once daily) for 40 d failed to alter the acute response to baclofen (T. Lemos and N. G. Bowery, unpublished observations).

9. Final Comments

Much has emerged from studies on the pharmacology of $GABA_B$ receptors in recent years, not least of which has been the advent of selective and potent $GABA_B$ receptor antagonists.

Surely the next step will be the discovery of the receptor structure(s), which will undoubtedly open the research flood-gates, facilitating the potential subtyping of $GABA_B$ receptors. Possibly the most significant goal is the introduction of $GABA_B$ receptor antagonists into clinical practice, since they appear to have considerable potential as effective drugs in CNS disorders.

Acknowledgments

The author is grateful to Carol Wilson and Rita Orgill for typing the manuscript and to the MRC and Wellcome Trust for financial support.

References

Albright, A. L., Cervi, A., and Singletary, J. (1991) Intrathecal baclofen for spasticity in cerebral palsy. *J. Am. Med. Assoc.* **265,** 1418–1422.
Aley, K. O. and Kulkarni, S. K. (1991) Baclofen analgesia in mice: a $GABA_B$-mediated response. *Methods Find. Exp. Clin. Pharmacol.* **13,** 681–686.
Alford, S. and Grillner, S. (1991) The involvement of $GABA_B$ receptors and coupled G-proteins in spinal GABAergic presynaptic inhibition. *J. Neurosci.* **11,** 3718–3726.

Alger, B. E. and Nicoll, R. A. (1982) Pharmacological evidence for two kinds of GABA receptor on rat hippocampal pyramidal cells studied in vitro. *J. Physiol.* **328**, 125–141.

Amano, M. and Kubo, T. (1993) Involvement of both GABA$_A$ and GABA$_B$ receptors in tonic inhibitory control of blood pressure at the rostral ventrolateral medulla of the rat. *Naunyn Schmiedebergs Arch. Pharmacol.* **348**, 146–153.

Andrade, R., Malenka, R. C., and Nicoll, R. A. (1986) A G protein couples serotonin and GABA$_B$ receptors to the same channels in hippocampus. *Science* **234**, 1261–1265.

Arenas, E., Marsal, J., and Alberch, J. (1990) GABA$_A$ and GABA$_B$ antagonists prevent the opioid inhibition of endogenous acetylcholine release evoked by glutamate from rat neostriatal slices. *Neurosci. Lett.* **120**, 201–204.

Azouvi, P., Roby-Brami, A., Biraber, A., Thiebaut, J. B., Thurel, C., and Bussel, B. (1993) Effects of intrathecal baclofen on the monosynaptic reflex in humans: evidence for a postsynaptic action. *J. Neurol. Neurosurg. Psychiatry* **56**, 515–519.

Bein, H. J. (1972) Pharmacological differentiation of muscle relaxants, in *Spasticity—A Topical Survey* (Birkmayer, W., ed.), Huber, Vienna, pp. 76–82.

Benardo, L. S. (1994) Separate activation of fast and slow inhibitory post-synaptic potentials in rat neocortex *in vitro*. *J. Physiol. (Lond.)* **476**, 203–215.

Benoliel, J. J., Bourgoin, S., Mauborgne, A., Pohl, M., Legrand, J.C., Hamon, M., and Cesselin, F. (1992) GABA, acting at both GABA$_A$ and GABA$_B$ receptors, inhibits the release of cholecystokinin-like material from the rat spinal cord *in vitro*. *Brain Res.* **590**, 255–262.

Bernasconi, R., Lauber, J., Marescaux, C., Vergnes, M., Markin, P., Rubic, V., Leonchardt, T., Reymann, N., and Bittiger, H. (1992) Experimental absence seizures: potential role of gamma-hydroxybutyric acid and GABA$_B$ receptors. *J. Neurol. Trans.* **35(Suppl.),** 155–177.

Bernasconi, R., Mathivet, P., Marescaux, C., Leonhardt, T., Martin, P., Mickel, S., and Froestl., W. (1994) NMDA receptors and No synthase (Nos) are involved in the increase of cerebral cGMP induced by the GABA$_B$ antagonists. *Br. J. Pharmacol.* **112,** 7P.

Bolser, D. C., Blythin, D. J., Chapman, R. W., Egan, R. W., Hey, J. A., Rizzo, C., Kuo, S.-C., and Kreutner, W. (1995) The pharmacology of SCH 50911 a novel: orally-active GABA-B receptor antagonist. *J. Pharmacol. Exp. Ther.* **274**, 1393–1398.

Bonanno, G. and Raiteri, M. (1993) Multiple GABA$_B$ receptors. *Trends Pharmacol. Sci.* **14**, 259–261.

Bowery, N. G. (1993) GABA$_B$ receptor pharmacology. *Annu. Rev. Pharmacol. Toxicol.* **33**, 109–147.

Bowery, N. G., Doble, A., Hill, D. R., Hudson, A. L., Shaw, J. S., Turnbull, M. J., and Warrington, R. (1981) Bicuculline-insensitive GABA receptors on peripheral autonomic nerve terminals. *Eur. J. Pharmacol.* **71,** 53–70.

Bowery, N. G., Hill, D. R., Hudson, A. L. Doble, A. Middlemiss, D. N., Shaw, J., and Turnbull, M. (1980) (–)Baclofen decreases neurotransmitter release in the mammalian CNS by an action at a novel GABA receptor. *Nature* **283**, 92–94.

Bowery, N. G., Hudson, A. L., and Price G. W. (1987) GABA$_A$ and GABA$_B$ receptor site distribution in the rat central nervous system. *Neuroscience* **20**, 365–383.

Burgard, E. C. and Sarvey, J. M. (1991) Long-lasting potentiation and epilepti-form activity produced by GABA$_B$ receptor activation in the dentate gyrus of rat hippocampal slice. *Neuroscience* **11,** 1198–209.

Carletti, R., Libri, V., and Bowery N. G. (1993) The $GABA_B$ antagonist CGP36742 enhances spatial learning performance and antagonises baclofen-induced amnesia in mice. *Br. J. Pharmacol.* **109,** 74p.

Castellano, C., Brioni, J. D., Nagahara, A. H., and McGaugh, J. L. (1989) Post-training systemic and intra-amygdala administration of the $GABA_B$ agonist baclofen impairs retention. *Behav. Neural Biol.* **52,** 170–179.

Castro-Lopes, J. M., Tavares, I., Tolle, T. R., Coito, A., and Coimbra, A. (1992) Increase in GABAergic cells and GABA levels in the spinal cord in unilateral inflammation of the hindlimb of the rat. *Eur. J. Neurosci.* **4,** 296–301.

Chapman, R. W., Hey, J. A., Rizzo, C. A. and Bolser, D. C. (1993) $GABA_B$ receptors in the lung. *Trends Pharmacol. Sci.* **14,** 26–29.

Chu, D. C. M., Albin, R. L., Young, A. B., and Penney, J. B. (1990) Distribution and kinetics of $GABA_B$ binding sites in rat central nervous system: a quantitative autoradiographic study. *Neuroscience* **34,** 341–357.

Colmers, W. F. and Williams, J. T. (1988) Pertussis toxin pretreatment discriminates between pre- and postsynaptic actions of baclofen in rat dorsal raphe nucleus in vitro. *Neurosci. Lett.* **93,** 300–306.

Crunelli, V. and Leresche, N. (1991) A role for $GABA_B$ receptors in excitation and inhibition of thalamocortical cells. *Trends Neurosci.* **14,** 16–21.

Curtis, D. R., Gynther, B. D., Beattie, D. T., Kerr, D. I. B., and Prager, R. H. (1988) Baclofen antagonism by 2-hydroxy-saclofen in the cat spinal cord. *Neurosci. Lett.* **92,** 97–101.

Cutting, D. A. and Jordan, C. C. (1975) Alternative approaches to analgesia: baclofen as a model compound. *Br. J. Pharmacol.* **54,** 171–179.

Davies, C. H., Davies, S. N., and Collingridge, G. L. (1990) Paired-pulse depression of monosynaptic GABA-mediated inhibitory postsynaptic responses in rat hippocampus. *J. Physiol.* **424,** 513–531.

Davies, J. (1981) Selective depression of synaptic excitation in cat spinal neurones by baclofen: an iontophoretic study. *Br. J. Pharmacol.* **72,** 373–384.

Deisz, R., Billard, J. M., Zieglgänsberger, W. (1992) Evidence for two types of $GABA_B$ receptors located pre- and postsynaptically in the rat neocortical slice in vitro. *J. Physiol.* **446,** 514P.

Deisz, R. A., Billard, J. M., and Zieglgänsberger, W. (1993) Pre and postsynaptic $GABA_B$ receptors of rat neocortical neurons differ in their pharmacological properties. *Neurosci. Lett.* **154,** 209–212.

Desarmenien, M., Feltz, P., Occhipinti, G., Santangelo, F., and Schlichter, R. (1984) Coexistence of $GABA_A$ and $GABA_B$ receptors on A and C primary afferents. *Br. J. Pharmacol.* **81,** 327–333.

DeSousa, N. J. Beninger, R., Jhamandas, K., and Boegman, R. J. (1994) Stimulation of $GABA_B$ receptors in the basal forebrain selectivity impairs working memory of rats in the double Y-maze. *Brain Res.* **641,** 29–38.

Dickenson, H. W., Allan, R. D., Ong, J., and Johnston, G. A. R. (1988) $GABA_B$ receptor antagonist and $GABA_A$ receptor agonist properties of a δ-aminovaleric acid derivative, Z-5-aminopent-2-enoic acid. *Neurosci. Lett.* **86,** 351–355.

Dolphin, A. C. (1990) G protein modulation of calcium current in neurons. *Annu. Rev. Physiol.* **52,** 243–255.

Dunlap, K. (1981) Two types of γ-aminobutyric acid receptor on embryonic sensory neurons. *Br. J. Pharmacol.* **74,** 579–585.

Dutar, P. and Nicoll, R. A. (1988a) A physiological role for GABA_B receptors in the central nervous system. *Nature* **332,** 156–158.

Dutar, P. and Nicoll, R. A. (1988b) Pre- and postsynaptic GABA_B receptors in the hippocampus have different pharmacological properties. *Neuron* **1,** 585–598.

Engberg, G. and Wissbrandt, H. (1993) Gamma-hydroxybutyric acid (GHBA) induces pacemaker activity and inhibition of substantia nigra dopamine neurons by activating GABA_B receptors. *Naunyn Schmiedebergs Arch. Pharmacol.* **348,** 491–497.

Erdö, S. L. and Bowery, N. G., eds. (1986) *GABAergic Mechanisms in the Mammalian Periphery,* Raven, New York.

Erdö, S. L. (1986) GABAergic mechanisms and their possible role in the oviduct and the uterus, in *GABAergic Mechanisms in the Mammalian Periphery* (Erdö, S. L. and Bowery, N. G., eds.), Raven, New York, pp. 205–222.

Fodstad, H. and Nilsson, S. (1993) Intractable singultus: a diagnostic and therapeutic challenge. *Brit. J. Neurosurg.* **7,** 255–260.

Fox, S., Krnjevic, K., Morris, M. E., Puil, E., and Werman, P. (1978) Action of baclofen on mammalian synaptic transmission. *Neuroscience* **3,** 445–515.

Fraser, D. D., Mudrick-Donnan, L. A., and MacVicar, B. A. (1994) Astrocytic GABA receptors. *Glia* **11,** 83–93.

Froestl, W., Mickel, S. J., Hall, R. G., von Sprecher, G., Strub, D., Baumann, P. A., Brugger, F., Gentsch, C., Jaekel, J., Olpe, H.-R., Rihs, G., Vassout, A., Waldmeier, P. C., and Bittiger, H. (1995a) A phosphinic acid analogues of GABA. 1. New potent and selective GABA_B agonists. *J. Med. Chem.* **38,** 3297–3312.

Froestl, W., Mickel, S. J., von Sprecher, G., Diel, P., Hall, R. G., Maier, L., Strub, D., Melillo, V., Baumann, P. A., Bernasconi, R., Gentsch, C., Hauser, K., Jaekel, J., Karlsson, G., Klebs, K., Maître, L., Marescaux, C., Pozza, M. F., Schmutz, M., Steinmann, M. W., van Riezen, H., Vassout, A., Mondadori, C., Olpe, H.-R., Waldmeier, P. C., and Bittiger, H. (1995b) Phosphinic acid analogues of GABA. 2. Selective, orally active GABA_B antagonists. *J. Med. Chem.* **38,** 3313–3331.

Fromm, G. H. (1992) Therapeutic applications of baclofen. *Pharmacol. Commun.* **2,** 132–137.

Fromm, G. G., Shibuya, T., Nakata, M., and Terrence, C.F. (1990) Effects of d-baclofen and l-baclofen on the trigeminal nucleus. *Neuropharmacology* **29,** 249–254.

Fromm, G. H. and Terence, C. F. (1987) Comparison of L-baclofen and racemic baclofen in trigeminal neuralgia. *Neurology* **37,** 1725–1728.

Frydenvang, K., Frolund, B., Kristiansen, U., and Krogsgaard-Larsen, P. (1996) Stereospecific GABA_B receptor antagonism, in *GABA: Receptors, Transporters and Metabolism* (Tanaka, C. and Bowery, N. G., eds.), Birkhauser, Basel, pp. 243–253.

Gähwiler, B. H. and Brown, D. A. (1985) GABA_B-receptor-activated K^+ current in voltage-clamped CA_3 pyramidal cells in hippocampal cultures. *Proc. Natl. Acad. Sci. USA* **82,** 1558–1562.

Gallagher, J. P., Stevens, D. R., and Shinnick-Gallagher, P. (1984) Actions of GABA and baclofen on neurons of the dorsolateral septal nucleus (DLSN) in vitro. *Neuropharmacology* **23,** 825,826.

Gemignani, A., Paudice, P., Bonanno, G., and Raiteri, M. (1994) Pharmacological discrimination between γ-aminobutyric acid Type B receptors regulating cholecystokinin and somatostatin release from rat neocortex synaptosomes. *Mol. Pharmacol.* **45,** 558–562.

Giotti, A., Luzzi, S., Spagnesi, S., and Zilletti, L. (1983a) GABA_A and GABA_B receptor-mediated effects in guinea-pig ileum. *Br. J. Pharmacol.* **78,** 469–478.

Giotti, A., Luzzi, S., Spagnesi, S., and Zilletti, L. (1983b) Homotaurine: a GABA$_B$ antagonist in guinea-pig ileum. *Br. J. Pharmacol.* **79,** 855–862.

Giotti, A., Luzzi, S., Maggi, C. A., Spagnesi, S., and Zilletti, L. (1985) Modulatory activity of GABA$_B$ receptors on cholinergic tone in guinea-pig distal colon. *Br. J. Pharmacol.* **84,** 883–895.

Gray, J. and Green, A. R. (1987) GABA$_B$ receptor-mediated inhibition of potassium-evoked release of endogenous 5-hydroxytryptamine from mouse frontal cortex. *Br. J. Pharmacol.* **91,** 517–522.

Harrison, N. L. (1990) On the presynaptic action of baclofen at inhibitory synapses between cultured rat hippocampal neurones. *J. Physiol.* **422,** 433–446.

Harrison, N. L., Lange, G. D., and Barker, J. L. (1988) (–) Baclofen activates presynaptic GABA$_B$ receptors on GABAergic inhibitor neurons from embryonic rat hippocampus. *Neurosci. Lett.* **85,** 105–109.

Henry, J. L. (1982) Effects of intravenously administered enantiomers of baclofen on functionally identified units in lumbar dorsal horn of the spinal cat. *Neuropharmacology* **21,** 1073–1083.

Hill, D. R. (1985) GABA$_B$ receptor modulation of adenylate cyclase activity in rat brain slices. *Br. J. Pharmacol.* **84,** 249–257.

Hill, D. R. and Bowery, N. G. (1981) ^{3}H-Baclofen and ^{3}H-GABA bind to bicuculline-insensitive GABA$_B$ sites in rat brain. *Nature* **290,** 149–152.

Hill, D. R., Bowery, N. G., and Hudson, A. L. (1984) Inhibition of GABA$_B$ receptor binding by guanyl nucleotides. *J. Neurochem.* **42,** 652–657.

Hosford, D. A., Clark, S., Cao, Z., Wilson, W. A., Lin, F.-H., Morrisett, R. A., and Huin, A. (1992) The role of GABA$_B$ receptor activation in absence seizures of lethargic (1h/1h) mice. *Science* **257,** 398–401.

Hosford, D. A., Wang, Y., Liu, C. C., and Snead, O. C. (1995) Characterization of the antiabsence effects of SCH 50911, a GABA$_B$ receptor antagonist, in the lethargic mouse, γ-hydroxybutyrate, and pentylenetetrazole models. *J. Pharmacol. Exp. Ther.* **274,** 1399–1403.

Hosli, L., Hosli, E., Redle, S., Rojas, J., and Schramek, H. (1990) Action of baclofen, GABA and antagonists on the membrane potential of cultured astrocytes of rat spinal cord. *Neurosci. Lett.* **117,** 307–312.

Howson, W., Mistry, J., Broekman, M., and Hills, J. M. (1993) Biological activity of 3-aminopropyl(methyl) phosphinic acid, a potent and selective GABA$_B$ agonist with CNS activity. *Bioorganic Med. Chem. Lett.* **3,** 515–518.

Humenuik, R. E., Ong, J., Kerr, D. I. B., and White, J. M. (1993) The role of GABA$_B$ antagonists in mediating the effects of ethanol in mice. *Psychopharmacology* **III,** 219–224.

Isaacson, J. S., Solis, J. M., and Nicoll, R. A. (1993) Local and diffuse synaptic actions of GABA in the hippocampus. *Neuron* **10,** 165–175.

Ito, Y., Ishige, K., Zaitsu, E., Anzai, K., and Fukuda, H. (1995) γ-Hydroxybutyric acid increases intracellular Ca2+ concentration and nuclear cyclic AMP-responsive element- and activator protein 1 DNA-binding activities through GABA$_B$ receptor in cultured cerebellar granule cells. *J. Neurochem.* **65,** 75–83.

Jarolimek, W., Bijak, M., and Misgeld, U. (P992) GABA and baclofen activate K$^+$ conductance of central neurons through different receptors. *Pharmacol. Commun.* **2,** 49.

Jessen, K. R. (1990) GABAergic neurons in the myenteric plexus, in *GABA Outside the CNS* (Erdö, S. L., ed.), Springer-Verlag, New York, pp. 19–27.

Jessen, K. R., Mirsky, R., Dennison, M. E., and Burnstock, G. (1979) GABA may be a neurotransmitter in the vertebrate peripheral nervous system. *Nature* **281**, 71–74.

Johnston, G. A. R. (1995) GABA receptor pharmacology, in *Pharmacological Sciences: Perspectives for Research and Therapy in the Late 1990s* (Cuello, A. C. and Collier, B., eds.), Birkhauser Verlag, Basel, pp. 11–16.

Kangra, I., Minchun, J., and Randic, M. (1991) Actions of (–) baclofen on rat dorsal horn neurons. *Brain Res.* **562**, 265–75.

Karbon, E. W., Duman, R. S., and Enna, S. J. (1984) GABA_B receptors and norepinephrine-stimuated cAMP production in rat brain cortex. *Brain Res.* **306**, 327–332.

Karlsson, G., Pozza, M., and Olpe, H.-R. (1988) Phaclofen: a GABA_B blocker reduces long-duration inhibition in the neocortex. *Eur. J. Pharmacol.* **148**, 485,486.

Kawai, K. and Unger, R. H. (1983) Effects of γ-aminobutyric acid on insulin, glucagon and somatostatin release from isolated perfused dog pancreas. *Endocrinology* **113**, 111–113.

Keberle, H. and Faigle, J. W. (1972) Synthesis and structure-activity relationships of the γ-aminobutyric acid derivatives, in *Spasticity—A Topical Survey* (Birkmayer, J. W., ed.), Hans Huber, Vienna, pp. 90–93.

Kerr, D. I. B. and Ong, J. (1995) GABA_B receptors. *Pharmacol. Ther.* **67**, 187–246.

Kerr, D. I. B., Ong, J., and Prager, R. H. (1986) Antagonism of peripheral GABA_B receptors by phaclofen, the phosphono-analogue of baclofen, in the guinea-pig isolated ileum. *Proc. Aust. Physiol. Pharmacol. Soc.* **17**, 114P.

Kerr, D. I. B., Ong, J., and Prager, R. H. (1990) Antagonism of GABA_B receptor-mediated responses in the guinea-pig isolated ileum and vas deferens by phosphono-analogues of GABA. *Br. J. Pharmacol.* **99**, 422–426.

Kerr, D. I. B., Ong, J., Prager, R. H., Gynther, B. D., and Curtis, D. R. (1987) Phaclofen: a peripheral and central baclofen antagonist. *Brain Res.* **405**, 150–154.

Kimura, T., Saunders, P. A., Kim, H. S., Rheu, H. M., Oh, K. W., and Ho, I. K. (1994) Interactions of ginsenosides with ligand binding of GABA_A and GABA_B receptors. *Gen. Pharmacol.* **25**, 193–199.

Kleinrok, A. and Kilbinger, H. (1983) γ-Aminobutyric acid and cholinergic transmission in the guinea-pig ileum. *Naunyn Schmiedebergs Arch. Pharmacol.* **322**, 216–220.

Knight, A. R. and Bowery, N. G. (1992) GABA receptors in rats with spontaneous generalized non-convulsive epilepsy. *J. Neural Transm.* **35(Suppl.)**, 189–196.

Knott, C., Maguire, J. J., and Bowery, N. G. (1993) Age-related regional sensitivity to pertussis toxin-mediated reduction in GABA_B receptor binding in rat brain. *Mol. Brain Res.* **18**, 353–357.

Krahn, A. and Penner, S. B. (1994) Use of baclofen for intractable hiccups in uremia. *Am. J. Med.* **96**, 391.

Lacey, M. G., Mercuri, N. B., and North, R. A. (1988) On the potassium conductance increase activated by GABA_B and dopamine D2 receptors in rat substantia nigra neurones. *J. Physiol.* **401**, 437–453.

Lalley, P. M. (1983) Biphasic effects of baclofen on phrenic motoneurons: possible involvement of two types of γ-aminobutyric acid (GABA) receptors. *J. Pharmacol. Exp. Ther.* **226**, 616–624.

Lambert, N. A., Harrison, N. L., Kerr, D. I. B., Ong, J., Prager, R. H., and Teyler, T. J. (1989) Blockade of the late IPSP in rat CA1 hippocampal neurons by 2-hydroxy-saclofen. *Neurosci. Lett.* **107**, 125–128.

Lambert, N. A. and Wilson, W. A. (1993) Discrimination of post and presynaptic GABA$_B$ receptor mediated responses by tetrahydroaminoacridine in area CA3 of the rat hippocampus. *J. Neurophysiol.* **69**, 630–635.

Lanza, M., Fassio, A., Gemignani, A., Bonanno, G., and Raiteri, M. (1993) CGP 52432: a novel potent and selective GABA$_B$ autoreceptor antagonist in rat cerebral cortex. *Eur. J. Pharmacol.* **237**, 191–195.

Levy, R. A. and Proudfit, H. K. (1977) The analgesic action of baclofen [-(4-chlorophenyl)-γ-aminobutyric acid]. *J. Pharmacol. Exp. Ther.* **202**, 437–445.

Libri, V., Constanti, A., and Bowery, N. G. (1995) GABA$_B$ receptor down-regulation facilitates muscarinic or metabotropic agonist-dependent burst firing in rat olfactory cortical neurones, in vitro. *Br. J. Pharmacol.* **116**, 332P.

Lin, F.-H., Cao, Z., and Hosford, D. A. (1993) Increased number of GABA$_B$ receptors in the lethargic (1h/1h) mouse model of absence epilepsy. *Brain Res.* **608**, 101–106.

Liu, Z., Vergnes, M., Depaulis, A., and Marescaux, C. (1991) Evidence for a critical role of GABAergic transmission within the thalamus in the genesis and control of absence seizures in the rat. *Brain Res.* **545**, 1–7.

Liu, Z., Vergnes, M., Depaulis, A., and Marescaux, C. (1992) Involvement of intrathalamic GABA$_B$ transmission in the control of absence seizures in the rat. *Neuroscience* **48,** 87–93.

Malcangio, M. and Bowery, N. G. (1993a) GABA$_B$ receptor-mediated inhibition of forskolin-stimulated cyclic AMP accumulation in rat spinal cord. *Neurosci. Lett.* **158,** 189–192.

Malcangio, M. and Bowery, N. G. (1993b) Gamma-aminobutyric acid$_B$ but not gamma-amino butyric and acid A receptor activation inhibits electrically evoked substance P-like immunoreactivity release from the rat spinal cord in vitro. *J. Pharmacol. Exp. Ther.* **266**, 1490–1496.

Malcangio, M. and Bowery, N. G. (1994) Spinal cord SP release and hyperalgesia in monoarthritic rats: involvement of the GABA$_B$ receptor system. *Br. J. Pharmacol.* **113,** 1561–1566.

Malcangio, M. and Bowery, N.G. (1996) Calcitonin gene-related peptide content, basal outflow and electrically evoked release from monoarthritic rat spinal cord in vitro. *Pain* (in press).

Malcangio, M., DaSilva, H., and Bowery, N. G. (1993) Plasticity of GABA$_B$ receptor in rat spinal cord detected by autoradiography. *Eur. J. Pharmacol.* **250**, 153–156.

Malcangio, M., Libri, V., Teoh, H., Constanti, A., and Bowery, N. G. (1995) Chronic (–)baclofen or CGP 36742 alters GABA$_B$ receptor sensitivity in rat brain and spinal cord. *Neuroreport* **6**, 339–403.

Marescaux, C., Vergnes, M., and Bernasconi, R. (1992) GABA$_B$ receptor antagonists: potential new anti-absence drugs. *J. Neural Transm.* **(35) Suppl,** 347–369.

Mondadori, C., Preiswerk, G., and Jaekel, J. (1992) Treatment with a GABA$_B$ receptor blocker improves the cognitive performance of mice, rats and rhesus monkeys. *Pharmacol. Commun.* **2,** 93–97.

Mott, D. D. and Lewis, D. L. (1994) The pharmacology and function of GABA$_B$ receptors. *Int. Rev. Neurobiol.* **36,** 97–223.

Mott, D. D. and Lewis, D. V. (1991) Facilitation of the induction of long term potentiation by GABA$_B$ receptors. *Science* **252**, 1718–1720.

Muhyaddin, M., Roberts, P. J., and Woodruff, G. N. (1982) Presynaptic γ-aminobutyric acid receptors in the rat anococcygeus muscle and their antagonism by 5-aminovaleric acid. *Br. J. Pharmacol.* **77**, 163–168.

Nakayasu, H., Nishikawa, M., Mizutani, H., Kimura, H., and Kuriyama, K. (1993) Immunoaffinity purification and characterization of γ-aminobutyric acid $(GABA)_B$ receptor from bovine cerebral crotex. *J. Biol. Chem.* **268,** 8658–8664.

Newberry, N. R. and Nicoll, R. A. (1984) Direct hyperpolarizing action of baclofen on hippocampal pyramidal cells. *Nature* **308,** 450–452.

Olpe, H.-R. and Karlsson, G. (1990) The effects of baclofen and two $GABA_B$ receptor antagonists on long term potentiation. *Naunyn Schmiedebergs Arch. Pharmakol.* **342,** 194–197.

Olpe, H.-R., Karlsson, G., Pozza, M. F., Brugger, F., Steinmann, M., Van Riezen, H., Fagg, G., Hall, R. G., Froestl, W., and Bittiger, H. (1990) CGP 35348: a centrally active blocker of $GABA_B$ receptors. *Eur. J. Pharmacol.* **187,** 27–38.

Olpe, H.-R., Steinmann, M. W., Ferrat, T., Pozza, M. F., Greiner, K., Brugger, F., Froestl, W., Mickel, S. J., and Bittiger, H. (1993) The actions of orally active $GABA_B$ receptor antagonists on GABAergic transmission in vivo and in vitro. *Eur. J. Pharmacol.* **233,** 179–186.

Olsen, R. W. and Tobin, A. J. (1990) Molecular biology of $GABA_A$ receptors. *FASEB J.* **4,** 1469–1480.

Ong, J. and Kerr, D. I. (1994) Suppression of $GABA_B$ receptor function in rat neocortical slices by amiloride. *Eur. J. Pharmacol.* **260,** 73–77.

Ong, J. and Kerr, D. I. B. (1983) $GABA_A$- and $GABA_B$-receptor-mediated modification of intestinal motility. *Eur. J. Pharmacol.* **86,** 9–17.

Ong, J. and Kerr, D. I. B. (1987) Comparison of GABA-induced responses in various segments of the guinea-pig intestine. *Eur. J. Pharmacol.* **134,** 349–353.

Ong, J. and Kerr, D. I. B. (1990) GABA receptors in peripheral tissues. *Life Sci.* **46,** 1489–1501.

Otis, T. S., De Koninck, Y., and Mody, I. (1993) Characterization of synaptically elicited $GABA_B$ responses using patch-clamp recordings in rat hippocampal slices. *J. Physiol.* **463,** 391–407.

Parkman, H. P., Stapelfeldt, W. H., Williams, C. L., Lennon, V. A,. and Szurszewski, J. H. (1993) Enteric GABA-containing nerves projecting to the guinea-pig inferior mesenteric ganglion modulate acetylcholine release. *J. Physiol.* **471,** 191–207.

Parry, K. P., Drinkenburg, W. H. I. M., and Bowery, N. G. (1996) Lack of alteration of $GABA_B$ receptor binding in the absence epileptic WAG/Rij strain of rat. *Br. J. Pharmacol.* (in press).

Penn, R. D. and Mangieri, E. A. (1993) Stiff-man syndrome treated with intrathecal baclofen. *Neurology* **43,** 2412.

Penn, R. D., Savoy, S. M., Corcos, D., Latash, M., Gottlieb, G., et al. (1989) Intrathecal baclofen for severe spinal spasticity. *N. Engl. J. Med.* **320,** 1517–1521.

Pfrieger, F. W., Gottmann, K., and Lux, H. D. (1994) Kinetics of $GABA_B$ receptor- mediated inhibition of calcium currents and excitatory synaptic transmission in hippocampal neurons in vitro. *Neuron* **12,** 97–107.

Pittaluga, A., Asaro, D., Pettegrinni, G., and Raiteri, M. (1987) Studies of ^{3}H-GABA and endogenous GABA release in rat cerebral cortex suggest the presence of autoreceptors of the $GABA_B$ type. *Eur. J. Pharmacol.* **144,** 45–52.

Potashner, S. J. (1978) Baclofen: effect on amino acid release. *Can. J. Physiol. Pharmacol.* **56,** 150–154.

Potashner, S. J. (1979) Baclofen: effects on amino acid release and metabolism in slices of guinea-pig cerebral cortex. *J. Neurochem.* **32,** 103–109.

Potier, B. and Dutar, P. (1993) Presynaptic inhibitory effect of baclofen on hippocampal inhibitory synaptic transmission involves a pertussis toxin-sensitive G-protein. *Eur. J. Pharmacol.* **231**, 427–433.

Premkumar, L. S. and Gage, P. W. (1994) Potassium channels activated by $GABA_B$ agonists and serotonin in cultured hippocampal neurons. *J. Neurophysiol.* **71**, 2570–2575.

Price, G. W., Blackburn, T. P., Hudson, A. L., and Bowery, N. G. (1984) Presynaptic $GABA_B$ sites in the interpeduncular nucleus. *Neuropharmacology* **23**, 861–862.

Price, G. W., Kelly, J. S., and Bowery, N. G. (1987) The location of $GABA_B$ receptor binding sites in mammalian spinal cord. *Synapse* **1**, 530–538.

Raiteri, M. (1992) Subtypes of $GABA_B$ receptor regulating the release of central neurotransmitters. *Pharmacol. Commun.* **2**, 1–3.

Raiteri, M., Giralt, M. T., Bonanno, G., Pittaluga, A., Fedele, E., and Fontana, G (1990) Release-regulating GABA autoreceptors in human and rat central nervous system, in *GABA_B Receptors in Mammalian Function* (Bowery, N. G., Bittiger, H., and Olpe H.-R., eds.), Wiley, Chichester, UK, pp. 81–98.

Ray, N. J., Jones, A. J., and Keen, P. (1991) $GABA_B$ receptor modulation of the release of substance P from capsaicin-sensitive neurons in the rat trachea *in vitro. Br. J. Pharmacol.* **102**, 801–804.

Rosenstein, R. E., Chuluyan, H. E., and Cardinali, D. P. (1990) Presynaptic effects of gamma-aminobutyric acid on norepinephrine release and uptake in rat pineal gland. *J. Neural Transm.* **82**, 131–140.

Reimann, W., Zwimstein, D., and Starke, K. (1982) γ-Aminobutyric acid can both inhibit and facilitate dopamine release in the cauclate nucleus of the rabbit. *J. Neurochem.* **39**, 961–969.

Richards, D. A., Lemos, T., Whitton, P. S., and Bowery N. G. (1995) Extracellular GABA in the ventrolateral thalamus of rats exhibiting spontaneous absence epilepsy: a microdialysis study. *J. Neurochem.* **65**, 1674–1680.

Robertson, B. and Taylor, R. (1986) Effects of γ-aminobutyric acid and (–) baclofen on calcium and potassium currents in cat dorsal root ganglion neurones in vitro. *Br. J. Pharmacol.* **89**, 661–672.

Saint, D. A., Thomas, T., and Gage, P. W. (1990) $GABA_B$ agonists modulate a transient potassium current in cultured mammalian hippocampal neurons. *Neurosci. Lett.* **188**, 9–13.

Santos, A. E., Carvalho, C. M., Macedo, T. A., and Carvalho, A. P. (1995) Regulation of intracellular $[Ca^{2+}]$ and GABA release by presynaptic $GABA_B$ receptors in rat cerebrocortical synaptosomes. *Neurochem. Int.* **27**.

Sawynok. J. (1989) GABAergic agents as analgesics, in *GABA: Basic Research and Clinical Applications* (Bowery, N. G. and Nistico, G., eds.), Pythagora, Rome, pp. 383–399.

Scherer, R. W., Ferkany, J. W. Enna, S. J. (1988) Evidence for pharmacologically distinct subsets of $GABA_B$ receptors. *Brain Res. Bull.* **21**, 439–443.

Schlicker, E., Classen, K., and Gothert, M. (1984) $GABA_B$ receptor-mediated inhibition of serotonin release in the rat brain. *Naunyn Schmeidebergs Arch. Pharmacol.* **326**, 99–105.

Schmid, K., Bohmer, G., and Gebauer, K. (1989) $GABA_B$ receptor mediated effects on central respiratory system and their antagonism by phaclofen. *Neurosci. Lett.* **99**, 305–310.

Scott, R. H., Wootton, J. F., and Dolphin, A. C. (1990) Modulaltion of neuronal T-type calcium channel currents by photoactivation of intracellular guanosine 5'-0(3-thio) triphosphate. *Neuroscience* **38**, 285–294.

Seabrook, G. R., Howson, W., and Lacey, M. G. (1990) Electrophysiological character-ization of potent agonists and antagonists at pre- and postsynaptic $GABA_B$ receptors on neurones in rat brain slices. *Br. J. Pharmacol.* **101,** 949–957.

Sekiguchi, M., Sakuta, H., Okamoto, K., and Sakai, Y. (1990) $GABA_B$ receptors expressed in *Xenopus* oocytes by guinea pig cerebral mRNA are functionally coupled with Ca^{2+} dependent Cl^- channels and with K^+ channels, through GTP-binding proteins. *Mol. Brain Res.* **8,** 301–309.

Shirakawa, J., Taniyama, K., and Tanaka, C. (1987) Gamma-aminobutyric acid-induced modulation of acetylcholine release from the guinea pig lung. *J. Pharmacol. Exp. Ther.* **243,** 364–369.

Snead, O. C. (1991) The γ-hydroxybutyrate model of absence seizures; correlation of regional brain levels of γ-hydroxybutyric acid and γ-butyrolactone with spike wave discharges. *Neuropharmacology* **30,** 161–67.

Snead, O. C. (1995) Basic mechanisms of generalized absence epilepsy. *Ann. Neurol.* **37,** 146–157.

Soltesz, I., Haby, M., Leresche, N., and Crunelli, V. (1988) The $GABA_B$ antagonist phaclofen inhibits the late K^+-dependent IPSP in cat and rat thalamic and hippocampal neurones. *Brain Res.* **448,** 351–354.

Stackman, R. W. and Walsh, T. J. (1994) Baclofen produces dose related working memory impairments after intraseptal injection. *Behav. Neural Biol.* **61,** 181–185.

Stefanski, R., Plaznik, A. Palejko, W., and Kostowski, W. (1990) Myorelaxant effect of baclofen injected to the nucleus accumbens septi. *J. Neural Transm. Parkinsons Dis. Dementia Sect.* **2,** 179–191.

Stuart, G. J. and Redman, S. J. (1992) The role of $GABA_A$ and $GABA_B$ receptors in presynaptic inhibition of 1a EPSPs in cat spinal motoneurones. *J. Physiol. (Lond.)* **447,** 675–692.

Swartzwelder, H. S., Lewis, D. V., Anderson, W. W., Wilson, W. A. (1987) Seizure-like events in brain slices: suppression by interictal activity. *Brain Res.* **410,** 362–366.

Taniyama, K., Takeda, K., Ando, H., Kuno, T., and Tanaka, C. (1991a). Expression of the $GABA_B$ receptor in *Xenopus* oocytes and inhibition of the response by activation of protein kinase C. *FEBS Lett.* **278,** 222–224.

Taniyama, K., Takeda, R., Ando, H., and Tanaka, C. (1991b). Expression or the $GABA_B$ receptor in *Xenopus* oocytes and desensitization by activation of protein kinase C. *Adv. Exp. Med. Biol.* **287,** 413–420.

Tareilus, E., Schoch, J., and Breer, H. (1994) $GABA_B$-receptor-mediated inhibition of calcium signals in isolated nerve terminals. *Neurochem. Int.* **24,** 349–361.

Teoh, H., Malcangio, M., and Bowery, N. G. (1996a) The effects of novel $GABA_B$ antagonists on the release of amino acids from spinal cord of the rat. *Br. J. Pharmacol.* **118,** 1153–1160.

Teoh, H., Malcangio, M., Fowler, L .J., and Bowery, N. G. (1996b) Evidence for release of glutamic acid, aspartic acid and substance P but not γ-aminobutyric acid from primary afferent fibres in rat spinal cord. *Eur. J. Pharmacol.* (in press).

Terence, C. F., Fromm, G. H., and Tenicela, R. (1985) Baclofen as an analgesic in chronic peripheral nerve disease. *Eur. Neurol.* **24,** 380–385.

Thalmann, R. H (1987) Pertussis toxin blocks a late inhibitory synaptic potential in hippocampal CA3 neurons. *Neurosci. Lett.* **82,** 41–46.

Thalmann, R. H. (1988) Evidence that guanosine triphosphate (GTP)-binding proteins control a synaptic response in brain: effect of pertussis toxin and GTP S on the late inhibitory postsynaptic potential of hippocampal CA3 neurons. *J. Neurosci.* **8,** 4589–4602.

Thompson, S. M. and Gahwiler, B. H. (1992) Comparison of the actions of baclofen at pre- and postsynaptic receptors in the rat hippocampus in vitro. *J. Physiol.* **451,** 329–345.

Turgeon, S. M. and Albin, R. L. (1993) Pharmacology, distribution, cellular localization, and development of $GABA_B$ binding in rodent cerebellum. *Neuroscience* **55,** 311–323.

Turski, L., Klockgether, T., Schwarz, M., Turski, W. A., and Sontag, K. H. (1990) Substantia nigra: a site of action of muscle relaxant drugs. *Ann. Neurol.* **28,** 341–348.

Vasko, M. R. and Harris, V. (1990) Gamma-aminobutyric acid inhibits the potassium-stimulated release of somatostatin from rat spinal cord slices. *Brain Res.* **507,** 129–137.

Vergnes, M., Marescaux, C., Micheletti, G., Reis, J., Depaulis, A., Rumbach, L., and Warter, J. M. (1982) Spontaneous paroxysmal electro-clinical patterns in a rat: a model of generalized non-convulsive epilepsy. *Neurosi. Lett.* **33,** 97–101.

Wada, T. and Fukuda, N. (1991) Pharmacologic profile of a new anxiolytic, DN-2327: effect of Ro15-1788 and interaction with diazepam in rodents. *Psychopharmacology* **103,** 314–322.

Wagner, P. G. and Dekin, M. S. (1993) $GABA_B$ receptors are coupled to a barium- insenstive outward rectifying potassium conductance in premotor respiratory neurons. *J. Neurophysiol.* **69,** 286–289.

Waldmeier, P. C., Wicki, P., Feldtrauer, J.-J., Mickel, S. J., Bittiger, H., and Baumann, P. A. (1994) GABA and glutamate release affected by $GABA_B$ receptor antagonists with similar potency: no evidence for pharmacologically different presynaptic receptors. *Br. J. Pharmacol.* **113,** 151,152.

Wall, M. J. and Dale, N. (1994) $GABA_B$ receptors modulate an omega-conotoxin-sensitive calcium current that is required for synaptic transmission in the *Xenopus* embryo spinal cord. *J. Neuroscience* **14,** 6248–6255.

Williams, S. R., Turner, J. P., and Crunelli, V. (1995) Gamma-hydroxybutyrate promotes oscillatory activity of rat and cat thalamocortical neurons by a tonic $GABA_B$ receptor mediated hyperpolarization. *Neuroscience* **66,** 133–141.

Wilson, P. R. and Yaksh, T. L. (1978) Baclofen is antinociceptive in the spinal intrathecal space of animals. *Eur. J. Pharmacol.* **51,** 323–330.

Woodward, R. M. and Miledi, R.(1992) Sensitivity of *Xenopus* oocytes to changes in extracellular pH: possible relevance to proposed expression of atypical mammalian $GABA_B$ receptors. *Brain Res.* **43,** 603–625.

Wullner, U., Klockgether, T., Sontag, K.-H. (1989) Phaclofen antagonizes the depressant effect of baclofen on spinal reflex transmission in rats. *Brain Res.* **596,** 341–344.

Xie, X. and Smart, T. G. (1992) γ-Hydroxybutyrate hyperpolarizes hippocampal neurones by activating $GABA_B$ receptors. *Eur. J. Pharmacol.* **212,** 291–294.

CHAPTER 8

Cellular and Biochemical Responses to GABA$_B$ Receptor Activation

Martin Cunningham and S. J. Enna

1. Introduction

The GABA$_B$ receptor was first identified with the characterization of a bicuculline-insensitive, GABA-mediated inhibition of transmitter release from peripheral and central nervous system (CNS) tissue (Bowery and Hudson, 1979; Bowery et al., 1980). The identification of baclofen as the prototypical GABA$_B$ receptor agonist provided a plausible mechanism of action for an agent used clinically for some time. These discoveries led to the development of potent and selective GABA$_B$ receptor agonists and antagonists which have, in turn, been crucial in characterizing the molecular, biochemical, electrophysiological, and behavioral responses associated with the GABA$_B$ receptor system (Bowery, 1993; Froestl et al., 1995a,b).

Given the widespread distribution of GABA and GABA$_B$ receptors, it is not surprising that GABA$_B$ agonists provoke a host of physiological responses. GABA$_B$ agonists inhibit airway smooth muscle contractility, vagally-mediated broncoconstriction, and intestinal peristalsis, suggesting possible utility for treating pulmonary and gastrointestinal disorders (Ong and Kerr, 1984; Belvisi et al., 1989; Chapman et al., 1993; Bolser et al., 1994). The efficacy of baclofen in the treatment of the rigidity and spasms of tetanus, and its beneficial effects in lessening the spasticity associated with multiple sclerosis, cerebral palsy, spinal cord injury, and trigeminal neuralgia have established the importance of GABA$_B$ receptors in controlling muscle tone (Parmar et al., 1989; Demaziere et al., 1991; Nockels and Young, 1992; Penn, 1992; Albright et al., 1993; Fromm et al., 1993). Laboratory and clinical studies have shown that GABA$_B$ agonists display anxiolytic, sedative, and antinociceptive properties (Zorn and Enna, 1985; Hoehn et al., 1988;

The GABA Receptors Eds.: S. J. Enna and N. G. Bowery
Humana Press Inc., Totowa, NJ

File et al., 1992; Sharma et al., 1993). Although $GABA_B$ receptor agonists are proconvulsant, antagonists suppress absence seizures in preclinical animal models, and improve learning and memory (Swartzwelder et al., 1987; Bernasconi et al., 1992; Marescaux et al., 1992; Snead, 1992; Snodgrass, 1992; Mondadori et al., 1993). Inasmuch as these findings suggest manipulation of $GABA_B$ receptor activity could yield a novel approach for treating a variety of clinical conditions, significant effort has been expended to characterize this system further.

Given the varied responses to $GABA_B$ agonists and antagonists, substantial research has been directed towards exploring the possible existence of multiple, pharmacologically and functionally distinct $GABA_B$ receptors. Early work revealed that, unlike $GABA_A$ receptor recognition sites which are located on a subunit of a chloride ion channel, $GABA_B$ receptors are coupled to G proteins (Enna, 1993). Guanyl nucleotides reduce the affinity of $GABA_B$ receptor binding sites and pertussis toxin inhibits $GABA_B$ receptor-mediated activity, actions characteristic of a G protein-coupled site (Hill et al., 1984; Asano et al., 1985; Andrade et al., 1986; Wojcik et al., 1989; Ticku and Delgade, 1989; Ohmori et al., 1990; Huston et al., 1990; Scholz and Miller, 1991; Knott et al., 1993; Amico et al., 1995). With the ever-increasing number of G protein subunits, associated effector enzymes, and ion channels, it is conceivable the responses to $GABA_B$ receptor agonists may be mediated, in part, by the differential regulation of intracellular functions by distinct subgroups of effectors. Evidence for this is provided by the finding that high-affinity $GABA_B$ receptor binding is reconstituted with only certain G_α subunits, and that $GABA_B$ receptors couple to voltage-sensitive calcium channels through only a select group of G_α proteins (Morishita et al., 1990; Campbell et al., 1993). Add to this the possibility of pharmacologically and molecularly distinct $GABA_B$ receptor recognition sites, the various isoforms of intracellular enzymes that may be influenced by G protein subunits, and the evidence that $GABA_B$ receptors may, in some circumstances, regulate the intracellular response to other neurotransmitter systems (coincident signaling), and it seems likely the $GABA_B$ system is composed of a family of receptors, each of which may be independently manipulated for therapeutic gain.

Contained in this chapter is a review of data concerning the cellular and biochemical responses associated with this receptor system, with the aim of establishing their potential importance in defining the physiological and clinical responses to $GABA_B$ receptor agonists and antagonists. Given the extensive literature in this and related fields, space does not allow a comprehensive treatment of this topic. Refer to other chapters in this volume for additional information, and to other reviews on the subject (Bowery, 1993; Bowery et al., 1993).

Table 1
Isoforms of G Protein Subunits
and Adenylate Cyclase (AC) Subtypes

G Proteins			
a	b	g	AC
i-1	1	1	I
i-2	2	2	II
i-3	3	3	III
o1	4	4	IV
o2	5	5	V
o3		s1	VI
oz		7	VII
gust		8	VIII
trod		9	
tcone		10	
s			
off			
11			
12			
13			
14			
15			
16			

2. Second Messenger Responses

To fully appreciate GABA$_B$ receptor-associated biochemical responses, it is essential to have some understanding of G protein-coupled effector systems. Molecular cloning experiments have identified at least eight different types of adenylate cyclase (Feinstein et al., 1991; Tang and Gilman, 1992; Iyengar, 1993; Pieroni et al., 1993), at least 16 different genes that encode for the α subunit of the G protein, five that encode for the β subunit, and 10 for the γ subunit (Simon et al., 1991; Iyengar, 1993) (Table 1). It has been shown that the α subunits of pertussis toxin-sensitive G proteins, G$_o$ and G$_i$, regulate neuronal potassium and calcium channels, as does GABA$_B$ receptor activation (Simon et al., 1991). All adenylate cyclases are found in brain, with different regions possessing different concentrations of these enzymes (Tang and Gilman, 1992; Pieroni et al., 1993; Mons et al., 1995). All adenylate cyclases are stimulated, at least to some extent, by G$_{s\alpha}$, although all do not appear to be inhibited by G$_{i\alpha}$ (Feinstein et al., 1991; Mons and Cooper, 1995). The mRNA for adenylate cyclase types I, III, and VIII predominate in olfactory bulb, those for types I, II, and VIII are found in the hippocampus, and those for types I, II, III, and VIII are found in the granular layer of the cerebellum (Pieroni et al., 1993).

Of particular relevance to the $GABA_B$ receptor system is the discovery that different forms of adenylate cyclase are subject to different types of regulation. Thus, types I, III, and VIII require calcium/calmodulin for activation, and type I is inhibited by the G protein $\beta\gamma$ complex. Types V and VI are unaffected by $\beta\gamma$, but types II, IV, and VII are stimulated by this complex in the presence of G_S (Gao and Gilman, 1991; Mons and Cooper, 1995). The ability of the $\beta\gamma$ subunit to stimulate some forms of adenylate cyclase appears to be unique for brain, suggesting it is an important mediator of neuronal activity (Birnbaumer, 1992; Hepler and Gilman, 1992; Tang et al., 1992; Taussig et al., 1993). Using cell lines transfected with different forms of cyclase, it was found that type I is fully stimulated by $G_{s\alpha}$, types II and IV are not, unless there is also present a high concentration of $G_{\beta\gamma}$ (Tang and Gilman, 1991; Bourne et al., 1992; Federman et al., 1992). It has also been found that phorbol esters enhance the activity of types II and VII cyclase and that this action is additive with the response to $G_{\beta\gamma}$ in the presence of $G_{s\alpha}$ (Bourne et al., 1992; Chen and Iyengar, 1993; Jacobowitz et al., 1993; Yoshimura and Cooper, 1993). It appears that phorbol esters stimulate the phosphorylation of $G_{i2-\alpha}$, selectively decreasing its ability to inhibit type II cyclase (Chen and Iyengar, 1993).

2.1. $GABA_B$ Receptors and Coincident Signaling

Consistent with the data indicating an affiliation of $GABA_B$ receptors with G proteins and a multiplicity of responses, $GABA_B$ agonists can either inhibit or activate adenylate cyclase in brain tissue, modifying cyclic AMP production (Hill et al., 1984; Wojcik and Neff, 1984; Asano et al., 1985; Hill, 1985; Watling and Bristow, 1986; Xu and Wojcik, 1986; Karbon and Enna, 1985; Bowery et al., 1989; Nishikawa and Kuriyama, 1989; Malcangio and Bowery, 1992). Thus, basal adenylate cyclase activity in brain membranes is inhibited by baclofen, as is forskolin-stimulated cyclic AMP accumulation in brain slices. Although baclofen has no significant effect on cyclic AMP production in brain slices on its own, when slices are exposed to a neurotransmitter or drug known to stimulate a receptor coupled to G_s, such as beta-adrenergic or adenosine receptor agonists, $GABA_B$ agonists greatly enhance the amount of second messenger produced (Karbon et al., 1984; Karbon and Enna, 1985; Watling and Bristow, 1986; Suzdak and Gianutsos, 1986; Schaad et al., 1989; Wojcik et al., 1989; Malcangio and Bowery, 1992). The generality of this interaction of $GABA_B$ receptors with a variety of substances that stimulate the liberation of $G_{\alpha s}$ (Table 2), and the regional distribution of the interaction in brain, suggest the coincident interaction of

Table 2
Effect of Baclofen on Neurotransmitter
and Drug-Induced cyclic AMP Accumulation
in Rat Brain Cortical Minces[a]

Condition	cyclic AMP Accumulation	
	Control	Baclofen
	% Conversion	
Basal	0.10	0.19
Histamine	0.21	0.67
Isproterenol	0.61	1.82
Norepinephrine	1.03	2.99
VIP	1.29	3.83
Adenosine	1.76	3.83
2-Cl-Adenosine	2.82	5.37

[a]Karbon and Enna (1985) *Mol. Pharm.*, **27**, 53–59.

GABA$_B$ receptors with other transmitter systems is of physiological importance (Karbon and Enna, 1985). It has been reported that baclofen increases cyclic AMP accumulation 2–3-fold in brain slices over the maximal responses obtained with histamine, isoproterenol, norepinephrine, vasoactive intestinal peptide, adenosine, and 2-chloroadenosine (Table 2). Since as baclofen is not an inhibitor of phosphodiesterases, the enzymes responsible for the destruction of cyclic AMP, this effect appears to be a result of an interaction of the effectors associated with these two receptor systems (coincident signaling).

Numerous studies have been conducted to define the biochemical mechanisms responsible for GABA$_B$ receptor-mediated coincident signaling. Early work suggested the involvement of calcium and phospholipase C (Duman et al., 1986). In addition, it was found that, like GABA$_B$ agonists, phorbol esters alone have no effect on cyclic AMP accumulation in brain slices, and yet they greatly enhance the response obtained with substances that stimulate production of this second messenger by liberation of G$_{\alpha s}$ (Karbon et al., 1986; Shenolikar et al., 1986). These data suggested that the coincident signal may normally be mediated through protein kinase C, which can be stimulated by products derived from phospholipase C catalyzed conversion of arachidonic acid (Duman et al., 1986). This model was inconsistent, however, with the finding that down-regulation of protein kinase C prevents phorbol ester-mediated augmentation of cyclic AMP production, but has no effect on the ability of baclofen to influence the accumulation of this second messenger (Shenolikar et al., 1986; Scherer et al., 1988). Given the existence of multiple forms of protein kinase C, the possibility remains that one or more of these is insensitive to phorbol esters, but is capable of mediating the response to $GABA_B$ activation, even when other isoforms of the enzyme are suppressed. More likely, it seems that protein kinase C mediates a coincident signaling response, and that this is independent of the pathway associated with $GABA_B$ receptors. Recent findings suggest that phorbol esters stimulate the phosphorylation of $G_{i2-\alpha}$, selectively decreasing the ability of this subunit to inhibit type II cyclase, thereby defining the mode of action of phorbol esters to enhance cyclic AMP accumulation when $G_{s\alpha}$ is liberated (Chen and Iyengar, 1993). There is no evidence that $GABA_B$ receptor activation results in the phosphorylation of $G_{i2-\alpha}$, which would be expected if it was associated with stimulation of protein kinase C.

A more plausible model of $GABA_B$ receptor-mediated coincident signaling involves the differential regulation of the various forms of adenylate cyclase (Fig. 1). Transmitters, drugs, and hormones that stimulate receptors coupled directly to G_s, liberate $G_{s\alpha}$, which only partially stimulates types II and IV cyclase. If, however, other G proteins are activated simultaneously, which liberate large quantities of $G_{\beta\gamma}$, types II and IV cyclase are stimulated further, producing a greater production of cyclic AMP than occurs when only the receptor coupled to G_s is involved. Because G_o represents 1–2% of brain membrane protein, it is potentially a major source of $G_{\beta\gamma}$ (Tang and Gilman, 1991). Accordingly, receptors coupled to pertussis toxin-sensitive sites, such as G_o and G_i, like the $GABA_B$ site, may liberate massive quantities of $G_{\beta\gamma}$, which, in the presence of $G_{s\alpha}$, would fully activate types II and IV cyclase, yielding the enhanced production of cyclic AMP observed with the combination of baclofen and any agent stimulating the release of $G_{o\alpha}$. Given the data indicating that G protein subunits influence ion channel activity directly, or indirectly by modifying the action of kinases, and the fact that $GABA_B$ receptors alter channel activity, the possible relationship between $GABA_B$ receptor recognition sites, different forms of G proteins, and different types of adenylate cyclase could provide the biochemical basis for the electrophysiological responses to $GABA_B$ agonists (Simon et al., 1991; *see also* Chapter 6 of this volume).

This mechanism, however, does not account for the fact that $GABA_B$ agonists inhibit forskolin-stimulated cyclic AMP accumulation in brain slices (Karbon and Enna, 1985). Within the context of the model, this response could be explained if baclofen is a nonselective $GABA_B$ agonist that stimulates receptors coupled to either G_i or G_o, liberating $G_{i\alpha}$ and G_α along with large quantities of $G_{\beta\gamma}$ (Fig. 1). Because neither $G_{i\alpha}$ nor $G_{o\alpha}$ stimulate adenylate cyclases, baclofen alone does not increase the production of cyclic AMP in brain slices. In the presence of $G_{s\alpha}$, the $G_{\beta\gamma}$ released by baclofen stimulation of G_o and G_i further activates some cyclases. On the other hand, $GABA_B$

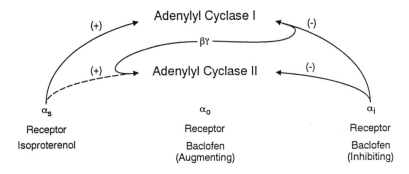

Fig. 1. Proposed model for multiple $GABA_B$ receptors in brain. Schematic representation of the possible relationship between $GABA_B$ receptors and receptors associated with G_s proteins, such as the beta adrenergic site. Illustrated is the concept that pharmacologically distinct $GABA_B$ receptors are associated with G_o and G_i. Although activation of G_s by a beta-adrenergic receptor agonist such as isoproterenol liberates sufficient α_s to fully stimulate adenylate cyclase I, there is only a partial stimulation of adenylate cyclase II (stippled arrow). If $GABA_B$ receptors affiliated with G_o are stimulated simultaneously with the adrenergic receptor system, larger quantities of $\beta\gamma$ are liberated which, together with α_s, fully stimulate adenylate cyclase II. If adenylate cyclases are activated in the absence of α_s, such as with forskolin stimulation, the liberation of α_i by those $GABA_B$ receptors coupled with G_i is most evident since there is a reduction in cyclase activity by $GABA_B$ agonists under this condition. Moreover, $\beta\gamma$ from either G_o or G_i can inhibit certain forms of adenylate cyclase, which could contribute to the overall inhibitor effect on the enzyme noted in the absence of α_s.

agonists inhibit forskolin-simulated cyclic AMP production because forskolin does not liberate $G_{s\alpha}$, which is essential for the $G_{\beta\gamma}$-mediated potentiation of cyclic AMP production, leaving only the inhibitory response to the baclofen-induced release of $G_{\alpha i}$. Evidence to support this is provided by the finding that certain $GABA_B$ receptor antagonists differentiate between the adenylate cyclase inhibitory responses to baclofen and the receptor-mediated enhancement in cyclic AMP production in brain slices, suggesting pharmacologically distinct sites that may be coupled to different forms of G protein (Cunningham and Enna, 1996) (Table 3). Three of the five selective $GABA_B$ receptor antagonists examined, SCH 50911, CGP 54626A, and CGP 52432, displayed greater than a 10-fold difference in their potencies to inhibit baclofen-mediated argumentation of cyclic AMP production compared to baclofen-mediated inhibition of forskolin-stimulated cyclic AMP accumulation. In all cases, these compounds were more potent in inhibiting the cyclic AMP-augmenting response to baclofen than in inhibiting the effect on

Table 3
Effects of GABA$_B$ Receptor Agonists and Antagonists on cyclic AMP
Accumulation in Rat Brain Cortical Slices[a]

Agonist	Effect on cyclic AMP	
	Isoproterenol (EC_{50}, NM)	Forskolin (EC_{50}, NM)
R(+)Baclofen	2.20	1.30
CGP 35024	1.62	0.63
CGP 44532	4.80	4.40
Antagonist	Reversal of baclofen effect on cyclic AMP	
CGP 36742	>100	>100
SCH 50911	2.6	36+
CGP 55845A	0.13	0.58
CGP 52432	0.11	3.25+
CGP 54626a	0.01	0.15+

[a]Adapted from Cunningham and Enna, *Brain Res.* (1996).

forskolin. Two GABA$_B$ receptor antagonists, CGP 36742 and CGP 55845A, and three GABA$_B$ agonists, baclofen, CGP 35024, and CGP 44532, displayed no significant differences in potencies between the two responses. These data are consistent with the notion of pharmacologically distinct GABA$_B$ receptors coupled to different forms of G protein.

Pharmacologically distinct subunits of GABA$_B$ receptors are not required, however, to support the G_i/G_o hypothesis. It has been established that receptors can interact with more than one G protein, as appears to be the case for alpha- and beta-adrenergic receptors, muscarinic, somatostatin, adenosine, dopamine, endothelin, prostaglandin, angiotensin II, and serotonin receptors among others (Kleuss et al., 1991, 1992, 1993; Coupry et al., 1992; Duzic and Lanier, 1992; Duzic et al., 1992; Ogino et al., 1992; Saudou et al., 1992; Charpentier et al., 1993; Conklin et al., 1993; Remaury et al., 1993; Chabre et al., 1994; Guiramand et al., 1995; Takigawa et al., 1995). It is possible that pharmacologically and molecularly identical receptor recognition sites couple to different effectors by interacting with distinct types of G protein complexes.

2.2. Guanylate Cyclase and Phospholipase C Activation

Less is known about the influence of GABA$_B$ receptors on second messengers other than cyclic AMP. Reports indicate that baclofen decreases cyclic GMP levels in cerebellar tissue, an effect reversed by the GABA$_B$ antagonist CGP 35348 (Mailman et al., 1978; Gumulka et al., 1979; Bernasconi et al., 1992). Baclofen has also been shown to influence phosphoinositide (PI) metabolism in certain species and tissues. Activation of GABA$_B$ receptors stimulates basal PI turnover in cultured rat and avian dorsal root ganglia (Dolphin et al., 1989; Harish and Role, 1992). No effect was observed on this second messenger in rat or mouse cortical slices (Godfrey et al., 1988; Crawford and Young, 1988). Baclofen attenuates histamine H$_1$ and serotonin$_2$ receptor-induced increases in PI turnover, but potentiates norepinephrine-mediated PI turnover and partially blocks the inhibitory effect of arachidonic acid on PI synthesis (Godfrey et al., 1988; Crawford and Young, 1988; Corradetti et al., 1987; Li et al., 1990). A similar pharmacology, G protein sensitivity, and time-course for transmitter-induced inhibition of calcium current and PI turnover have been reported, suggesting that GABA$_B$ receptor-mediated PI turnover activates protein kinase C and inhibits calcium conductance by channel phosphorylation (Harish and Role, 1992). Inhibition of phospholipase C attenuates the ability of baclofen to reduce muscimol-stimulated chloride transport across cerebellar membrane vesicles (Hahner et al., 1991). While the physiological significance of these findings remains obscure, the weight of evidence favors the notion that some GABA$_B$ receptors are associated with G proteins regulating phospholipase C. The interaction between GABA$_B$ and noradrenergic receptors with respect to phosphoinositide metabolism is reminiscent of the coincident signaling that occurs with cyclic AMP production. This reinforces the notion that GABA$_B$ receptors influence multiple biochemical pathways, depending upon the cell type and the presence of other receptors and effectors.

3. Protein Kinases

Protein kinases play a central role in the regulation of cellular activity. GABA$_B$ agonists influence the intracellular concentrations of calcium, diacylglycerol, IP$_3$, cyclic AMP, and cyclic GMP; it is likely that activation of GABA$_B$ receptors alters the activity of kinases. Such an effect could explain many of the actions of GABA$_B$ agonists on neuronal excitability, since ion channels are regulated by phosphorylation. Under certain conditions, activation of protein kinase C reduces some responses to GABA$_B$ agonists. For example, stimulation of protein kinase C suppresses the inhibition by baclofen of potassium-evoked, calcium-dependent norepinephrine or acetylcholine release from cerebellar cortical slices (Taniyama et al., 1992). Moreover, protein kinase C activation reduces the electrophysiological response to GABA$_B$ agonists and the effect of baclofen on depolarization-induced, calcium-activated rubidium efflux in cultured spinal neurons (Worley et al.,

1987; Kamatchi and Ticku, 1990; Thompson and Gähwiler, 1992; Swartz, 1993; Pitter and Alger, 1994). An explanation of these findings is provided by the discovery that stimulation of protein kinase C and protein kinase A, but not protein kinase G, desensitizes $GABA_B$ receptors expressed in *Xenopus* oocytes (Taniyama et al., 1991). Like other transmitter receptors, it appears the sensitivity of the $GABA_B$ site is determined by its state of phosphorylation, which is a function of receptor activity.

A $GABA_B$ receptor-mediated effect on kinase activity may be involved in the coincident signaling response to baclofen. For example, stimulation of kinase A activates DARPP-32, a protein phosphatase inhibitor that blocks protein kinase G-dependent type 1 phosphatase activity, enhancing the action of protein kinase C. This leads to disinhibition of adenylate cyclase, since $G_{i2-\alpha}$ is more actively phosphorylated. In this way, stimulation of protein kinase C could enhance the response to $GABA_B$ agonists (Chen and Iyengar, 1993). This is consistent with the finding that like baclofen, phorbol esters, which stimulate protein kinase C, increase the production of cyclic AMP only in the presence of an agent known to activate $G_{s\alpha}$ (Karbon et al., 1986). However, the importance of a linkage between $GABA_B$ receptor function and activation or inhibition of protein kinases remains to be established.

4. Ion Channels

A chief characteristic of $GABA_B$ receptor activation is its effect on calcium and potassium transport. $GABA_B$ receptor agonists inhibit voltage-sensitive calcium currents in isolated sensory and central neurons (Mott and Lewis, 1991; Bowery, 1993). The kinetics of this inhibition have been studied in both hippocampal neurons and isolated hippocampal synaptosomes. The results indicate that inhibition of presynaptic calcium currents by baclofen occurs with a time-course consistent with an effect of G proteins on calcium channels, rather than one involving second messengers (Pfreiger et al., 1994; Tareilus et al., 1994). This action is blocked by pertussis toxin, but it appears to be mediated by either G_o or G_i. Indeed, antibodies and antisense oligonucleotides complimentary to $G_{\alpha o}$, but not $G_{\alpha i}$, block baclofen-mediated inhibition of calcium currents, supporting the notion that at least some $GABA_B$ receptors are linked to G_o (Campbell et al., 1993). Moreover, depletion of calcium channel β subunits enhances the response to baclofen, leading to speculation that under normal circumstances there is a competition between $G_{o\alpha}$ and the β subunits for calcium channel α subunits (Campbell et al., 1995). It is possible this $G_{o\alpha}$ isoform may mediate other baclofen-mediated effects, such as those associated with potassium ion conductance.

Various studies have shown that $GABA_B$ agonists influence multiple types of calcium currents, depending on the cell type examined and the experimental model employed (Bowery, 1993; Mott and Lewis, 1991). In mammalian hippocampal neurons, baclofen suppresses high-threshold N-type, L-type, P-type, and Q-type channels through voltage-dependent and voltage-independent mechanisms (Scholz and Miller, 1991; Toselli and Taglietti, 1993; Hirata et al, 1995). In cerebellum, baclofen modulates L-type and P-type channels, but in spinal ganglion neurons it inhibits N-type channels (Sweeney and Dolphin, 1992; Mintz and Bean, 1993; Amico et al., 1995).

As for potassium channels, the long-latency inhibitory, postsynaptic potential noted following GABA$_B$ receptor activation is caused by an increase in inward potassium conductance (Hirsch and Burnod, 1987; Dutar and Nicoll, 1988; Lovinger et al., 1992; Jarolimek et al., 1993). This effect is blocked by GABA$_B$ receptor antagonists and is calcium-independent (Andrade et al., 1986; Jarolimek et al., 1993; Olpe et al., 1993). As with calcium channels, GABA$_B$ receptors regulate inwardly rectifying potassium channels through pertussis toxin-sensitive G proteins (Thalmann, 1988; Mott and Lewis, 1991; Okuhara and Beck, 1994). Inward rectifiers are a class of potassium-selective ion channels that preferentially conduct inward potassium currents at voltages negative to the potassium equilibrium potential. Although it is yet to be established which members of this group are regulated by GABA$_B$ receptors. Although it has been demonstrated that purified or recombinant forms of G$_{\beta\gamma}$ activate G protein-gated potassium channels, it remains unclear whether this is the mechanism by which GABA$_B$ receptors influence these sites (Logothetis et al., 1987; Reuveny et al., 1994).

The possible physiological significance of GABA$_B$-mediated coincident signaling is evidenced by studies on potassium currents. The decrease in calcium-dependent potassium currents (I_{AHP}) in response to increased intracellular cyclic AMP is an index of adenylate cyclase activity in hippocampal CA3 pyramidal cells (Gerber and Gähwiler, 1994). Baclofen enhances evoked I_{AHP} and antagonizes the action of isoproterenol to reduce I_{AHP}. Inhibition of protein kinase A diminishes the ability of baclofen to enhance the I_{AHP}. These results suggest that GABA$_B$ and β-adrenoceptor signals converge at the level of adenylate cyclase, consistent with the model proposed for GABA$_B$ coincident signaling and cyclic AMP formation (Fig. 1).

5. Neurotransmitter Release

A major consequence of GABA$_B$ receptor activation is inhibition of neurotransmitter release. GABA$_B$ receptor agonists inhibit the evoked release of GABA, glutamic acid, serotonin, CCK, PGE$_2$, substance P, dopamine, norepinephrine, LHRH, acetylcholine, and somatostatin (Taniyama et al., 1985; Conzelmann et al., 1986; Gray and Green, 1987; Masotto et al., 1989; Huston et al., 1990; Waldmeier and Baumann, 1990; Bonanno et al., 1991;

Bonanno and Raiteri, 1992, 1993; Malcangio and Bowery, 1993; Mayfield and Zahniser, 1993; Oset-Gasque et al., 1993; Pende et al., 1993; Waldmeier and Wiki, 1994). While there are some contradictory findings, it appears the $GABA_B$ binding site in brain represents the presynaptic $GABA_B$ receptor responsible for controlling transmitter release (Bonanno and Raiteri, 1992; Lanza et al., 1993; Fassio et al., 1994; Waldmeier and Wiki, 1994). This conclusion is based on the finding that the rank order of potencies of $GABA_B$ receptor agonists and antagonists to influence transmitter release are similar to that found for inhibiting $GABA_B$ binding. Exceptions to this have been reported, suggesting the existence of $GABA_B$ receptors that may be molecularly and pharmacologically distinct from those labeled in the binding assay, but which are coupled to effectors controlling the transmitter release process. This issue will not be conclusively resolved until it is possible to directly compare $GABA_B$ receptor structures at a molecular level.

The precise manner in which $GABA_B$ receptors regulate neurotransmitter release is yet to be defined. Given what is known about the effector systems influenced by $GABA_B$ receptor activation, it is possible to envision various possibilities. It has been established that $GABA_B$ receptor-mediated inhibition of calcium-dependent neurotransmitter release is diminished by pertussis toxin, indicating the involvement of a G_i/G_o protein (Huston et al., 1990, 1993; Shibuya and Douglas, 1993). Moreover, activation of protein kinase C attenuates baclofen-mediated inhibition of neurotransmitter release (Taniyama et al., 1992). Since $GABA_B$ receptors influence intracellular levels of calcium, and this ion is crucial for the functioning of the vesicular release process, this could well be the primary mechanism of action of baclofen in regulating transmitter release (Klapstein and Colmers, 1992; Mayfield and Zahinser, 1993; Oset-Gasque et al., 1993; Kardos et al., 1994). In this case, activation of a presynaptic $GABA_B$ receptor would liberate G protein subunits that directly reduce ion channel activity, decreasing the inward flux of calcium necessary for the vesicular release process. The findings with protein kinase C activation suggest a crucial role for phosphorylation in this response. Candidate proteins include the $GABA_B$ receptor recognition site itself, a G protein subunit, the calcium ion channel or some key enzyme, perhaps adenylate cyclase, that catalyzes a reaction necessary for expressing the receptor response to $GABA_B$ agonists (Katada et al., 1985; Harish and Role, 1992; Iyengar, 1993; Rhee et al., 1993; Bartschat and Rhodes, 1995; Inoue and Imanaga, 1995; Ishikawa et al., 1995; Tareilus and Breer, 1995).

6. Summary and Conclusions

Activation of $GABA_B$ receptors initiates a number of biochemical processes resulting in a modification of cellular activity. The variety of physiological and behavioral responses to GABA$_B$ agonists and antagonists reflects the presence of GABA$_B$ receptors in numerous organs and tissues, including the brain, it also appears these receptors are coupled to a number of different effecter systems, perhaps within the same organ, tissue, or cell, each of which could influence cellular activity in a unique manner. Many of the cellular and biochemical changes observed following administration of a GABA$_B$ agonist or antagonist are secondary responses not directly mediated by a GABA$_B$ receptor/effector system. Examples include alteration in serotonin and dopamine synthesis after baclofen administration (Nishikawa et al., 1989; Arias-Montano et al., 1991; Waldmeier, 1991).

Data indicating pharmacologically distinct subsets of GABA$_B$ receptors point to the possibility of developing receptor subtype-specific agonists and antagonists. Such drugs would make possible the selective modification of individual cellular responses to GABA$_B$ receptor activation, which could yield more clinically useful agents. Beyond the receptor recognition sites, the identification of GABA$_B$ effectors will provide new targets for manipulating this transmitter system. Progress has been hindered by the lack of information on the molecular structure of the GABA$_B$ receptor and of the tools needed to study the receptor at the molecular level. Although there has been some success in this regard (Ohmori et al., 1990; Ohmori and Kuriyama, 1991; Nakayasu et al., 1992, 1993; *see also* Chapter 9 of this volume), the receptor structure and the genes encoding for this site have yet to be unequivocally identified. Nonetheless, there are sufficient data already to support the notion that GABA$_B$ receptors, or receptor functions, may be targeted selectively, opening the possibility of a new class of therapeutic agents.

Acknowledgments

Preparation of this manuscript was made possible, in part, by a grant from Marion Merrill Dow Corp. We thank Maxine Floyd for her secretarial assistance.

References

Albright, A. L., Barrow, W. B., Fasick, M. P., Polinko, P., and Janosky, J. (1993) Continuous intrathecal baclofen infusion for spasticity of cerebral origin. *J. Am. Med. Assoc.* **270,** 2475–2477.

Amico, C., Marchetti, C., Nobile, M., and Usai, C. (1995) Pharmacological types of calcium channels and their modulation by baclofen in cerebellar granules. *J. Neurosci.* **15,** 2839–2848.

Andrade, R., Malenka, R. C., and Nicoll, R. R. (1986) A G protein couples serotonin and GABAB receptors to the same channels in hippocampus. *Science* **234,** 1261–1265.

Arias-Montano, J. A., Martinez-Fong, D., and Aceves, J. (1991) Gamma-aminobutyric acid (GABAB) receptor-mediated inhibition of tyrosine hydroxylase activity in the stratum of rat. *Neuropharmacology* **30,** 1047.

Asano, T., Ui, M., and Ogasawara, N. (1985) Prevention of the agonist binding to gamma-aminobutyric acid B receptors by guanine nucleotides and islet-activating protein, pertussis toxin, in bovine cerebral cortex. Possible coupling of the toxin-sensitive GTP binding proteins to receptors. *J. Biol. Chem.* **260,** 12,653–12,658.

Bartschat, D. K. and Rhodes, T. E. (1995) Protein kinase C modulates calcium channels in isolated presynaptic nerve terminals of rat hippocampus. *J. Neurochem.* **64,** 2064–2072.

Belvisi, M. G., Ichinose, M., and Barnes, P. J. (1989) Modulation of non-adrenergic, noncholinergic neural bronchoconstriction in guinea pig airways via GABA$_B$ receptors. *Br. J. Pharmacol.* **97,** 1225–1231.

Bernasconi, R., Lauber, J., Marescaux, C., Vergnes, M., Markin, P., Rubic, V., Leonchardt, T., Reymann, N., and Bettiger, H. (1992) Experimental absence seizures: potential role of gamma-hydroxybutyric acid and GABAB receptors. *J. Neuron Trans.* **35(Suppl.),** 155–177.

Birnbaumer, L. (1992) Receptor-to-effector signaling through G proteins: roles for beta gamma dimers as well as alpha subunits. *Cell* **71,** 1069–1072.

Bolser, D. C., DeGennaro, F. C., O'Reilly, S., Chapman, R. W., Kreutner, W. S., Egan, R. W., and Hey, J. A. (1994) Peripheral and central sites of action of GABA-B agonists to inhibit the cough reflex in the cat and guinea pig. *Br. J. Pharmacol.* **113,** 1344–1348.

Bonanno, G., Gemignani, A., Fedele, E., Fontana, G., and Raiteri, M. (1991) Gamma-aminobutyric acid B receptors mediate inhibition of somatostatin release from cerebrocortex nerve terminals. *J. Pharmacol. Exp. Ther.* **259,** 1153–1157.

Bonnano, G. and Raiteri, M. (1992) Functional evidence for multiple gamma-aminobutyric acid B receptor subtypes in the rat cerebral cortex. *J. Pharmacol. Exp. Ther.* **262,** 114–118.

Bonnano, G. and Raiteri, M. (1993) Gamma-anninobutyric acid (GABA) autoreceptors in rat cerebral cortex and spinal cord represent pharmacologically distinct subtypes of the GABAB receptor. *J. Pharmacol. Exp. Ther.* **265,** 765–770.

Bourne, H. R., Lustig, K. D., Wong, V. H., and Conklin, B. R. (1992) Detection of coincident signals by G proteins and adenylyl cyclase. *Cold Spring Harb. Symp. Quant. Biol.* **57,** 145–148.

Bowery, N. G. (1993) GABA$_B$ receptor pharmacology. *Ann. Rev. Pharmacol.* **33,** 109–147.

Bowery, N. G. Bittiger, H., and Olpe, H.-R. eds. (1993) GABA$_B$ *Receptors in Mammalian Function,* John Wiley, New York.

Bowery, N. G., Hill, D. R., Hudson, A. L., Doble, A., Middlemiss, D. N., Shaw, J., and Turnbull, M. (1980) (–)Baclofen decreases neurotransmitter release in the mammalian CNS by an action at a novel GABA receptor. *Nature* **283,** 92–94.

Bowery, N. G., Hill, D. R., and Moratalla, R. (1989) Neurochemistry and autoradiography of GABA$_B$ receptors in mammalian brain: second messenger system(s), in *Allosteric Modulation of Amino Acid Receptor: Therapeutic Implications* (Barnard, E. A. and Cost, A., eds.), Raven, New York, pp. 159–172.

Bowery, N. G. and Hudson, A. L. (1979) γ-Aminobutyric acid reduces the evoked release of ^{3}H-noradrenaline from sympathetic nerve terminals. *Br. J. Pharmacol.* **66,** 108P.

Campbell, V., Berrow, N., and Dolphin, A. C. (1993) GABAB receptor modulation of CA2+ currents in rat sensory neurones by the G protein G (O): antisense oligonucleotide studies. *J. Physiol. Lond.* **470,** 1–11.

Campbell, V., Berrow, N., Brickley, K., Page K., Wade, R., and Dolphin, A. C. (1995) Voltage-dependent calcium channel beta-subunits in combination with alpha 1 subunits, have a GTPase activating effect to promote the hydrolysis to GTP by G alpha 0 in rat frontal cortex. *FEBS Lett.* **370**, 135–140.

Chabre, O., Conklin, B. R., Brandon, S., Bourne, H. R., and Limbird, L. E. (1994) Coupling of the alpha 2A-adrenergic receptor to multiple G-proteins. A simple approach for estimating receptor-G-protein coupling efficacy in a transient expression system. *J. Biol. Chem.* 5730–5734.

Chapman, R. W., Hey, J. A., Rizzo, C. A., Kreutner, W., and Bolser, D. C. (1993) GABA$_B$ receptors in the lung. *Trends Pharmacol. Sci.* **14**, 26–29.

Charpentier, N., Prezeau, L., Carrette, J., Bertorelli, R., Le Cam, G., Manzoni, O., Bockaert, J., and Homburger, V. (1993) Transfected G$_o$ 1 alpha inhibits the calcium dependence of beta-adrenergic stimulated cAMP accumulation in C6 glioma cells. *J. Biol. Chem.* **268**, 8980–8989.

Chen, J. and Iyengar, R. (1993) Inhibition of cloned adenylyl cyclases by mutant-activated Gi-alpha and specific suppression of type 2 adenylyl cyclase inhibition by phorbol ester treatment. *J. Biol. Chem.* **168**, 12,253–12,256.

Conklin, B. R., Rarfel, Z., Lustig, K. D., Julius, D., and Bourne, H. R. (1993) Substitution of three amino acids switches receptor specificity of Gq alpha to that of Gi alpha. *Nature* **363**, 274–276.

Conzelmann, U., Meyer, D. K., and Sperk, G. (1986) Stimulation of receptors of gamma-aminobutyric acid modulates the release of cholecystokinin-like immunoactivity from slices of rat neostriatum. *Br. J. Pharmacol.* **89**, 845–852.

Corradotti, R., Ruggiero, M., Chiarugi, V. P., and Pepeu, G. (1987) GABA-receptor stimulation enhances norepinephrine-induced polyphosphoinositide metabolism in rat hippocampal slices. *Brain Res.* **411**, 196–199.

Coupry, I., Duzic, E., and Lanier, S. M. (1992) Factors determining the specificity of signal transduction by guanine nucleotide-binding protein-coupled receptors. II. Preferential coupling of the alpha 2C-adrenergic receptor for the guanine nucleotide- binding protein, Go. *J. Biol. Chem.* **267**, 9852–9857.

Crawford, M. L. and Young, J. M. (1988) GABAB receptor-mediated inhibition of histamine H1-receptor-induced inositol phosphate fotmation in slices of rat cerebral cortex. *J. Neurochem.* **51**, 1441–1447.

Cunningham, M. D. and Enna, S. J. (1996) Evidence for pharmacologically distinct GABA$_B$ receptors associated with cAMP production in rat brain. *Brain Res.* **720**, 220–224.

Demaziere, J., Saissy, J. M., Vitris, M., Seck, M., Marcoux, L., and Ndiaye, M. (1991) Intermittent intrathecal baclofen for severe tetanus. *Lancet* **337**, 427.

Dolphin, A. C., McGuirk, S. M., and Scott, R. H. (1989) An investigation into the mechanisms of inhibition of calcium channel currents in cultured sensory neurones of the rat by guanine nucleotide analogues and (–)-baclofen. *Br. J. Pharmacol.* **97**, 263–273.

Duman, R. S., Karbon, E. W., Harrington, C., and Enna, S. J. (1986) An examination of the involvement of phospholipases A2 and C in the alpha-adrenergic and gamma-aminobutyric acid receptor modulation of cyclic AMP accumulation in rat brain slices. *J. Neurochem.* **47**, 800–810.

Dutar, P. and Nicoll, R. A. (1988) A physiological role for GABAB receptors in the central nervous system. *Nature* **332**, 156–158.

Duzic, E., Coupry, I., Downing, S., and Lanier, S. M. (1992) Factors determining the specificity of signal transduction by guanine nucleotide-binding protein-coupled receptors. I. Coupling of alpha 2-adrenergic receptor subtypes to distinct G-proteins. *J. Biol. Chem.* **267**, 9844–9851.

Duzic, E. and Lanier, S. M. (1992) Factors determining the specificity of signal transduction by guanine-nucleotide binding protein-coupled receptors. III Coupling of alpha 2-adrenergic receptor subtypes in a cell type-specific manner. *J. Biol. Chem.* **267**, 24,095–24,052.

Enna, S. J. (1993) Gamma-aminobutyric acid A receptor-subunits in the mediation of selective drug action. *Curr. Opin. Neurol. Neurosurg.* **6**, 597–601.

Fassio, A., Bonanno, G., Cavazzani, P. and Raiteri, M. (1994) Characterization of the GABA autoreceptor in human neocortex as as pharmacological subtype of the GABAB receptor. *Eur. J. Pharmacol.* **263**, 311–314.

Federman, A. D., Conklin, B. R., Schrader, K. A., Reed, R. R., and Bourne, H. R. (1992) Hormonal stimulation of adenylyl cyclase through Gi-protein beta gamma subunits. *Nature* **356**, 154–161.

Feinstein, P. G., Schrader, K. A., Bakalyav, H. A., Tang, W. J., Krupinski, J., Gilman, A. G., and Reed, R. R. (1991) Molecular cloning and characterization of a Ca2+/calmodulin-insensitive adenylyl cyclase from rat brain. *Proc. Natl. Acad. Sci. USA* **88**, 10,173–10,177.

File, S. E., Charkovsky, A., and Hitchcott, P. K. (1992) Effects of nitrendipine, chlordiazepoxide, flumazenil and baclofen on the increased anxiety resulting from ethanol withdrawal. *Prog. Neuropsychopharmacol. Biol. Psychiat.* **16**, 87–93.

Froestl, W., Mickel, S. J., Hall, R. G., von Sprecher, G., Strub, D., Baumann, P. A., Brugger, F., Gentsch, C., Jaekel, J., Olpe, H.-R., Rihs, G., Vassout, A., Waldmeier, P. C., and Bittiger, H. (1995a) Phosphinic acid analogues of GABA. 1. New potent and selective GABA$_B$ agonists. *J. Med. Chem.* **38**, 3297–3312.

Froestl, W., Mickel, S. J., von Sprecher, G., Diel, P. J., Hall, R. G., Maier, L ., Strub, D., Melillo, V., Baumann, P. A., Bernasconi, R., Gentsch, C., Hauser, K., Jaekel, J., Karlsson, G., Klebs, K., Maitre, L., Marescaux, C., Pozza, M. F., Schmutz, M., Steinmann, M. W., van Riezen, H., Vassout, A., Mondadori, C., Olpe, H.-R., Waldmeier, P. C., and Bittiger, H. (1995b) Phosphinic acid analogues of GABA. 2. Selective, orally active GABA$_B$ antagonists. *J. Med. Chem.* **38**, 3313–3331.

Fromm, G. H., Aumentado, D., and Terrence, C. F. (1993) A clinical and experimental investigation of the effects of tizanidine in trigeminal neuralgia. *Pain* **53**, 265–271.

Gao, B. and Gilman, A. G. (1991) Cloning and expression of a widely distributed (type IV) adenylyl cyclase. *Proc. Natl. Acad. Sci. USA* **88**, 10,178–10,182.

Gerber, U. and Gähwiler, B. H. (1994) GABAB and adenosine receptors mediate enhancement of the K^+ current, IAHP, by reducing adenylyl cyclase activity in rat CA3 hippocampal neurons. *J. Neurophysiol.* **72**, 2360–2367.

Godfrey, P. P., Grahame-Smith, D. G., and Gray, J. A. (1988) GABAB receptor activation inhibits 5-hydroxytryptamine-stimulated inositol phospholipid turnover in mouse cerebral cortex. *Eur. J. Pharmacol.* **152**, 185–188.

Gray, J. A. and Green, A. R. (1987) GABAB-receptor mediated inhibition of potassium-evoked release of endogenous 5-hydroxytryptamine from mouse frontal cortex. *Br. J. Pharmacol.* **91**, 517–522.

Guiramand, J., Montmayeur, J. P., Ceraline, J., Bhatia, M., and Borrelli, E. (1995) Alternative splicing of the dopamine D$_2$ receptor directs specificity of coupling to G-proteins. *J. Biol. Chem.* **270**, 7354–7358.

Gumulka, S. W., Dinnendahl, V., and Schowhofer, P. S. (1979) Baclofen and cerebellar cycle GMP levels in mice. *Pharmacology* **19**, 75–81.

Hahner, L., McQuilken, S., and Harris, R. A. (1991) Cerebellar GABAB receptors modulate function of GABA receptors. *FASEB J.* **5**, 2466–2472.

Harish, O. E. and Role, L. W. (1992) Activation of phosphoinositide turnover and protein kinase C by neurotransmitters that modulate calcium channels in embryonic chick sensory neurons. *Int. J. Dev. Neurosci.* **10**, 421–433.

Hepler, J. R. and Gilman, A. G. (1992) G proteins. *Trends Biochem. Sci.* **17**, 383–387.

Hill, D. R. (1985) GABAB receptor modulation of adenylate cyclase activity in rat brain slices. *Br. J. Pharmacol.* **84**, 249–257.

Hill, D. R., Bowery, N. G., and Hudson, A. L. (1984) Inhibition of GABAB receptor binding by guanyl nucleotides. *J. Neurochem.* **42**, 652–657.

Hirata, K., Ohno-Shosaku, T., Sawada, S., and Yamamoto, C. (1995) Baclofen inhibits GABAergic transmission after treatment with type-specific calcium channel blockers in cultural rat hippocampal neurons. *Neurosci. Lett.* **187**, 205–208.

Hirsch, J. C. and Burnod, Y. (1987) A synaptically evoked late hyperpolarization in the rat dorsolateral geniculate neurons in vitro. *Neuroscience* **23**, 457–468.

Hoehn, K., Reid, A., and Sawynok, J. (1988) Pertussis toxin inhibits antinociception produced by intrathecal injection of morphine, noradrenaline and baclofen. *Eur. J. Pharmacol.* **146**, 65–72.

Huston, E., Cullen, G., Sweeney, M. I., Pearson, H., Fazeli, M. S., and Dolphin, C. (1993) Pertussis toxin treatment increases glutamate release and dihydropyridine binding sites in cultured rat cerebellar granule neurons. *Neuroscience* **52**, 787–798.

Huston, E., Scott R. H., and Dolphin, A. C. (1990) A comparison of the effect of calcium channel ligands and GABA_B agonists and antagonists on transmitter release and somatic calcium channel currents in cultured neurons. *Neuroscience* **38**, 721–729.

Inoue, M. and Imanaga, I. (1995) Phosphatase is responsible for run down, and probably G protein-mediated inhibition of inwardly rectifying K^+ currents in guinea pig chromaffin cells. *J. Gen. Physiol.* **105**, 249–266.

Ishikawa, Y., Amano, I., Eguchi, T., and Ishida, H. (1995) Mechanism of isoproterenol-induced heterologous desensitization of mucin secretion from rat submandibular glands. Regulation of phosphorylation of Gi proteins controls the cell response to the subsequent stimulation. *Biochim. Biophys. Acta* **1265**, 173–180.

Iyengar, R. (1993) Multiple families of G_s-regulated adenylyl cyclases. *Adv. Second Messenger Phosphoprot. Res.* **28**, 27–36.

Jacobowitz, O., Chen, J., Premont, R. T., and Iyengar, R. (1993) Stimulation of specific types of G_s-stimulated adenylyl cyclases by phorbol ester treatment. *J. Biol. Chem.* **268**, 3829–3832.

Jarolimek, W., Demmelhuber, J., Bijak, M., and Misgeld, U. (1993) CGP55845A blocks baclofen, gamma-aminobutyric acid and inhibitory postsynaptic potassium currents in guinea pig CA3 neurons. *Neurosci. Lett.* **154**, 31–34.

Kamatchi, G. L. and Ticku, M. K. (1990) Functional coupling of presynaptic GABAB receptors with voltage-gated CA^{2+} channel: regulation by protein kinases A and C in cultured spinal cord neurons. *Mol. Pharmacol.* **38**, 342–347.

Karbon, E. W., Duman, R. S., and Enna, S. J. (1984) GABAB receptors and norepinephrine stimulated cAMP production in rat brain cortex. *Brain Res.* **306**, 327–332.

Karbon, E. W. and Enna, S. J. (1985) Characterization of the relationship between gammaaminobutyric acid B agonists and transmitter-coupled cyclic nucleotide-generating systems in rat brain. *Mol. Pharmacol.* **27**, 53–59.

Karbon, E. W., Shenolikar, S., and Enna, S. J. (1986) Phorbol esters enhance neurotransmitter stimulated cyclic AMP production in rat brain slices. *J. Neurochem.* **47,** 1566–1575.

Kardos, J., Elster, L., Damgaard, I., Krogsgaard-Larsen, P., and Schousbe, A. (1994) Role of GABAB receptors in intracellular Ca2+ homeostasis and possible interaction between GABA and GABAB receptors in regulation of transmitter release in cerebellar granule neurons. *J. Neurosci. Res.* **39,** 645–655.

Katada, T., Gilman, A. G., Watanabe, Y., Bauer, S., and Jakobs, H. (1985) Protein kinase C phosphorylates the inhibitory guanine-nucleotide-binding regulatory component and apparently suppresses its function in hormonal inhibition of adenylate cyclase. *Eur. J. Biochem.* **151,** 431–437.

Klapstein, G. J. and Colmers, W. F. (1992) 4-Aminopyridine and low Ca^{2+} differentiate presynaptic inhibition mediated by neuropeptide Y, baclofen and 2-chloroadenosine in rat hippocampal CA1 in vitro. *Br. J. Pharmacol.* **105,** 470–474.

Kleuss, C., Hescheler, J., Ewel, C., Rosenthal, W., Schultz, G., and Wittig, B. (1991) Assignment of G-protein subtypes to specific receptors inducing inhibition of calcium currents. *Nature* **353,** 43–48.

Kleuss, C., Scherubl, H., Hescheler, J., Schultz, G., and Wittig, B. (1992) Different beta-subunits determine G-protein interaction with transmembrane receptors. *Nature* **358,** 424–426.

Kleuss, C., Scherubl, H., Hescheler, J., Schultz, G., and Wittig, B. (1993) Selectivity in signal transduction determined by gamma subunits of heterotrimeric G proteins. *Science* **254,** 832–834.

Knott, C., Maguire, J. J., and Bowery, N. C. (1993) Age-related regional selectivity to pertussis toxin-mediated reduction in GABAB receptor binding in rat brain. *Brain Res.* **18,** 353–357.

Lanza, M., Fassio, A, Gemingnani, A., Bonalmo, G., and Raiteri, M. (1993) CGP52432: a novel potent and selective GABAB autoreceptor antagonist in rat cerebral cortex. *Eur. J. Pharmacol.* **237,** 191–195.

Li, X. H., Song, L., and Jope, R. S. (1990) Modulation of phosphoinositide metabolism in rat brain slices by excitatory amino acids, arachidonic acid, and GABA. *Neurochem. Res.* **15,** 725–738.

Logothetis, D. E., Kurachi, Y., Galper, J., Neer, E. J., and Clapham, D. E. (1987) The beta gamma subunits of GTP-binding proteins activate the muscarinic K^+ channel in heart. *Nature* **325,** 321–326.

Lovinger, D. M., Harrison, N. L., and Lambert, N. A. (1992) The actions of 3-aminopropanephosphinic acid at GABAB receptors in rat hippocampus. *Eur. J. Pharmacol.* **211,** 337–341.

Mailman, R. B., Mueller, R. A., and Breese, G. R. (1978) The effect of drugs which alter GABA-ergic function on cerebellar guanosine-3',5'-monophosphate content. *Life Sci.* **23,** 623–627.

Malcangio, M. and Bowery, N. G. (1992) Effect of (–)-baclofen on cAMP formation in rat spinal cord slices. *Br. J. Pharmacol.* **106,** 31P.

Marescaux, C., Vergnes, M., and Bernasconi, R. (1992) GABAB receptor antagonists: potential new anti-absence drugs. *J. Neurol. Trans. Suppl.* **35,** 179–188.

Masotto, C., Wisniewski, G., and Negro-Vilar, A. (1989) Different gamma- amino–butyric-acid receptor subtypes are involved in the regulation of opiate-dependent and independent luteinizing hormone-releasing hormone secretion. *Endocrinology* **125,** 548–553.

Mayfield, R. D. and Zahniser, N. R. (1993) Endogenous GABA release from rat striatal slices: effects of the GABAB receptor antagonist 2-hydroxy-saclofen. *Synapse* **14**, 16–23.

Mintz, I. M. and Bean, B. P. (1993) GABAB receptor inhibition of P-type Ca2+ channels in central neurons. *Neuron* **10**, 889–898.

Mondadori, C., Jaekel, J., and Preiswork, G. (1993) CGP 36742: the first orally active GABAB blocker improves the cognitive performance of mice, rats, and rhesus monkeys. *Behav. Neurol. Biol.* **60**, 62–68.

Mons, N. and Cooper, D. M. (1995) Adenylate cyclases: critical foci in neuronal signaling. *Trends Neurosci.* **18**, 536–542.

Mons, N., Harry, A., Dubourg, P., Premont, R. T., Iyengar, R., and Cooper, D. M. (1995) Immunohistochemical localization of adenylyl cyclase in rat brain indicates a highly selective concentration at synapses. *Proc. Natl. Acad. Sci. USA* **92**, 8473–8477.

Morishita, R., Kato, K., and Asano, T. (1990) GABAB receptors couple to G proteins G$_o$, G$_o$* and G$_{i1}$ but not to G$_{i2}$. *FEBS Lett.* **271**, 231–235.

Mott, D. D. and Lewis, D. V. (1991) Facilitation of the induction of long-term potentiation by GABAB receptors. *Science* **252**, 1718–1720.

Nakayasu, H., Mizutani, H., Hanai, K., Kimura, H., and Kuriyama, K. (1992) Monoclonal antibody to GABA binding protein, a possible GABAB receptor. *Biochem. Biophys. Res. Comm.* **182**, 722–726.

Nakayasu, H., Nishikawa, M., Mizutani, H., Kimura, H., and Kuriyama, K. (1993) Immunoaffinity purification and characterization of gamma-aminobutyric acid (GABA)B receptor from bovine cerebral cortex. *J. Biol. Chem.* **268**, 8658–8664.

Nishikawa, M. and Kuriyama, K. (1989) Functional coupling of cerebral γ-aminobutyric acid (GABA$_B$) receptors with the adenylate cyclase system: effect of phaclofen. *Neurochem. Int.* **14**, 85–90.

Nishikawa, T., Scatton, B., Inomoto, T., Shinohava, K., and Takahashi, K. (1989) Modulation of striatal serotonin metabolism by baclofen, a gamma-aminobutyric acid B receptor agonist. *Tokai J. Exp. Clin. Med.* **14**, 375–380.

Nockels, R. and Young, W. (1992) Pharmacologic strategies in the treatment of experimental spinal cord injury. *J. Neurotrauma* **9**, S211–S217.

Ogino, Y., Fraser, C. M., and Costa, T. (1992) Selective interaction of beta 2- and alpha 2-adrenergic receptors with stimulatory and inhibitory guanine nucleotide-binding proteins. *Mol. Pharmacol.* **42**, 6–9.

Ohmori, Y., Hirouchi, M., Taguchi, J., and Kuriyama, K. (1990) Functional coupling of the gamma-aminobutyric acid B receptor with calcium ion channel and GTP-binding protein and its alteration following solubilization of the gamma-aminobutyric acid B receptor. *J. Neurochem.* **54**, 80–85.

Ohmori, Y. and Kuriyama, K. (1991) Pharmacological and biochemical characteristics of partially purified GABA$_B$ receptor. *Neurochem. Res.* **16**, 357–362.

Okuhara, D. Y. and Beck, S. G. (1994) 5-HT 1A receptor linked to inward-rectifying potassium current in hippocampal CA3 pyramidal cells. *J. Neurophysiol.* **71**, 2161–2167.

Olpe, H. R., Steinmann, M. W., Ferrat, T., Pozza, M. F., Greiner, K., Brugger, F., Froestl, W., Mickel, S. J. and Bittiger, H. (1993) The actions of orally active GABAB receptor antagonists on GABAergic transmission in vivo and in vitro. *Eur. J. Pharmacol.* **233**, 179–186.

Ong, J. and Kerr, D. I. B. (1984) Evidence for a physiological role of GABA in the control of guinea pig intestinal motility. *Neurosci. Lett.* **50**, 339–343.

Oset-Gasque, M. J., Parramon, M., and Gonzalez, M. P. (1993) GABAB receptors modulate catecholamine secretion in chromaffin cells by a mechanism involving cyclic AMP formation. *Br. J. Pharmacol.* **110**, 1586–1592.

Parmar, B. S., Shah, K. H., and Gandhi, I. C. (1989) Baclofen in trigeminal neuralgia—a clinical trial. *Indian J. Dent. Res.* **1**, 109–113.

Pende, M., Lanza, M., Bonnano, G., and Railteri, M. (1993) Release of endogenous glutamic and aspartic acids from cerebrocortex synaptosomes and its modulation through activation of a gamma-aminobutyric acid B (GABAB) receptor subtype. *Brain Res.* **604**, 325–330.

Penn, R. D. (1992) Intrathecal baclofen for spasticity of spinal origin: seven years of experience. *J. Neurosurg.* **77**, 236–240.

Pfrieger, F. W., Gottmann, K., and Lux, H. D. (1994) Kinetics of GABAB receptor-mediated inhibition of calcium currents and excitatory synaptic transmission in hippocampal neurons in vitro. *Neuron* **12**, 979– 107.

Pieroni, J. P., Jacobowitz, O., Chen, J., and Iyengar, R. (1993) Signal recognition and integration by G_s-stimulated adenylyl cyclase. *Curr. Opin. Neurobiol.* **3**, 345–351.

Pitler, T. A. and Alger, B. E. (1994) Differences between presynaptic and postsynaptic GABAB mechanisms in rat hippocampal pyramidal cells. *J. Neurophysiol.* **72**, 2317–2332.

Remaury, A., Larrouy, D., Daviaud, D., Rouot, B., and Paris, H. (1993) Coupling of the alpha 2-adrenergic receptor to the inhibitory G-protein G_i and adenylate cyclase in HT29 cells. *Biochem. J.* **292**, 283–288.

Reuveny, E., Slesinger, P. A., Inglese, J., Morales, J. M., Iniguez-Lluhi, J. A., Lefkowitz, R. J., Bourne, H. R., and Jan, Y. N., and Jan, L. Y. (1994) Activation of the cloned muscarinic potassium channel by G protein beta gamma subunits. *Nature* **370**, 143–146.

Rhee, S. G., Lee, C. W., and Jhon, D. Y. (1993) Phospholipase C isozymes and modulation by cAMP-dependent protein kinase. *Adv. Second Mess. Phosphoprot. Res.* **28**, 57–64.

Saudou, F., Boschert, U., Amlaiky, N., Plassat, J. L., and Hen, R. (1992) A family of drosphila serotonin receptors with distinct intracellular signalling properties and expression patterns. *EMBO J.* **11**, 7–17.

Schaad, N. C., Schorderet, M., and Mogistretti, P. J. (1989) Accumulation of cyclic AMP elicited by vasoactive intestinal peptide is potentiated by noradrenaline, histamine, adenosine, baclofen, phorbol esters, and ouabain in mouse cerebral cortical slices: studies on the role of arachidonic acid metabolites and protein kinase C. *J. Neurochem.* **53**, 1941–1951.

Scherer, R. W., Karbon, E. W., Ferkany, J. W., and Enna, S. J. (1988) Augmentation of neurotransmitter receptor-stimulated cyclic AMP accumulation in rat brain: differentiation between the effects of baclofen and phorbol esters. *Brain Res.* **451**, 361–365.

Scholz, K. P. and Miller, R. J. (1991) GABAB receptor-mediated inhibition of Ca^{+2} currents and synaptic transmission in cultured rat hippocampal neurones. *J. Physiol. Lond.* **444**, 669–686.

Sharma, R., Mathur, R., and Nayar, U. (1993) GABAB mediated analgesia in tonic pain in monkeys. *Indian J. Physiol. Pharmacol.* **37**, 189–193.

Shenolikar, S., Karbon, E. W., and Enna, S. J. (1986) Phorbol esters down-regulate protein kinase C in rat brain cerebral cortical slices. *Biochem. Biophys. Res. Comm.* **139**, 251–258.

Shibuya, I. and Douglas, W. W. (1993) Indications from Mn-quenching of Fura-2 fluorescence in melanotrophs that dopamine and baclofen close Ca channels that are spontaneously open but not those opened by high [K+]O; and that Cd preferentially blocks the latter. *Cell Calcium* **14**, 33–44.

Simon, M. I., Strathmann, M. P., and Gautam, N. (1991) Diversity of G proteins in signal transduction. *Science* **252**, 802–808.

Snead, O. C. (1992) Evidence for GABAB-mediated mechanisms in experimental generalized absence seizures. *Eur. J. Pharmacol.* **21**, 343–349.

Snodgrass, S. R. (1992) GABA and epilepsy: their complex relationship and the evolution of our understanding. *J. Child Neurol.* **7**, 77–86.

Suzdak, P. D. and Gianutsos, G. (1986) Effect of chronic imipramine or baclofen and GABA-B binding and cyclic AMP production in cerebral cortex. *Eur. J. Pharmacol.* **131**, 129–133.

Swartz, K. J. (1993) Modulation of Ca^{2+} channels by protein kinase C in rat central and peripheral neurons: disruption of G protein-mediated inhibition. *Neuron* **11**, 305–320.

Swartzwelder, H. S., Lewis, D. V., Anderson, W. W., and Wilson, W. A. (1987) Seizure-like events in brain slices: suppression by interictal activity. *Brain Res.* **410**, 362–366.

Sweeney, M. I. and Dolphin, A. C. (1992) 1,4-Dihydropyridines modulate GTP hydrolysis by G$_o$ in neuronal membranes. *FEBS Lett.* **310**, 66–70.

Takigawa, M., Sakurai, T., Kasuya, Y., Abe, Y., Masaki, T., and Goto, K. (1995) Molecular identification of guanine-nucleotide-binding regulatory proteins which couple to endothelin receptors. *Eur. J. Biochem.* **228**, 102–108.

Tang, W. J. and Gilman, A. G. (1991) Type-specific regulation of adenylyl cyclase by G protein beta-gamma subunits. *Science* **254**, 1500–1503.

Tang, W. J. and Gilman, A. G. (1992) Adenylyl cyclases. *Cell* **70**, 869–872.

Tang, W. J., Iniguez-Lluhi, J. A., Mumby, S., and Gilman, A. G. (1992) Regulation of mammalian adenylyl cyclase by G-protein alpha and beta gamma subunits. *Cold Spring Harb. Symp. Quant. Biol.* **57**, 135–144.

Taniyama, K., Hanada, S., and Tanaka, C. (1985) Autoreceptors regulate gamma-[^{3}H] aminobutyric acid release from the guinea pig small intestine. *Neurosci. Lett.* **55**, 245–248.

Taniyama, K., Niwa, M., Kataoka, Y., and Yamashita, K. (1992) Activation of protein kinase C suppresses the gamma-aminobutyric acid B receptor-mediated inhibition of the vesicular release of noradrenaline and acetylcholine. *J. Neurochem.* **58**, 1239–1245.

Taniyama, K., Takeda, K., Ando, H., Tanaka, C. (1991) Expression of the GABAB receptor in *Xenopus* oocytes and desensitization bXy activation of protein kinase C. *Adv. Exp. Med. Biol.* **287**, 413–420.

Tareilus, E. and Breer, H. (1995) Presynaptic calcium channels: pharmacology and regulation. *Neurochem. Int.* **26**, 539–558.

Tareilus, E., Schoch, J., and Breer, H. (1994) GABAB-receptor-mediated inhibition of calcium signals in isolated nerve terminals. *Neurochem. Int.* **24**, 349–361.

Taussig, R., Quarmby, L. M., and Gilman, A. G. (1993) Regulation of purified type I and type II adenylyl cyclases by G protein beta gamma subunits. *J. Biol. Chem.* **268**, 9–12.

Thalmann, R. H. (1988) Evidence that guanosine triphosphate (GTP)-binding proteins control a synaptic response in brain: effect of pertussis toxin and GTP gamma S on the late inhibitory postsynaptic potential of hippocampal CA3 neurons. *J. Neurosci.* **8**, 4589–4602.

Thompson, S. M. and Gähwiler, B. H. (1992) Comparison of the actions of baclofen at pre- and postsynaptic receptors in the rat hippocampus in vitro. *J. Physiol Lond.* **451**, 329–345.

Ticku, M. K. and Delgado, A. (1989) GABAB receptor activation inhibits Ca^{2+}-mediated potassium channels in symptosomes: involvement of G-proteins. *Life Sci.* **44**, 1271–1276.

Toselli, M. and Taglietti, V. (1993) Baclofen inhibits high-threshold calcium currents with two distinct modes in rat hippocampal neurons. *Neurosci. Lett.* **164,** 134–136.

Waldmeier, P. C. (1991) The GABAB antagonist, CGP35348 antagonizes the effects of baclofen, gamma-butyrolactone and HA966 on rat striatal dopamine synthesis. *Naunyn Schmiedebergs Arch. Pharmacol.* **343,** 173–178.

Waldmeier, P. C. and Baumann, P. A. (1990) Presynaptic GABA receptors. *Ann. N.Y. Acad. Sci.* **604,** 136–151.

Waldmeier, P. C. and Wiki, P. (1994) GABA release in rat cortical slices is unable to cope with demand if the autoreceptor is blocked. *Naunyn Schmiedebergs Arch. Pharmacol.* **349,** 583–587.

Watling, K. J. and Bristow, D. R. (1986) $GABA_B$ receptor-mediated enhancement of vasoactive intestinal peptide-stimulated cyclic AMP production in slices of rat cerebral cortex. *J. Neurochem.* **46,** 1756–1762.

Wojcik, W. J. and Neff, N. H. (1984) Gamma-aminobutyric acid B receptors are negatively coupled to adenylate cyclase in brain, and in the cerebellum these receptors may be associated with granule cells. *Mol. Pharmacol.* **25,** 24–28.

Wojcik, W. J., Ulivi, M., Paez, X., and Costa, E. (1989) Islet-activating protein inhibits the beta-adrenergic receptor facilitation elicited by gamma-aminbutyric-acid B receptors. *J. Neurochem.* **53,** 753–758.

Worley, P. F., Baraban, J. M., McCarren, M., Snyder, S. H., and Alger, B. E. (1987) Cholinergic phosphatidylinositol modulation of inhibitory, G protein-linked neurotransmitter actions: electrophysiological studies in rat hippocampus. *Proc. Natl. Acad. Sci. USA* **84,** 3467–3471.

Xu, J. and Wojcik, W. J. (1986) Gamma aminobutyric acid B receptor-mediated inhibition of adenylate cyclase in cultured cerebellar granule cells: blockade by islet-activating protein. *J. Pharmacol. Exp. Ther.* **239,** 568–573.

Yoshimura, M. and Cooper, D. M. (1993) Type-specific stimulation of adenyl cyclase by protein kinase C. *J. Biol. Chem.* **268,** 4604–4607.

Zorn, S. H. and Enna, S. J. (1985) The effect of mouse spinal cord transection on the antinociceptive response to the gamma-aminobutyric acid agonists THIP (4,5,6,7-tetrahydroisoxazolo[5,4-c]pyridine-3-ol) and baclofen. *Brain Res.* **338,** 380–383.

CHAPTER 9

Biochemical and Molecular Properties of GABA$_B$ Receptors

Kinya Kuriyama and Masaaki Hirouchi

1. Introduction

γ-Aminobutyric acid (GABA) is known as one of the major inhibitory neurotransmitters in the brain. GABA receptors are many, and are pharmacologically classified into two major subtypes, GABA$_A$ and GABA$_B$. The GABA$_A$ receptor is well-characterized pharmacologically. Muscimol and bicuculline, which are, respectively, an agonist and an antagonist for the GABA$_A$ receptor, bind selectively to the GABA$_A$. Various central acting drugs, such as benzodiazepines and barbiturates, also have binding sites within the GABA$_A$ receptor complex (Doble and Martin, 1992). In addition, the GABA$_A$ receptor consists of heterogeneous subunits, and functions as a Cl$^-$ channel (Burt and Kamatchi, 1991; *see also* Chapter 2 of this volume).

Baclofen binds to a novel GABA receptor, the GABA$_B$ site, activation of which induces the suppression of neurotransmitter release (Bowery et al., 1980). [^{3}H]Baclofen binding in the rat brain is inhibited by GABA, but not by bicuculline, an antagonist of the classical GABA$_A$ receptor; GABA and baclofen inhibit [^{3}H]GABA binding (Hill and Bowery, 1981). In addition, Cl$^-$ channel activity is not associated with the GABA$_B$ receptor, and activation of GABA$_B$ receptors results in the suppression of cyclic AMP formation (Wojcik and Neff, 1984; *see also* Chapter 8 of this volume). These results clearly indicate that the GABA$_B$ receptor has the distinct mechanism for signal transduction, compared to the GABA$_A$ site.

Recently, it has also been postulated that a GABA$_C$ receptor, which is insensitive to bicuculline and baclofen, exists as a new subtype of GABA receptors (Johnston, 1986; *see also* Chapter 11 of this volume). The pharmacological properties of this receptor correspond to a site possessing GABA

The GABA Receptors Eds.: S. J. Enna and N. G. Bowery
Humana Press Inc., Totowa, NJ

receptor ρ subunits (Shimada et al., 1992). This ρ subunit is abundantly expressed in the retina and is homologous to other $GABA_A$ receptor subunits. The $GABA_C$ receptor in the retina may consist of homooligomers to form the Cl^- channel. The exact nature of the $GABA_C$ receptor, however, remains to be clarified (*see also* Chapter 11 of this volume).

Electrophysiological studies have demonstrated that $GABA_B$ receptors induce slow inhibitory postsynaptic potentials (IPSP), and $GABA_A$ receptors mediate fast IPSPs (Bormann, 1988). $GABA_B$ receptors directly hyperpolarize neuronal cells postsynaptically, with activation of $GABA_B$ receptors causing an increase in K^+ conductance (Newberry and Nicoll, 1984; Dutar and Nicoll, 1988a,b). Also, $GABA_B$ receptors inhibit voltage-dependent Ca^{2+} channels by acting through a GTP-binding protein (G protein) (Holz et al., 1986). It is presumed, therefore, that $GABA_B$ receptors also inhibit Ca^{2+} channels presynaptically, which may explain their ability to block neurotransmitter release.

This accumulated evidence clearly indicates that $GABA_A$ and $GABA_B$ receptors, ionotropic and metabotropic types, respectively, are present in the mammalian central nervous system. In this chapter, recent studies on $GABA_B$ receptors are reviewed, with emphasis on those relating to the biochemical, molecular, and pharmacological properties of this site.

2. Molecular Pharmacological Studies on $GABA_B$ Receptors

The binding characteristics of $GABA_B$ receptors have been studied using baclofen-sensitive [³H]GABA binding or [³H]baclofen binding. The $GABA_B$ receptor binding is a useful tool for estimating the potency of $GABA_B$ receptor ligands, and is, therefore, important for developing selective and sensitive agonists and antagonists for this site.

$GABA_B$ receptor binding is inhibited by GTP and its analogs, which decrease the affinity of the $GABA_B$ site (Hill et al., 1984). Treatment of synaptic membranes with N-ethylmaleimide or islet-activating protein (IAP) prevents this inhibition by GTP analogs (Asano et al., 1985, 1986). In contrast, GTPase activity is increased by stimulation of $GABA_B$ receptors, and this increase is also abolished by IAP (Ohmori et al., 1990).

Baclofen inhibits both forskolin- and GTP-stimulated adenylate cyclase activities in the rat brain (Wojcik and Neff, 1984). In cerebellum, this inhibition, mediated by the $GABA_B$ receptor stimulation, may be associated with granule cells and is blocked by IAP (Xu and Wojcik, 1986). These results indicate that the $GABA_B$ receptor is negatively coupled to adenylate cyclase through an IAP-sensitive G protein.

Activation of $GABA_B$ receptors also potentiates neurotransmitter receptor-stimulated cyclic AMP formation (Karbon et al, 1984; Karbon and Enna, 1985; Cunningham and Enna, Chapter 6 of this volume). For example, baclofen induces a further increase in isoproterenol-stimulated cyclic AMP formation in the rat cerebral cortex, although forskolin-stimulated cyclic AMP formation is inhibited by baclofen under these conditions. This facilitation, elicited by $GABA_B$ receptor stimulation in slices of the rat cerebral cortex and hippocampus, is blocked by IAP (Wojcik et al., 1989). The affinity of both low- and high-affinity binding sites on the beta adrenergic receptor is increased by preincubation with $GABA_B$ receptor agonists (Scherer et al., 1989). As a possible molecular mechanism, a cross-regulation of intracellular-mediated system between beta adrenergic and $GABA_B$ receptors has been suggested. In brief, the $\beta\gamma$ subunits liberated from G_i coupling to $GABA_B$ receptor may synergize with the activated $G_{s\alpha}$ to stimulate adenylate cyclase II (AC II). In cells expressing predominantly adenylate cyclase I (AC I), it has been postulated that the $GABA_B$ receptor stimulation may inhibit the cyclic AMP formation through the AC I cascade. Alternatively, in cells expressing predominantly AC II, the $GABA_B$ receptor stimulation may enhance the cyclic AMP formation through the AC II cascade (Tang and Gilman, 1991; Federman et al., 1992; Andrade, 1993; *see also* Chapter 8 of this volume).

Stimulation of the $GABA_B$ receptor, however, fails to enhance cyclic AMP accumulation induced by norepinephrine in the rat spinal cord (Malcangio and Bowery, 1993). $GABA_B$ receptor antagonists abolish baclofen-mediated inhibition of adenylate cyclase in the rat cerebellar granule cells in culture (Holopainen et al., 1992), $GABA_B$ receptor-mediated inhibition of forskolin-stimulated cyclic AMP accumulation in the rat spinal cord is not eliminated by such agents (Malcangio and Bowery, 1993). Because CGP 35348, a $GABA_B$ receptor antagonist, blocks the suppressive effect of baclofen on the spontaneous discharges of motoneurons in the spinal cord (Olpe and Karlsson, 1990; Brugger et al., 1993), it appears the antinociception induced by $GABA_B$ receptor stimulation may not be related to cyclic AMP accumulation, which appears to be modulated by a distinct group of $GABA_B$ receptors, as is the inhibition of the $GABA_B$ autoreceptor.

Ligand binding to the $GABA_B$ receptor in the bovine cerebral cortical membranes is inhibited by IAP (Asano et al., 1985). This effect is regionally selective in brain during postnatal development, although $GABA_B$ receptor binding decreases equally in the presence of GTPγS (Knott et al., 1993). $GABA_B$ receptors in the bovine brain couple to G_o and G_{i1} but not G_{i2} (Morishita et al., 1990). This also suggests the existence of multiple $GABA_B$ receptors. Moreover, it is possible that the coupling of $GABA_B$ receptors with

G proteins and adenylate cyclases in the spinal cord may form a different combination than those in the cerebral cortex.

The existence of multiple GABA$_B$ receptors has also been inferred from the results of pharmacological studies on GABA$_B$ receptor-mediated inhibition of neurotransmitter release. GABA$_B$ receptors (heteroreceptors) modulate the release of various neurotransmitters, such as noradrenaline (Bowery et al., 1980), 5-hydroxytryptamine, cholecystokinin, and somatostatin (Bowery et al., 1980; Gray and Green, 1987; Conzelmann et al., 1986; Bonanno et al., 1991). Moreover, stimulation of GABA$_B$ receptors causes inhibition of glutamate release (Travagli et al., 1991; Bonanno and Raiteri, 1992). In the case of the GABA$_B$ heteroreceptor, application of a GABA$_B$ receptor antagonist facilitates the induction of long-term potentiation, which requires the transient activation of the *N*-methyl-D-aspartate (NMDA) receptor system (Olpe and Karlsson, 1990; Mott and Lewis, 1991). During high frequency transmission, the release of GABA is depressed by a GABA$_B$ autoreceptor, and the NMDA receptor is sufficiently activated to induce long-term potentiation (Davies et al., 1991). These findings indicate that the GABA$_B$ receptor has an important role in synaptic plasticity. In fact, facilitation of long-term potentiation by CGP 35348, a GABA$_B$ receptor antagonist, occurs after applying nonprimed trains of stimuli with an increasing duration to the Schaffer collateral/commissural fibers (Olpe et al., 1993).

GABA$_A$ receptors modulate the synaptic release of GABA, serving as autoreceptors (Kuriyama et al., 1984). Similarly, GABA$_B$ autoreceptors have been found in nerve endings of the rat cerebral cortex (Pittaluga et al., 1987; Waldmeier et al., 1988). GABA$_B$ receptors modulating GABA release have different pharmacological properties than GABA$_B$ receptors modulating glutamate release (Bonanno and Raiteri, 1992). For example, phaclofen reduces the effect of baclofen on the releases of GABA and somatostatin-like immunoreactivity (SRIF-LI), but not on the release of glutamate in the rat brain cerebral cortex. In contrast, CGP 35348, a GABA$_B$ receptor antagonist, increases the releases of glutamate and SRIF-LI, but not that of GABA. These findings suggest the existence of GABA$_B$ receptor heterogeneity, such as a phaclofen-sensitive, CGP 35348-insensitive type, and a phaclofen-insensitive, CGP 35348-sensitive type, or a phaclofen-sensitive, CGP 35348-sensitive type. Presumably, all of these subtypes are stimulated by baclofen. These subtypes appear to be localized on GABA-ergic, glutamatergic, and somatostatinergic axon terminals, respectively. Furthermore, modulation of GABA release in the rat brain cerebral cortex and spinal cord appears to be mediated by distinct subtypes of the GABA$_B$ receptor (Raiteri et al., 1989; Seabrook et al., 1991; Bonanno and Raiteri, 1993a). The GABA$_B$ receptor in the spinal cord is sensitive to CGP 35348, but not to baclofen and phaclofen, although the $GABA_B$ receptors in both cerebral cortex and spinal cord are sensitive to 3-aminopropane phosphinic acid (APPA), a $GABA_B$ receptor agonist (Bonanno and Raiteri, 1993a). Based on these findings, Bonanno and Raiteri have proposed the existence of multiple $GABA_B$ receptors (Bonanno and Raiteri, 1993b).

$GABA_B$ receptor stimulation has no effect on phosphatidylinositol turnover (Brown et al., 1984), but the increase in inositol formation induced by histamine or serotonin is reduced by the activation of $GABA_B$ receptors (Crawford and Young, 1988; Godfrey et al., 1988). Stimulation of $GABA_B$ receptors inhibits GTP-stimulated accumulation of inositol-1,4,5-triphosphate (Ohmori and Kuriyama, 1989). The $GABA_B$ receptor-mediated inhibition of inositol phosphate formation is blocked by phaclofen and IAP. It is uncertain, however, whether $GABA_B$ receptor stimulation directly affects phosphatidylinositol turnover in the brain.

3. Biochemical Studies on GABA_B Receptor: Purification and Characterization of GABA_B Receptor

Identification of $GABA_B$ receptors with differing pharmacological properties suggests the existence of $GABA_B$ receptor subtypes. Because the precise identification of $GABA_B$ receptors requires that the site be purified, we have undertaken attempts to isolate this protein.

Solubilization of the $GABA_B$ receptor from crude synaptic membranes taken from bovine cerebral cortex has been attempted using various detergents, such as 3-(3-cholamidopropyl)-dimethylammonine-1-propane-sulfonate (CHAPS) (Ohmori and Kuriyama, 1990). Although the treatment of synaptic membranes with CHAPS resulted in the solubilization of the $GABA_B$ receptor, the coupling with G proteins was eliminated (Ohmori et al., 1990).

Neurotransmitter receptors, such as those associated with acetylcholine, dopamine, and adenosine, may be purified using ligand-affinity column chromatography (Haga and Haga, 1983; Ramwani and Mishra, 1986; Nakata, 1989). The purification of the $GABA_A$ receptor was achieved using benzodiazepine-coupled affinity column chromatography (Taguchi and Kuriyama, 1984). A similar approach was attempted using a ligand for the $GABA_B$ receptor, establishing the usefulness of a baclofen-affinity column (Ohmori and Kuriyama, 1990). When the solubilized fraction from the bovine cerebral cortex was applied to a baclofen-immobilized gel, most of the binding activity of the $GABA_B$ receptor was adsorbed to the affinity column. The fraction eluted by the application of baclofen displayed baclofen-sensitive [^{3}H]GABA binding (Kuriyama et al., 1992). It was difficult to obtain the $GABA_B$ receptor as a homogenous protein by this procedure, but there was an 11,000-fold increase in purification compared to the original solubilized fraction.

The development of a monoclonal antibody against the $GABA_B$ receptor has been attempted using the eluate from the baclofen-affinity gel (Nakayasu et al., 1992). A monoclonal antibody, which was identified as an IgM type, has been identified. This antibody revealed the presence of an 80 kDa protein on the immunoblot from crude synaptic membrane of the bovine cerebral cortex. Moreover, $GABA_B$ receptor binding activity in the crude synaptic membrane and in the solubilized fractions was inhibited to a similar extent when exposed to the monoclonal antibody. This 80 kDa protein was specifically adsorbed on the immunoabsorbent agarose beads conjugated with the antibody. This immunoabsorbent agarose was found useful for the immunoaffinity purification of $GABA_B$ receptor (Nakayasu et al., 1993).

After the solubilized fractions were mixed with the immunoaffinity gel, they were packed into a small column and washed with a high-salt buffer. The antigenic protein was eluted by the application of an acidic buffer and displayed a molecular weight of 80 kDa on SDS-polyacrylamide gel electrophoresis. This protein had baclofen-sensitive [^{3}H]GABA binding, which was inhibited by GABA and 2-hydroxy saclofen, but not by bicuculline. In addition, this 80 kDa protein was reconstituted with partially purified G protein, which contained both G_i and G_o, but not G_s, and adenylate cyclase. In this reconstituted system, forskolin-stimulated cyclic AMP accumulation was suppressed by GABA and baclofen, both of which were inhibited by 2-hydroxy saclofen, a $GABA_B$ receptor antagonist. Since this inhibition of forskolin-stimulated cyclic AMP accumulation was not detected in a reconstituted system lacking either the 80 kDa protein or the G protein preparation, it was concluded that the 80 kDa protein obtained by immunoaffinity column purification was a $GABA_B$ receptor coupled to G_i/G_o protein and adenylate cyclase.

The eluate from the baclofen-affinity gel was examined on immunoblot using the monoclonal antibody. It showed the presence of two major bands (79 and 80 kDa proteins) and a few minor bands (about 65–80 kDa proteins); the protein staining by colloidal gold suggested the presence of many proteins (Hirouchi et al., 1995). In the reconstituted system with G_i/G_o and adenylate cyclase, this eluate from the baclofen column mediated GABA and baclofen-induced suppressions on forskolin-stimulated cyclic AMP accumulation similar to that found in the reconstituted system with the 80 kDa protein from the immunoaffinity column. These results suggest that the monoclonal antibody-sensitive 80 kDa protein in the eluate from the baclofen-column is capable of inhibiting cyclic AMP formation via activation of G_i/G_o. These findings support the presence of multiple $GABA_B$ receptors (Bonano and Raiteri, 1993b).

Data on the mRNA-coding GABA$_B$ receptor are still incomplete. Various neurotransmitter receptors have been expressed on *Xenopus* oocytes injected with brain mRNAs. Likewise, the functional expression of GABA$_B$ receptors has been detected using *Xenopus* oocytes injected with guinea pig cerebral mRNA and rat cerebellar mRNA (Sekiguchi et al., 1990; Taniyama et al., 1991). We have also found APPA-induced responses in the oocytes injected with mouse brain mRNA, although the efficacy of expression was quite low (Kuriyama et al., 1993; Taniyama et al., 1991). A high concentration of baclofen altered the sensitivity of *Xenopus* oocytes (Woodward and Miledi, 1992). These difficulties hinder the use of the oocyte system for expressing the GABA$_B$ receptor.

Treatment with antisense oligonucleotide for seven transmembrane-spanning receptors selectively prevents the muscarinic m2 and GABA$_B$ receptor-mediated inhibition of cyclic AMP formation in rat cerebellar granule cells, while the antisense oligonucleotide encoding alpha-2 adrenergic receptor does not affect the GABA$_B$ receptor-mediated response (Holopainen and Wojcik, 1993). These data suggest that the GABA$_B$ receptor may have a sequence similar to the muscarinic site, although there is no direct evidence that this antisense oligonucleotide traps the mRNA for the GABA$_B$ receptor. Multiple approaches are being used to search for the mRNA encoding the GABA$_B$ receptor, including amino acid sequence analysis of the purified protein; its isolation should be forthcoming.

4. Conclusion

It has been well-established that the GABA$_B$ receptor is a metabotropic receptor coupled to G$_i$/G$_o$ proteins. The molecular weight of the native receptor is approximately 80 kDa, with the possibility of multiple sites. Presynaptic inhibition by GABA$_B$ autoreceptors and/or heteroreceptors suggests the possible utility of GABA$_B$ receptor agonists and antagonists for modulating neurotransmitter release and as a new class of therapeutic agents (Bittiger et al., 1993). Delineation of the primary structure of the GABA$_B$ receptor is of paramount importance in addressing these issues.

Acknowledgment

This work is supported, in part, by research grants from the Ministry of Education, Science, and Culture, Japan.

References

Andrade, R. (1993) Enhancement of β-adrenergic responses by G$_i$-linked receptors in rat hippocampus. *Neuron* **10,** 83–88.

Asano, T. and Ogasawara, N. (1986) Uncoupling of γ-aminobutyric acid B receptors from GTP-binding proteins by N-ethylmaleimide: effect of N-ethylmaleimide on purified GTP-binding proteins. *Mol. Pharmacol.* **29,** 244–249.

Asano, T., Ui, M., and Ogasawara, N. (1985) Prevention of the agonist binding to γ-aminobutyric acid B receptors by guanine nucleotides and islet-activating protein, pertussis toxin, in bovine cerebral cortex. *J. Biol. Chem.* **260,** 12,653–12,658.

Bittiger, H., Froestl, W., Mickel, S. J., and Olpe, H. R. (1993) GABA_B receptor antagonists: from synthesis to therapeutic applications. *Trends Pharmacol. Sci.* **14,** 391–394.

Bonanno, G., Gemignani, A., Fedele, E., Fontana, G., and Raiteri, M. (1991) γ-Aminobutyric acid (GABA_B) receptors mediate inhibition of somatostatin release from cerebrocortex nerve terminals. *J. Pharmacol. Exp. Ther.* **259,** 1153–1159.

Bonanno, G. and Raiteri, M. (1992) Functional evidence for multiple γ-aminobutyric acids receptor subtypes in the rat cerebral cortex. *J. Pharmacol. Exp. Ther.* **262,** 114–118.

Bonanno, G. and Raiteri, M. (1993a) γ-Aminobutyric acid (GABA) autoreceptors in rat cerebral cortex and spinal cord represent pharmacologically distinct subtypes of the GABA_B receptor. *J. Pharmacol. Exp. Ther.* **265,** 765–770.

Bonanno, G., and Raiteri, M. (1993b) Multiple GABA_B receptors. *Trends Pharmacol. Sci.* **14,** 259–261.

Bormann, J. (1988) Electrophysiology of GABA_A and GABA_B receptor subtypes. *Trends Neurosci.* **11,** 112–116.

Bowery, N. G., Hill, D. R., Hudson, A. L., Doble, A., Middlemiss, D. N., Shaw, J., and Turnbull, M. (1980) (–)-Baclofen decreases neurotransmitter release in the mammalian CNS by an action at a novel GABA receptor. *Nature* **283,** 92–94.

Brown, E., Kendall, D. A., and Nahorski, S. R. (1984) Inositol phospholipid hydrolysis in rat cerebral cortical slices: I. Receptor characterization. *J. Neurochem.* **42,** 1379–1387.

Brugger, F., Wicki, U., Olpe, H. R., Froestl, W., and Mickel, S. (1993) The action of new potent GABA_B receptor antagonists in the hemisected spinal cord preparation of the rat. *Eur. J. Pharmacol.* **235,** 153–155.

Burt, D. B. and Kamatchi, G. L. (1991) GABA_A receptor subtypes: from pharmacology to molecular pharmacology. *FASEB J.* **5,** 2916–2923.

Conzelmann, U., Meyer, D. K., and Sperk, G. (1986) Stimulation of receptors of γ-aminobutyric acid modulates the release of cholecystokinin-like immunoreactivity from slices of rat neostriatum. *Br. J. Pharmacol.* **89,** 845–852.

Crawford, M. L. A. and Young, J. M. (1988) GABA_B receptor-mediated inhibition of histamine H_1-receptor-induced inositol phosphate formation in slices of rat cerebral cortex. *J. Neurochem.* **51,** 1441–1447.

Davies, C. H., Starkey, S. J., Pozza, M. F., and Collingridge, G. L. (1991) GABA_B autoreceptors regulate the induction of LTP. *Nature* **349,** 609–611.

Doble, A. and Martin, I. L. (1992) Multiple benzodiazepine receptors: no reason for anxiety. *Trends Pharmacol. Sci.* **13,** 76–81.

Dutar, P. and Nicoll, R. A. (1988a) A physiological role for GABA_B receptors in the central nervous system. *Nature* **332,** 156–158.

Dutar, P. and Nicoll, R. A. (1988b) Pre- and postsynaptic GABA_B receptors in the hippocampus have different pharmacological properties. *Neuron* **1,** 585–591.

Federman, A. D., Conklin, B. R., Schrader, K. A., Reed, R. R., and Bourne, H. R. (1992) Hormonal stimulation of adenylyl cyclase via G_i protein βγ subunits. *Nature* **356,** 159–161.

Godfrey, P. P., Grahame-Smith, D. G., and Gray, J. A. (1988) $GABA_B$ receptor activation inhibits 5-hydroxytryptamine-stimulated inositol phospholipid turnover in mouse cerebral cortex. *Eur. J. Pharmacol.* **152,** 185–188.

Gray, J. A. and Green, A. R. (1987) $GABA_B$ receptor mediated inhibition of potassium-evoked release of endogenous 5-hydroxytryptamine from mouse frontal cortex. *Br. J. Pharmacol.* **91,** 517–522.

Haga, K. and Haga, T. (1983) Affinity chromatography of the muscarinic acetylcholine receptor. *J. Biol. Chem.* **258,** 13,575–13,579.

Hill, D. R. and Bowery, N. G. (1981) ^{3}H-Baclofen and ^{3}H-GABA bind to bicuculline-insensitive $GABA_B$ sites in rat brain. *Nature* **290,** 149–152.

Hill, D. R., Bowery, N. G., and Hudson, A. L. (1984) Inhibition of $GABA_B$ receptor binding by guanyl nucleotides. *J. Neurochem.* **42,** 652–657.

Hirouchi, M., Mizutani, H., Nishikawa, M., Nakayasu, H., and Kuriyama, K. (1996) Functional analysis on $GABA_B$ receptor using a reconstituted system with purified $GABA_B$ receptor, G_i/G_o protein and adenylyl cyclase, in *GABA: Receptors, Transporters and Metabolism* (Tanaka, C. and Bowery, N. G., eds.), Birkhauser, Basel, pp. 227–235.

Holopainen, I., Rau, C., and Wojcik, W. J. (1992) Proposed antagonists at $GABA_B$ receptors that inhibit adenylyl cyclase in cerebellar granule cell cultures of rat. *Eup. J. Pharmacol. Mol. Pharmacol. Sec.* **227,** 225–228.

Holopainen, I. and Wojcik, W. J. (1993) A specific antisense oligonucleotide to mRNAs encoding receptors with seven transrmembrane spanning regions decreases muscarinic m2 and γ-aminobutyric acid$_B$ receptors in rat cerebellar granule cells. *J. Pharmacol. Exp. Ther.* **264,** 423–430.

Holz, G. G., Rane, S. G., and Dunlap, K. (1986) GTP-binding proteins mediate transmitter inhibition of voltage-dependent calcium channels. *Nature* **319,** 670–672.

Johnston, G. A. R. (1986) Multiplicity of GABA receptors, in *Benzodiazepine/GABA receptors and chloride channels. Receptor biochemistry and methodology,* vol. 5 (Olsen, R. W. and Venter, J. C., eds.), Liss, New York, pp. 57–71.

Karbon, E. W., Duman, R. S., and Enna, S. J. (1984) $GABA_B$ receptors and norepinephrine-stimulated cAMP production in rat brain cortex. *Brain Res.* **306,** 327–332.

Karbon, E. W. and Enna, S. J. (1985) Characterization of the relationship between γ-aminobutyric acid B agonists and transmitter-coupled cyclic nucleotide-generating systems in rat brain. *Mol. Pharmacol.* **27,** 53–59.

Knott, C., Maguire, J. J., and Bowery, N. G. (1993) Age-related regional sensitivity to pertussis toxin-mediated reduction in $GABA_B$ receptor binding in rat brain. *Mol. Brain Res.* **18,** 353–357.

Kuriyama, K., Kanmori, K., Taguchi, J., and Yoneda, Y. (1984) Stress-induced enhancement of suppression of [^{3}H]GABA release from striatal slices by presynaptic autoreceptor. *J. Neurochem.* **42,** 943–950.

Kuriyama, K., Mizutani, H., and Nakayasu, H. (1992) Purification and identification of 61 kilodalton GABA (γ-aminobutyric acid)$_B$ receptor from bovine brain. *Mol. Neuropharmacol.* **2,** 155–157.

Kuriyama, K., Nakayasu, H., Hirouchi, M., Mizutani, H., Tsujimura, A., Hashimoto-Gotoh, T., and Kimura, H. (1993) Purification and expression of $GABA_B$ receptor. *J. Neurochem.* **61 (Suppl),** S236.

Malcangio, M. and Bowery, N. G. (1993) $GABA_B$ receptor-mediated inhibition of forskolin-stimulated cyclic AMP accumulation in rat spinal cord. *Neurosci. Lett.* **158,** 189–192.

Morishita, R., Kato, K., and Asano, T. (1990) GABA$_B$ receptors couple to G proteins G$_o$, G$_o$*, and G$_{i1}$ but not to G$_{i2}$. *FEBS Lett.* **271**, 231–235.

Mott, D. D. and Lewis, D. V. (1991) Facilitation of the induction of long-term potentiation by GABA$_B$ receptors. *Science* **252**, 1718–1720.

Nakata, H. (1989) Purification of A$_1$ adenosine receptor from rat brain membranes. *J. Biol. Chem.* **264**, 16,545–16,551.

Nakayasu, H., Mizutani, H., Hanai, K., Kimura, H., and Kuriyama, K. (1992) Monoclonal antibody to GABA binding protein, a possible GABA$_B$ receptor. *Biochem. Biophys. Res. Commun.* **182**, 722–726.

Nakayasu, H., Nishikawa, M., Mizutcmi, H., Kimura, H., and Kuriyama, K. (1993) Immunoaffinity purification and characterization of γ-aminobutyric acid (GABA)$_B$ receptor from bovine cerebral cortex. *J. Biol. Chem.* **268**, 8658–8664.

Newberry, N. R. and Nicoll, R. A. (1984) Direct hyperpolarizing action of baclofen on hippocampal pyramidal cells. *Nature* **308**, 450–452.

Ohmori, Y., Hirouchi, M., Taguchi, J., and Kuriyama, K. (1990) Functional coupling of γ-aminobutyric acid$_B$ receptor with calcium ion channel and GTP-binding protein and its alteration following solubilization of the γ-aminobutyric acid β receptor. *J. Neurochem.* **54**, 80–85.

Ohmori, Y. and Kuriyama, K. (1989) Negative coupling of γ-aminobutyric acid (GABA)$_B$ receptor with phosphatidylinositol turnover in the brain. *Neurochem. Int.* **15**, 359–363.

Ohmori, Y. and Kuriyama, K. (1990) Solubilization and partial purification of GABA$_B$ receptor from bovine brain. *Biochem. Biophys. Res. Commun.* **172**, 22–27.

Olpe, H. R. and Karlsson, G. (1990) The effects of baclofen and two GABA$_B$-receptor antagonists on long-term potentiation. *Naunyn Schmiedeberg's Arch. Pharmacol.* **342**, 194–197.

Olpe, H. R., Worner, W., and Ferrat, T. (1993) Stimulation parameters determine role of GABA$_B$ receptors in long-term potentiation. *Experentia* **49**, 542–546.

Pittaluga, A., Asaro, D., Pellegrini, G., and Raiteri, M. (1987) Studies on [^{3}H]GABA and endogenous GABA release in rat cerebral cortex suggest the presence of autoreceptors of the GABA$_B$ type. *Eur. J. Pharmacol.* **144**, 45–52.

Raiteri, M., Pellegrini, G., Cantoni, C., and Bonanno, G. (1989) A novel type of GABA receptor in rat spinal cord? *Naunyn Schmiedeberg's Arch. Pharmacol.* **340**, 666–670.

Ramwani, J., and Mishra, R. K. (1986) Purification of bovine striatal dopamine D-2 receptor by affinity chromatography. *J. Biol. Chem.* **261**, 8894–8898.

Scherer, R. W., Ferkany, J. W., Karbon, E. W., and Enna, S. J. (1989) γ-Aminobutyric acid β receptor activation modifies agonist binding to β-adrenergic receptors in rat brain cerebral cortex. *J. Neurochem.* **53**, 989–991.

Seabrook, G. R., Howson, W., and Lacey, M. G. (1991) Subpopulations of GABA-mediated synaptic potentials in slices of rat: dorsal striatum are differentially modulated by presynaptic GABA$_B$ receptors. *Brain Res.* **562**, 332–334.

Sekiguchi, M., Sakuta, H., Okamoto, K., and Sakai, Y. (1990) GABA$_B$ receptors expressed in *Xenopus* oocytes by guinea pig cerebral mRNA are functionally coupled with Ca^{2+}-dependent Cl$^-$ channels and with K$^+$ channels, through GTP-binding proteins. *Mol. Brain Res.* **8**, 301–309.

Shimada, S., Cutting, G., and Uhl, G. R. (1992) γ-Aminobutyric acid A or C receptor? γ-Aminobutyric acid ρ1 receptor RNA induces bicuculline-, barbiturate-, and benzodiazepine-insensitive γ-aminobutyric acid responses in *Xenopus* oocytes. *Mol. Pharmacol.* **41**, 683–687.

Taguchi, J. and Kuriyama, K. (1984) Purification of γ-aminobutyric acid (GABA) receptor from rat brain by affinity column chromatography using a new benzodiazepine, 1012-S, as an immobilized ligand. *Brain Res.* **323,** 219–226.

Tang, W. J. and Gilman, A. G. (1991) Type specific regulation of adenylyl cyclase by G protein βγ subunits. *Science* **254,** 1500–1503.

Taniyama, K., Takeda, K., Ando, H., Kuno, T., and Tanaka, C. (1991) Expression of the GABA_B receptor in *Xenopus* oocytes and inhibition of the response by activation of protein kinase C. *FEBS Lett.* **278,** 222–224.

Travagli, R. A., Ulivi, M., and Wojcik, W. J. (1991) γ-Aminobutyric acid-B receptors inhibit glutamate release from cerebellar cells: consequences of inhibiting cyclic AMP formation and calcium influx. *J. Pharmacol. Exp. Ther.* **258,** 903–909.

Waldmeier, P. C., Wicki, P., Feldtrauer, J. J., and Baumann, P. A. (1988) Potential involvement of a baclofen-sensitive autoreceptor in the modulation of the release of endogenous GABA from rat brain slices in vitro. *Naunyn Schmiedeberg's Arch. Pharmacol.* **337,** 289–295.

Wojcik, W. J., and Neff, N. H. (1984) γ-Aminobutyric acid B receptors are negatively coupled to adenylate cyclase in brain, and in the cerebellum these receptors may be associated with granule cells. *Mol. Pharmacol.* **25,** 24–28.

Wojcik, W. J., Ulivi, M., Paez, X., and Costa, E. (1989) Islet-activating protein inhibits the β-adrenergic receptor facilitation elicited by γ-aminobutyric acid β receptors. *J. Neurochem.* **53,** 753–758.

Woodward, R. M. and Miledi, R. (1992) Sensitivity of *Xenopus* oocytes to changes in extracellular pH: possible relevance to proposed expression of atypical mammalian GABA_B receptors. *Mol. Brain Res.* **16,** 204–210.

Xu, J. and Wojcik, W. J. (1986) Gamma aminobutyric acid B receptor-mediated inhibition of adenylate cyclase in cultured cerebellar granule cells: blockade by islet-activating protein. *J. Pharmacol. Exp. Ther.* **239,** 568–573.

CHAPTER 10

Chemistry of GABA$_B$ Modulators

Wolfgang Froestl and Stuart J. Mickel

1. Introduction

An important step toward understanding the diverse roles of the ubiquitous inhibitory neurotransmitter g-aminobutyric acid (GABA) was Bowery's discovery that baclofen **1** (Fig. 1) stereospecifically decreases neurotransmitter release in the mammalian central nervous system (CNS) by action at a novel GABA receptor, an effect that was not blocked by bicuculline or other GABA antagonists (Bowery et al., 1980; Hill and Bowery, 1981).

Baclofen was synthesized for the first time in September, 1962, by Keberle as a lipophilic derivative of GABA, in an attempt to enhance the blood-brain barrier penetrability of the endogenous lead structure (Keberle et al., 1968). The drug is now widely prescribed as an antispastic agent and muscle relaxant for the treatment of multiple sclerosis and trigeminal neuralgia (Marsden, 1989; Fromm, 1991). In particular, for very severe cases of spasticity, intrathecal administration of baclofen proves to be the best treatment currently available (Penn et al., 1989; Penn, 1992; Ochs, 1993).

It would surpass the scope of this review to discuss extensively the different synthetic schemes devised for the preparation of either racemic or *(R)*-(–)-baclofen. Two elegant chiral syntheses were published recently, as were methods for either resolution or chromatographic separation of racemic baclofen (Allan et al., 1990; Herdeis and Hubmann, 1992; Schoenfelder et al., 1993; Vaccher et al., 1993a). The superb syntheses developed by Meyers and Mulzer for the preparation of the potent antidepressant *(R)*-(–)-Rolipram (3-cyclo-pentyloxy-4-methoxypyrrolidin-2-one) may be applied for *(R)*-(–)-baclofen (Meyers and Snyder, 1993; Mulzer, 1994).

2. GABA$_B$ Receptor Agonists

For a generation of medicinal chemists, baclofen, which was the very first compound of several series of lipophilic GABA derivatives, remained

The GABA Receptors Eds.: S. J. Enna and N. G. Bowery
Humana Press Inc., Totowa, NJ

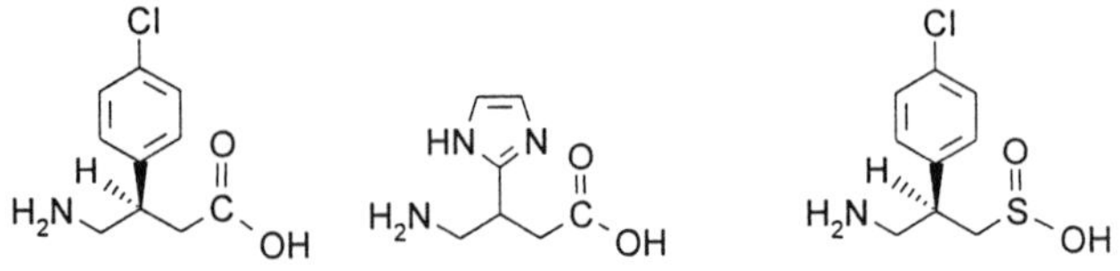

1 (R)-(-)-Baclofen   2   3 (R)-(-)-Siclofen

Fig. 1. Structures of GABA$_B$ receptor agonists.

the most potent agonist for the GABA$_B$ receptor. An exhaustive overview of structural modifications of baclofen up to 1992 was provided by Kerr and Ong (1992). Neither 3-heteroaryl-GABA analogs nor compounds mimicking a possible bioactive conformation produced GABA$_B$ agonists displaying superior affinity to the GABA$_B$ receptors (Berthelot et al., 1991; Mann et al., 1991). A recent patent claimed that some heterocyclic baclofen analogs, e.g., 4-amino-3-(2-imidazolyl)-butanoic acid 2 (Fig. 1), were superior to baclofen in suppressing bicuculline-induced epileptogenesis in vitro (Debaert et al., 1992).

An interesting result was communicated by chemists of Schering-Plough (Carruthers et al., 1995). They found that the sulfinic acid analog of baclofen, siclofen 3 (Fig. 1), showed properties of a GABA$_B$ receptor agonist in functional in vitro assays; however, the sulfonic acid analog of baclofen, saclofen 39 (*see* Fig. 5, later in this chapter), showed properties of a GABA$_B$ receptor antagonist (Kerr et al., 1989a). Comparison of the circular dichroism curves of both enantiomers of siclofen with those of the baclofen enantiomers suggested that the biological activity of siclofen resides in the *(R)*-(−)-enantiomer, as is the case with baclofen. The IC$_{50}$ values were for *(R,S)*-siclofen: 1.2 μM, for *(R)*-(−)-siclofen: 0.2 μM and for *(S)*-(+)-siclofen: 90 μM (measured by inhibition of binding of [³H]GABA to GABA$_B$ receptors of rat cortex) (Carruthers et al., 1995).

A new series of potent and selective GABA$_B$ receptor agonists was discovered by replacing the carboxylic acid groups of GABA, GABOB (i.e., γ-amino-β-hydroxy-butyric acid) or baclofen, respectively, by potentially isosteric phosphinic acid residues, an idea that was explored first for naturally occurring α-amino acids (Baylis et al, 1984; Dingwall et al., 1987, 1989).

The affinity of the novel phosphinic acid derivatives of GABA, γ-amino-propyl-phosphinic acid CGP27492 (4, Fig. 2) and γ-aminopropyl-methyl-phosphinic acid CGP35024 (5, identical to SK&F97541, Fig. 2), to GABA$_B$ receptors was superior to that of the endogenous neurotransmitter and to that of baclofen (inhibition of binding of [³H]baclofen to GABA$_B$ receptors from synaptosomal membranes of cat cerebellum, Table 1) (Froestl et al., 1992; Howson et al., 1993). The new compounds showed weak or no affinity for

4 R = H
5 R = Me
6 R = CHF$_2$
7 R = CH$_2$OH
8 R = OH

9 R = H (*R,S*)-OH
10 R = Me (*R,S*)-OH
11 R = Me (*S*)-(-)-OH
12 R = Me (*R*)-(+)-OH

Fig. 2. Structures of novel GABA$_B$ receptor agonists.

GABA$_A$ receptors (Table 1). Because of its 15 times higher potency, its high specific binding, and the possibility for carrying out filtration assays, [^{3}H]CGP27492 has now replaced [^{3}H]baclofen as a radioligand for GABA$_B$ receptor binding assays (Bittiger et al., 1988; Hall et al., 1995).

2.1. Chemistry of Novel GABA$_B$ Receptor Agonists

The syntheses of GABA$_B$ agonists 4–7, 9–12 (Fig. 2), 13–18 (Fig. 3), and 23, 24, 26, and 27 (Fig. 4) have all been described, as have the syntheses of the GABA$_B$ receptor antagonists 20 and 21 (Fig. 3) (Dingwall et al., 1989; Froestl et al., 1995a,b).

Scheme 1 depicts the synthetic procedures used to obtain 3-aminopropyl-phosphinic acids 4–7 and 9–12 (Fig. 2) and the unsaturated derivatives 23, 24, 26, and 27 (Fig. 4). Starting from inexpensive inorganic hypophosphorus acid, the key reagent, ethyl diethoxymethylphosphinate (Gallagher's reagent, 28), was obtained by acid-catalyzed condensation with triethylorthoformate, allowing selective protection of one of the two P—H bonds (Gallagher and Honegger, 1980). Alkylation with alkylhalides, concomitant cleavage of the P—H protecting group and the ester under strongly acidic conditions, and subsequent re-esterification of the intermediate phosphinic acids, using ethyl chloroformate, gave the various ethyl phosphinates 29. The introduction of the 3-aminopropyl side chain was achieved via base-catalyzed conjugate addition to acrylonitrile, followed by hydrogenation of the intermediate nitriles over Raney nickel in the presence of ammonia. The aminopropyl-phosphinic acid esters were then hydrolyzed under acidic conditions to give the final products 5–7 (Fig. 2). 4 (CGP27492, Fig. 2) was obtained by conjugate addition of the anion of reagent 28 to acrylonitrile, followed by hydrogenation and simultaneous acidic hydrolysis of the ester and the diethoxymethyl protecting group.

Table 1
Inhibition of Binding of [^{3}H]Baclofen to GABA$_B$ Receptors of Cat Cerebellum,
of [^{3}H]CGP27492 to GABA$_B$ Receptors of Rat Cortex,
and of [^{3}H]Muscimol to GABA$_A$ Receptors of Rat Cortex

Compound	[^{3}H]Baclofen IC$_{50}$ (nM)	[^{3}H]CGP27492 IC$_{50}$ (nM)	[^{3}H]Muscimol IC$_{50}$ (nM)
GABA	25	17	128
(R,S)-baclofen	35	107	1,047,000
(R)-(−)-baclofen	15	32	964,000
(S)-(+)-baclofen	1770	84,000	1,564,000
4 CGP27492	2.4	5.4	1700
5 CGP35024	6.6	16.3	Inactive[a]
6 CGP47656	n.t.[b]	89	135,000
7 CGP45120	n.t.[b]	1050	n.t.[b]
8 CGP34854	1500[c]	4000	Inactive[a]
9 CGP35583	18	21	14,500
10 CGP34938	29	77	Inactive[a]
11 CGP44532	27	45	Inactive[a]
12 CGP44533	180	152	Inactive[a]
13 CGP35832	39	42	Inactive[a]
14 CGP39153	25	n.t.[b]	n.t.[b]
15 CGP39154	5600	n.t.[b]	n.t.[b]
16 CGP35997	360	n.t.[b]	Inactive[a]
17 CGP35914	880	n.t.[b]	n.t.[b]
18 CGP38218	10,000	n.t.[b]	n.t.[b]
19 CGP49713	n.t.[b]	65	Inactive[a]
22 *trans*-ACA	2300[d]	3250	90
23 CGP38593	560	280	6800
24 CGP44530	1350	665	Inactive[a]
25 *cis*-ACA	n.t.[b]	>100,000	2800
26 CGP70522	n.t.[b]	4410	6600
27 CGP70523	n.t.[b]	16,600	242,000

[a]At a concentration of $10^{-5}M$.
[b]Not tested.
[c][^{3}H](−)Baclofen (Drew et al., 1990).
[d][^{3}H]GABA (Falch et al., 1986).

In order to introduce a hydroxy group into position 2 of the 3-amino-propyl side chain, ethyl phosphinates **29** were converted to their corresponding highly reactive silylated P(III) intermediates by reaction with trimethylsilyl-chloride in the presence of triethylamine, under anhydrous conditions. Reaction with racemic or *(R)*- or *(S)*-epichlorohydrin, catalyzed by zinc chloride

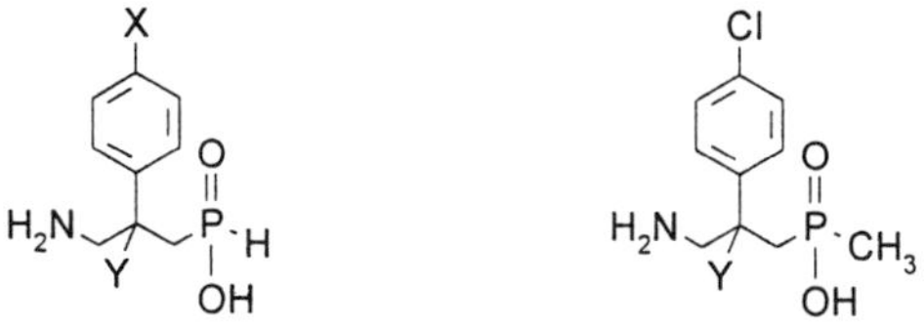

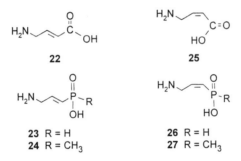

13 (*R,S*)   X = Cl   Y = H
14 (*R*)-(-)   X = Cl   Y = H
15 (*S*)-(+)   X = Cl   Y = H
16 (*R,S*)   X = F   Y = H
17 (*R,S*)   X = H   Y = H
18 (*R,S*)   X = CF₃   Y = H
19 (*R,S*)   X = Cl   Y = OH

20 (*R,S*)   Y = H
21 (*R,S*)   Y = OH

Fig. 3. Structures of novel GABA_B receptor agonists.

22

25

23 R = H
24 R = CH₃

26 R = H
27 R = CH₃

Fig. 4. Structures of novel GABA_B receptor agonists.

in the absence of solvent gave, regiospecifically, the trimethylsilyl-ethers of ethyl (3-chloro-2-hydroxypropyl) phosphinates, which were then hydrolyzed to chlorohydrins **30**. Nucleophilic displacement of the chlorine atom with ethanolic ammonia proceeded via a clean S_N2 process to give amino-phosphinic acid esters with complete retention of the stereochemistry at the chiral carbon. Finally, acidic hydrolysis yielded (3-amino-2-hydroxypropyl)-phosphinic acids **9–12** (Fig. 2). An X-ray analysis of the methanesulfonate salt of **11** provided an unambiguous proof of the retention of the stereochemistry during all these synthetic transformations (Froestl et al., 1995a).

Displacement of the chlorine atom of the chiral intermediates **30** obtained via reaction with optically pure epichlorohydrins—still 1:1 mixtures of diastereoisomers caused by phosphorus chirality—with potassium

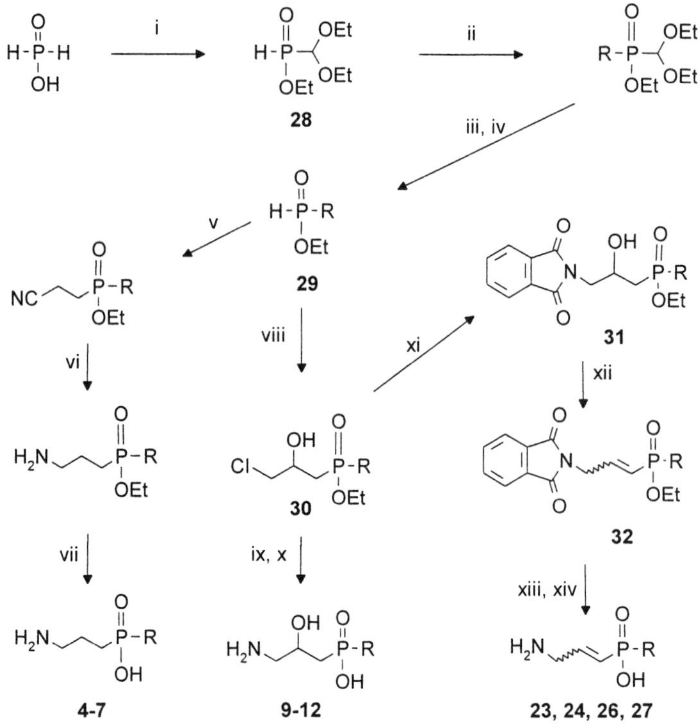

Scheme 1. Reagents and conditions: (i) HC(OEt)$_3$, CF$_3$COOH, rt, 72 h; (ii) NaH, THF, rt, 2 h, RX, rt, 24 h; (iii) 4M HCl, reflux, 24 h; (iv) ClCO$_2$Et, Et$_3$N, DCM, 10°C → rt, 2 h; (v) Na, EtOH, CH$_2$ = CHCN, 10°C, 1 h, rt, 1 h, reflux, 1 h; (vi) H$_2$ Raney nickel, 10% NH$_3$ in EtOH, 70°C, 100 bar, 2 h; (vii) 5M HCl, reflux, 24 h; propylene oxide, MeOH, 4°C, 24 h; (viii) (a) Me$_3$SiCl, Et$_3$N, rt, 24 h; (b) THF, 10 mol% ZnCl$_2$, (R,S)- or (R)- or (S)-epichlorohydrin, rt → 70°C, 24 h; (c) 1% HOAc in MeOH, rt, 24 h; (ix) 20 equiv. NH$_3$ in EtOH, rt, 96 h; (x) conc. HCl, reflux, 2 h; propylene oxide, MeOH; (xi) potassium phthalimide, 18-crown-6, toluene, 60°C, 120 h; (xii) Ph$_3$P, EtOOCN = NCOOEt, THF, toluene, 5°C → rt, 16 h; (xiii) chromatography; (xiv) conc. HCl, reflux, 5 h; propylene oxide, MeOH, rt, 5°C, 16 h.

phthalimide, proceeded also via a clean S$_N$2 process yielding phthalimides **31**. Elimination of water under Mitsonobu conditions gave *cis*- and *trans*-phthalimido-phosphinic acid esters **32** in a 1:1 ratio. After separation by chromatography, each individual geometrical isomer of **32** was hydrolyzed under acidic conditions to give unsaturated phosphinic acid derivatives **23, 24, 26**, and **27** (Fig. 4).

Scheme 2 outlines the syntheses of phosphinic acid and methylphosphinic acid analogs of baclofen **13–18** and **20** (Fig. 3). Generation of the

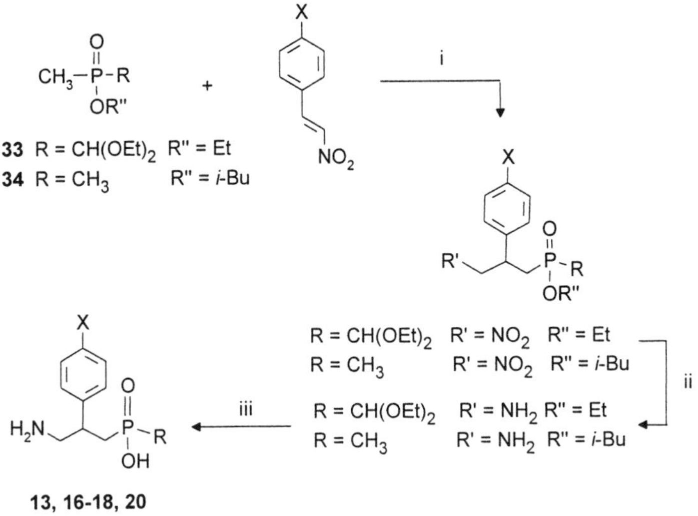

13, 16-18, 20

Scheme 2. Reagants and conditions: (i) LDA, THF, −78°C, 1 h, add to −78°C solution of 4-X-C$_6$H$_4$CH = CHNO$_2$, 30 min; (ii) H$_2$, Raney nickel, 10% NH$_3$ in EtOH, rt, 1 bar, 3 h; (iii) conc. HCl, 100°C, 24 h; propylene oxide, EtOH, rt, 24 h.

anions of either ethyl diethoxymethyl methyl-phosphinate **33** or *iso*-butyl dimethyl-phosphinate **34** by deprotonation with LDA and conjugate addition to 4-substituted β-nitrostyrenes gave the intermediate 3-nitropropylphosphinic acid esters (Dingwall et al., 1989; Froestl et al., 1995b). Reduction of the nitro group by hydrogenation over Raney nickel gave amino-phosphinic acid esters, which were hydrolyzed under acidic conditions to yield **13, 16–18**, and **20** (Fig. 3).

The enantiomerically pure *(R)*- and *(S)*-[3-amino-2-(4-chlorophenyl)-propyl]-phosphinic acids (**14** and **15**, Fig. 3) were prepared via resolution of the phthalimide derivative of racemic **13** by fractional crystallization of the diastereomeric salts with (+) and (−)-α-methyl-benzylamine.

An interesting disubstitution pattern was reported with the structure of the novel GABA$_B$ antagonist 2-hydroxysaclofen **40** (Fig. 5) (Kerr et al., 1988; Curtis et al., 1988). The synthesis of its phosphinic acid analogs **19** and **21** is shown in Scheme 3.

1,2-propadienyl-phosphinic acid, prepared from hypophosphorus acid and propargylalcohol, was esterified by treatment with ethylchloroformate to give the corresponding ethyl ester (Belakhov et al., 1983). The P—H bond was protected by Lewis acid catalyzed reaction with triethylorthoacetate to give allene **35**, a very reactive Michael acceptor. Addition of 4-chlorophenyl-

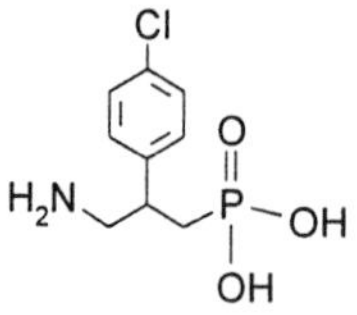

38 Phaclofen

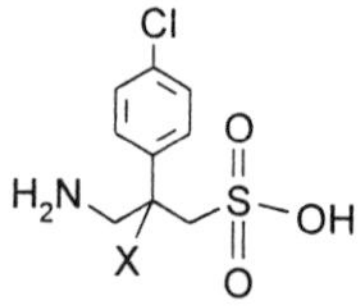

39 X = H Saclofen
40 X = OH 2-OH-Saclofen

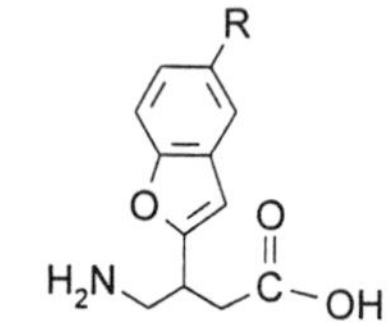

41 3-(Benzo[b]furan-2-yl)-GABA

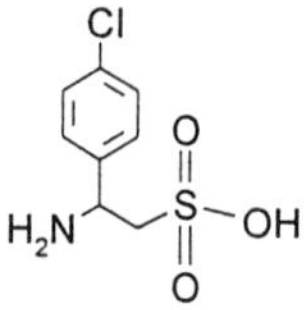

42 2-Amino-2-(*p*-chlorophenyl)-ethane-sulfonic acid

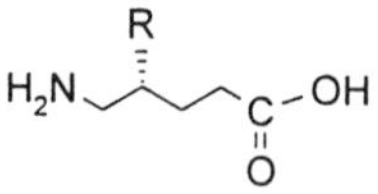

43 R = H DAVA
45 R = OH (R)-(-)-4-OH-DAVA

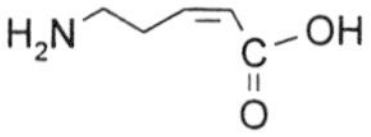

44 *Z*-5-Aminopent-2-enoic acid

Fig. 5. Structures of $GABA_B$ receptor antagonists.

cuprate furnished the allylic compound **36** without rearrangement, provided that the temperature during the alkylation was maintained strictly at –78°C. The regiospecific introduction of the 3-amino and 2-hydroxy groups was achieved, using the osmium catalyzed oxyamination procedure described by Herranz et al. (1978), to give Boc-protected ester **37** as a 1:1 mixture of diastereoisomers. All three protecting groups were cleaved simultaneously, using trimethylsilylbromide to give the $GABA_B$ agonist **19** (Fig. 3). Deprotection of the ketal protecting group of intermediate **36** was possible under very mild conditions by reaction with anhydrous HCl generated from the reaction of trimethylsilylchloride with ethanol in dichloromethane. The intermediate phosphinate was deprotonated by treatment with *n*-butyllithium at –78°C and alkylated with methyliodide. Oxyamination and treatment with trimethylsilylbromide, followed by methanolysis, gave the $GABA_B$ antagonist **21** (Fig. 3) in good yield.

2.2. Structure–Activity Relationships

2.2.1. Affinity to $GABA_B$ Receptors In Vitro

The affinities of some of the phosphinic acid analogs of GABA to $GABA_B$ receptors were surprisingly high. For the sake of direct comparison, Table 1 shows the IC_{50} values of selected compounds for the inhibition of binding of [^{3}H]baclofen to $GABA_B$ receptors of cat cerebellum, the inhibition of binding of the new ligand [^{3}H]CGP27492 to $GABA_B$ receptors of rat

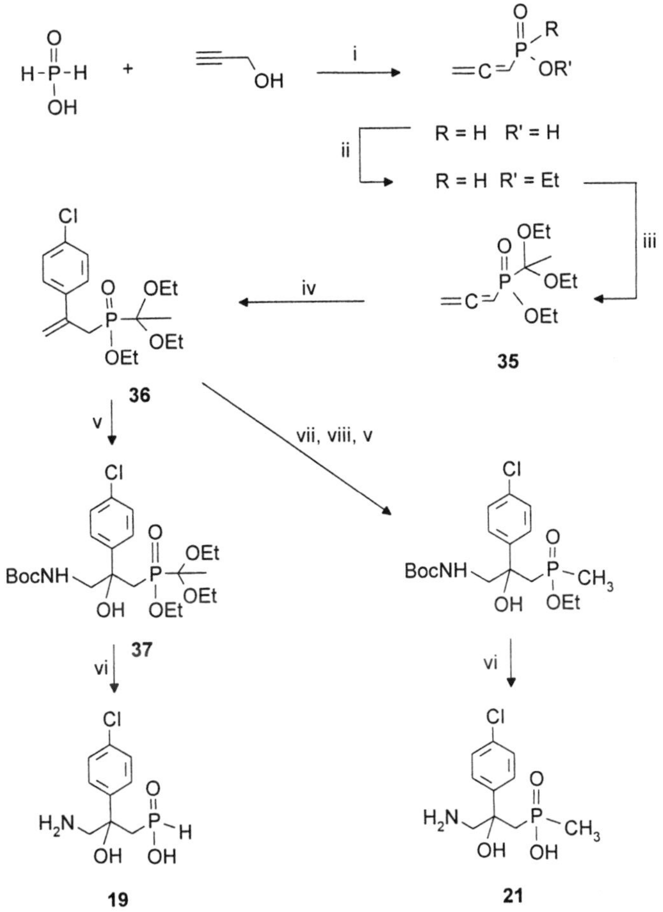

Scheme 3. Reagents and conditions: (i) toluene, reflux, 24 h; (ii) ClCOOEt, Et$_3$N, DCM/THF, 2:1, −5°C, 2 h, rt, 16 h: (iii) MeC(OEt)$_3$, BF$_3$ · Et$_2$O, rt, 24 h; (iv) 4-ClC$_6$H$_4$MgI · CuBr · Me$_2$S, Et$_2$O, −45°C, 3 h, −20°C, 2 h; (v) BocNH$_2$, MeOH, 0°C, t-BuOCl, 0°C, 15 min, NaOH, MeOH, 0°C → rt; AgNO$_3$, MeCN, 3 mol% OsO$_4$, t-BuOH, H$_2$O, rt, 24 h; (vi) Me$_3$SiBr, DCM, rt, 24 h; propylene oxide, MeOH, rt, 24 h; (vii) Me$_3$SiCl, 10% EtOH/DCM, rt, 24 h; (viii) n-BuLi, THF, −78°C, 10 min, CH$_3$I, −78°C, 5 min; NH$_4$Cl/H$_2$O, −78°C rt.

cortex and the inhibition of binding of [^{3}H]muscimol to GABA$_A$ receptors of rat cortex (Froestl et al., 1995a).

The size of the substituent R at the phosphorus of the phosphinic acid analogs of GABA (Fig. 2) determines whether the compound acts as a GABA$_B$ receptor agonist or a GABA$_B$ receptor antagonist. Electrophysiological experiments demonstrated that compounds with substituents R equal to H, Me, and CH_2OH (**4, 5,** and **7,** Fig. 2) showed effects of $GABA_B$ receptor agonists; homologous alkylphosphinic acids with substituents $R \geq C_2H_5$, e.g., **46–50** (Fig. 6), were $GABA_B$ antagonists (Froestl et al., 1995b). Compound **6** (R = CHF_2) with a substituent, the size of which is between a methyl and an ethyl group, showed properties of a $GABA_B$ receptor partial agonist, as was shown in GABA release experiments (Froestl et al., 1995a). When $GABA_B$ agonists interact with $GABA_B$ autoreceptors, they cause an inhibition of the electrically induced release of [^{3}H]GABA from rat cortical slices. **6** inhibited [^{3}H]GABA release when the slices were stimulated at a frequency of 0.125 Hz (IC_{50} = 10.6 μM), however, upon stimulation at a frequency of 2 Hz, it increased the release of [^{3}H]GABA (EC_{150} = 62 μM, i.e., the concentration causing a 50% increase to controls), an effect displayed by many $GABA_B$ receptor antagonists of this class of compounds (Froestl et al., 1995a,b).

The most potent $GABA_B$ receptor agonists in vitro were 3-amino-propyl-phosphinic acid **4** and 3-aminopropyl-methylphosphinic acid **5** followed by the 2-hydroxy-substituted derivatives **9–12**. The affinity to $GABA_B$ receptors is higher when the 2-hydroxy group is oriented in the *(S)*-configuration, as in **11**. Falch et al. (1986) obtained similar results with a series of hydroxylated GABA derivatives. They reported IC_{50}s for 4-amino-3-*(R)*-(–) -hydroxy-butyric acid and for 4-amino-3-*(S)*-(+)-hydroxy-butyric acid of 0.35 μM and 2.4 μM, respectively, i.e., inhibition of binding of [^{3}H]GABA from rat brain after blockade of the $GABA_A$ receptors by isoguvacine. Despite opposite suffixes *(R)* or *(S)*, the absolute stereochemical orientations of the more potent compounds in both series are identical, because in the Cahn Ingold Prelog nomenclature the phosphinic acid assumes a higher priority than the carboxylic acid.

The baclofen substitution pattern also produced potent $GABA_B$ agonists, the *(R)*-(–)enantiomer **14** being more potent than the *(S)*-(+)-enantiomer **15** by a factor of 225, as compared to a factor of 120 for *(R)*-(–)-baclofen vs *(S)*-(+)-baclofen. Substituents other than chlorine on the aromatic ring caused a significant loss of affinity, an effect also found in the baclofen series, suggesting that the chlorine residue may interact with the active site of the $GABA_B$ receptor (Kerr and Ong, 1992; Wermuth, personal communication). The phosphinic acid analog **19** of 2-hydroxy-saclofen did not show superior affinity to $GABA_B$ receptors, compared to the deshydroxy derivative **13**. As its synthesis was considerably more laborious, the resolution of the racemate **19** was not carried out. Both *methyl*phosphinic acid analogs, either of baclofen **20** (CGP36278, IC_{50} = 9 μM; Fig. 3) or of 2-hydroxy-saclofen **21** (CGP49650, IC_{50} = 6 μM; Fig. 3) showed properties of $GABA_B$ receptor antagonists (Froestl et al., 1995b).

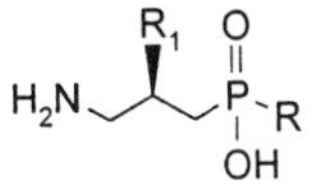

$$\text{H}_2\text{N} \diagdown \diagdown \overset{\displaystyle \text{R}_1}{\underset{\displaystyle \underset{\text{OH}}{|}}{\overset{\text{O}}{\overset{||}{\underset{}{\text{P}}}}}\text{-R}$$

46	R = C$_2$H$_5$	R$_1$ = H	CGP36216
47	R = CH(OEt)$_2$	R$_1$ = H	CGP35348
48	R = n-C$_4$H$_9$	R$_1$ = H	CGP36742
49	R = CH$_2$C$_6$H$_{11}$	R$_1$ = H	CGP46381
50	R = CH$_2$C$_6$H$_{11}$	R$_1$ = OH	CGP51176

Fig. 6. Structures of GABA$_B$ receptor antagonists.

The interaction of unsaturated phosphinic acid analogs of GABA (Fig. 4) with GABA$_A$ and GABA$_B$ receptors were of particular interest. The *trans*-α,β-unsaturated derivative of GABA, *trans*-aminocrotonic acid 22, interacted with a similar potency with GABA$_A$ receptors as GABA; its affinity to GABA$_B$ receptors was considerably weaker than that of GABA by a factor of about 200 (Table 1, inhibition of binding of [³H]CGP27492) (Johnston et al., 1975; Falch et al., 1986). A *trans*-double bond in the series of phosphinic acid analogs of GABA caused a loss of affinity to GABA$_B$ receptors by factors of 40–50 compared to the saturated compounds (**23** compared to **4** and **24** compared to **5**, Table 1, inhibition of binding of [³H]CGP27492). *Cis*-aminocrotonic acid **25**, a selective agonist of the putative GABA$_C$ receptors (Johnston, 1994), had only weak affinity for GABA$_A$ receptors (30 times less than its *trans* isomer **22**) and did not interact with GABA$_B$ receptors. The phosphinic acid derivatives of GABA with a *cis* double bond lost affinity for GABA$_B$ receptors by factors of 15–25, in comparison to their *trans* isomers.

2.2.2. Structure–Activity Relationships In Vivo

The rotarod test, in which rodents have to keep their balance on a rotating cylinder, was used to assess the antispastic and muscle relaxant effects of the novel GABA$_B$ agonists in vivo. The results are presented in Table 2 for sc and po administration. The racemic phosphinic acid analog of baclofen **13** was equipotent to racemic baclofen when administered sc, but was inactive after oral administration. This finding may be a result of oxidation of the P—H bond of **13** under in vivo conditions to the corresponding phosphonic acid, which is phaclofen **38** (Fig. 5), a weak GABA$_B$ antagonist (Kerr et al., 1987). CGP27492 (**4**), although very potent in many in vitro paradigms, did not show muscle-relaxant effects, even after sc administration, which may also be a result of the metabolic lability of its P—H bond. Oxidation of **4** leads to the corresponding 3-aminopropylphosphonic acid (**8**, Fig. 2), a weak GABA$_B$ receptor antagonist (Drew et al., 1990; Froestl et al., 1995a). This may explain the observations made in some biochemical and electrophysiological experiments that **4** showed properties of a GABA$_B$ receptor

Table 2
Deterioration of Rotarod Performance of Rats
after Treatment with Selected GABA$_B$ Agonists
(EC$_{50}$s in µmol/kg, sc and po)

Compound	sc[a]	po[b]
(R,S)-Baclofen	24	52
(R)-(–)-Baclofen	9	16
(S)-(+)-Baclofen	>200	>200
13 CGP35832	19	>215
4 CGP27492	>813	n.t.[c]
5 CGP35024	2	9
6 CGP47656	22	101
11 CGP44532	2	36
12 CGP44533	13	135

[a]Observed 0.5–1 h after sc administration (i.e., at time point of maximal effect = minimal EC$_{50}$).
[b]Observed 1.5–2 h after po administration (i.e., at time point of maximal effect = minimal EC$_{50}$).
[c]Not tested.

partial agonist (Pratt et al., 1989; Ong et al., 1990). The most potent compound in the rotarod test was **5**. However, toxic effects were observed at relatively low doses after sc and po administration. The GABA$_B$ receptor partial agonist **6** also produced strong muscle relaxant effects comparable to those of baclofen, but also showed prohibitive toxic effects.

The requirements for a valuable antispastic agent were fulfilled by CGP44532 (**11**), which proved to be more potent than racemic baclofen. **11** showed a significantly larger therapeutic window than any other new GABA$_B$ agonist. In cases of severe spasticity, the doses of baclofen required by some individuals exceed the tolerated doses. The most frequent side effects at high doses of baclofen are sedation, vertigo, nausea, and gastrointestinal side effects causing vomiting and diarrhea. Extensive comparative studies in three groups of four Rhesus monkeys each (single blind paradigm, baclofen vs **11** vs placebo) demonstrated that **11** produced pronounced muscle relaxation, but no sedation. The monkeys were capable of reacting fully to external stimuli, such as noise or offered food, but did not show any gastrointestinal side effects.

3. GABA$_B$ Receptor Antagonists

Selective GABA$_B$ antagonists have been elusive for many years. Kerr et al. (1987) introduced phaclofen **38** (Fig. 5), the phosphonic acid analog of baclofen, as the first peripheral and central baclofen antagonist. Phaclofen showed an IC_{50} value of 130 μM (inhibition of binding of [^{3}H]CGP27492). Three efficient syntheses have been communicated for the preparation of phaclofen (Chiefari et al., 1987; Hall, 1989; Robinson et al, 1989). Racemic phaclofen was resolved using chiral chromatographic techniques (Frydenvang et al., 1994). The GABA_B receptor affinity and antagonist effects of phaclofen also reside in the *(R)*-(–)-enantiomer, as is the case with baclofen, suggesting that both ligands bind to the GABA_B recognition site in a similar fashion. The IC_{50} value for *(R)*-(–)-phaclofen was 76 μM, for *(S)*-(+), >1 mM.

Some compounds with similar structures (Fig. 5) were more potent than phaclofen: saclofen **39** (IC_{50} = 26 μM); 2-hydroxy-saclofen **40** (IC_{50} = 12 μM) and 2-benzo[b]furan-2-yl-GABA **41** (IC_{50} = 10 μM; all IC_{50}s: inhibition of binding of [^{3}H]CGP27492) (Berthelot et al., 1987; Curtis et al., 1988; Kerr et al., 1988, 1989a,b; Beattie et al., 1989). Saclofen, for which three different synthetic approaches were reported, was also resolved; the *(R)*-(–)-enantiomer showed significantly higher affinity for GABA_B receptors (IC_{50} = 33 μM) than the *(S)*-(+)-enantiomer (IC_{50} > 100 μM, i.e., inhibition of binding of [^{3}H]GABA) (Abbenante and Prager, 1990, 1992a; Li et al., 1991; Vaccher et al., 1993b; Carruthers et al., 1995).

Several syntheses for 2-hydroxy-saclofen **40** have been disclosed (Abbenante and Prager, 1990, 1992b). Recent electrophysiological studies revealed that **40** may act as a GABA_B receptor partial agonist, whose effects were blocked by phaclofen, but not bicuculline (Caddick et al., 1995). Both enantiomers of 2-hydroxy-saclofen **40** have been prepared by chiral synthesis (Kerr et al., 1995; Prager et al., 1995). *(S)*-(+)-2-hydroxy-saclofen hydrochloride was the active GABA_B receptor antagonist. However, its absolute stereochemistry is identical to *(R)*-(–)-baclofen, *(R)*-(–)-siclofen, *(R)*-(–)-phaclofen, or *(R)*-(–)-saclofen, since the 2-hydroxy substituent assumes highest priority under the Cahn Ingold Prelog sequence rule. However, none of these compounds was able to penetrate the blood brain barrier. The lower homolog of saclofen, 2-amino-*(p*-chlorophenyl)-ethanesulfonic acid **42** (Fig. 5), showed some central effects, but was approximately five times weaker than CGP35348 (**47**, Fig. 6) (Ong et al., 1991).

Various other analogs of GABA and baclofen, exerting properties of weak GABA_B receptor antagonists, have been described (Kerr and Ong, 1992). GABA_B receptor antagonistic properties have also been reported for δ-aminovaleric acid (DAVA, **43**), for its conformationally restricted analog, Z-5-amino-pent-2-enoic acid (**44**), as well as for its hydroxylated derivatives, *(S)*-(–)-2-OH-DAVA and *(R)*-(–)-4-OH-DAVA (**45**, Fig. 5) (Muhyaddin et al., 1982; Dickenson et al., 1988; Kristiansen et al., 1992). However, these compounds also showed significant affinity for GABA_A receptors, e.g., *(R)*-(–)-4-OH-DAVA (**45**): IC_{50} = 8 μM for GABA_B receptors and IC_{50} = 82 μM for GABA_A receptors.

A new series of selective $GABA_B$ receptor antagonists, capable of penetrating the blood brain barrier after systemic (including oral) administration, was discovered during the course of a medicinal chemistry program designed to improve upon the pharmacology of substituted 3-aminopropylphosphinic acids (**4** and **5**, Fig. 2). The structures of the most interesting $GABA_B$ receptor antagonists are shown in Fig. 6. 3-Aminopropylethylphosphinic acid CGP36216 (**46**) displayed a significantly lower affinity for $GABA_B$ receptors ($IC_{50} = 2 \mu M$) than its lower homolog 3-aminopropyl-methylphosphinic acid, (**5**, $IC_{50} = 16$ nM, Table 1), which, however, showed the properties of a $GABA_B$ receptor *agonist* (Froestl et al., 1995b). By far the best-characterized $GABA_B$ receptor antagonist is CGP 35348, 3-aminopropyl-diethoxymethyl-phosphinic acid (**47**, $IC_{50} = 27 \mu M$), which crossed the blood-brain barrier after iv or ip administration (Bittiger et al., 1990; Olpe et al., 1990). The first orally active $GABA_B$ receptor antagonists were 3-aminopropyl-*n*-butyl phosphinic acid CGP36742 (**48**, $IC_{50} = 38 \mu M$), the corresponding cylohexyl-methyl-phosphinic acid CGP46381 (**49**, $IC_{50} = 4 \mu M$) and 3-amino-2-*(R)*-(+)-hydroxypropyl-cyclohexylmethylphosphinic acid CGP51176 (**50**, $IC_{50} = 6$ μM; all IC_{50}s: inhibition of binding of [^{3}H]CGP27492) (Bittige et al., 1992a; Olpe et al., 1993; Lingenhoehl and Olpe, 1993). The new $GABA_B$ receptor antagonists were all prepared according to Scheme 1. Full experimental details are now available (Froestl et al., 1995b).

Despite weak affinities for $GABA_B$ receptors, compounds **47–50** showed remarkable and very different in vivo activities in a multitude of psychopharmacological tests. CGP36742 (**48**) showed pronounced learning- and memory-enhancing effects in mice, adult and old rats, and Rhesus monkeys (Mondadori et al., 1992, 1993; Carletti et al., 1993). CGP35348 (**47**), CGP36742 (**48**), and CGP46381 (**49**) suppressed spontaneous 3 Hz spike and wave discharges in various animal models of absence epilepsy (Hosford et al., 1992; Klebs et al., 1992; Marescaux et al., 1992; Snead, 1992). **49** was, however, inactive in learning and memory paradigms. CGP51176 (**50**) showed remarkable antidepressant effects in the chronic stress model of Wilner (Papp, personal communication). The broad spectrum of pharmacological activity of these chemically quite similar $GABA_B$ receptor antagonists may originate from their different affinities for presynaptic $GABA_B$ receptor subtypes controlling the release of excitatory and inhibitory neurotransmitters in different ratios (Bonanno and Raiteri, 1993; Gemignani et al., 1994).

More recently, researchers at Schering reported a novel structural class of $GABA_B$ receptor antagonists, 2,5 disubstituted-1,4-morpholines (Fig. 7) and -thiomorpholines (Kuo et al., 1994). The synthesis of SCH 50911 **52** is outlined in Scheme 4. The IC_{50} values for **51** were 6 μM, for **52**, 2 μM and for **53**, >100 μM, (measured by inhibition of binding of [^{3}H]GABA in presence

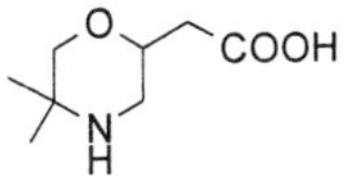

	51 Racemate
	52 (+)-Enantiomer SCH50911
	53 (-)-Enantiomer

Fig. 7. Structure of a new class of GABA$_B$ receptor antagonists.

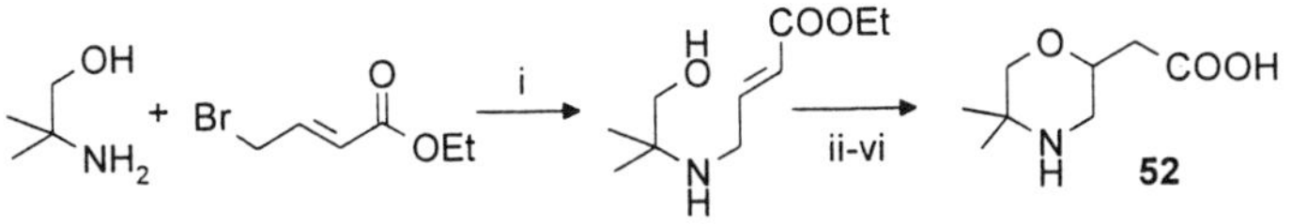

Scheme 4. Reagents and conditions: (i) Hüning's base, DCM, rt, 24 h; (ii) DBU, toluene, reflux, 18 h; (iii) 6N HCl, reflux, 18 h; (iv) ClCOOCH$_2$C$_6$H$_5$, DMAP, DCM, Et$_3$N, rt, 6 h; (v) HPLC on Daicel Chiralcel; (vi) 1N NaOH, MeOH, THF, rt, 18 h; H$_2$, 10% Pd/C, MeOH, rt, 1 bar, 18 h; 1N HCl.

of isoguvacine). The new GABA$_B$ receptor antagonists prevented absence-type seizures in lethargic mice and seizures induced by either γ-hydroxybuty-rate or pentylenetetrazole in rats (Bolser et al., 1995; Hosford et al., 1995).

3.1. Chemistry of Potent GABA$_B$ Receptor Antagonists

Despite extensive work on structure activity relationships by varying the substituents on the phosphorus and the carbon atoms of the novel 3-amino-propyl-alkyl-, cycloalkyl-, or arylalkyl-phosphinic acids (Fig. 6), their affini-ties to GABA$_B$ receptors never surpassed the micromolar range. A significant, and unexpected, improvement in the potency of this class of compounds was discovered by substituting the nitrogen of various 3-aminopropylphosphinic acids with selected benzyl substituents (Froestl et al., 1992, 1993a,b; Bittiger et al, 1993). This finding was very unusual, since it was well-known from many baclofen analogs, i.e., GABA$_B$ receptor agonists, that any substitution on the nitrogen invariably led to a significant loss of affinity. For example, baclofen showed an affinity for GABA$_B$ receptors of 35 nM (inhibition of binding of [³H]baclofen; Table 1), the IC$_{50}$ of N-monobenzylbaclofen (CGP11970) was only 16 μM. However, substitution on the nitrogen of the weak GABA$_B$ re-ceptor antagonist CGP35348 (**47**, Fig. 8, IC$_{50}$ = 27 μM) with a 4-chlorobenzyl residue led to CGP51783 (**54**, Fig. 8), displaying an enhanced affinity for GABA$_B$ receptors (IC$_{50}$ = 1 μM; Table 3). By applying the same substitution to the very potent GABA$_B$ receptor agonist CGP27492 (**4**, Fig. 8, IC$_{50}$ = 5 nM, inhibition of binding of [³H]CGP27492, Table 1), affinity was lost, as was the case with the baclofen series: CGP52880 (**55**, Fig. 8) displayed an IC$_{50}$ of 110 nM and showed properties of a GABA$_B$ receptor agonist in electrophysiologi-

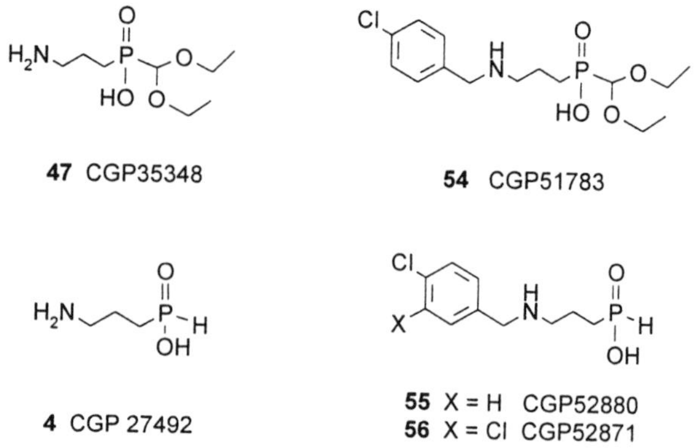

47 CGP35348

54 CGP51783

4 CGP 27492

55 X = H CGP52880
56 X = Cl CGP52871

Fig. 8. Antagonists gain, agonists lose affinity for GABA$_B$ receptors on *N*-substitution.

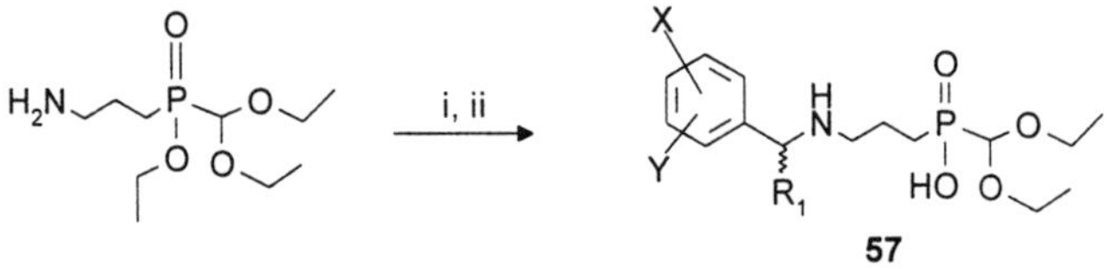

57

Scheme 5. Reagents and conditions: (i) NaCNBH$_3$, HOAc, MeOH, rt, 24 h, 2*M* HCl; (ii) LiOH, EtOH/H$_2$O, reflux, 24 h, H$_3$PO$_4$.

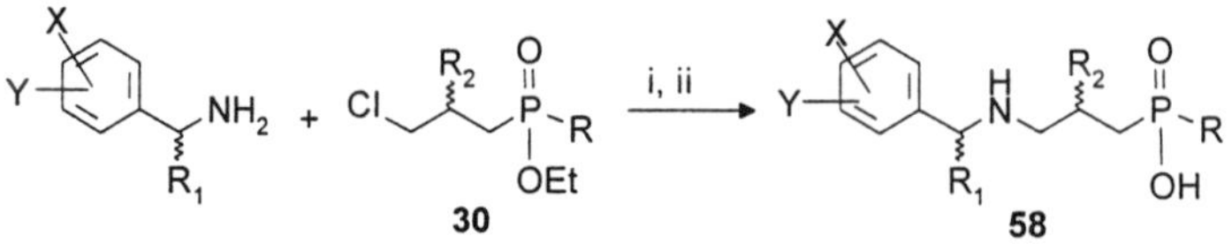

30   **58**

Scheme 6. Reagents and conditions: (i) Hünig's base, EtOH, reflux, 7–10 d; (ii) HCl/H$_2$O, reflux, 24 h.

cal paradigms. However, substitution of **4** with a 3,4-dichlorobenzyl residue gave the weak GABA$_B$ receptor antagonist CGP52871 (**56**, Fig. 8), with an IC$_{50}$ of 1.1 µ*M*. This is another example of a sharp transition from a GABA$_B$ receptor agonist to a GABA$_B$ receptor antagonist, comparable to the transitions from baclofen **1** to phaclofen **38** or from 3-aminopropyl methylphosphinic acid **5** to its homologous ethylphosphinic acid **46**. Apart from steric requirements, these findings may also imply that the GABA$_B$ agonist and antagonist binding sites are located within different regions of the G protein-coupled receptor (Schwartz, 1994).

Table 3
Inhibition of Binding of [^{3}H]CGP27492 to GABA$_B$ Receptors
of Rat Cortex by Compounds of Structures
of General Formula **57** (Scheme 5, R$_1$ = H)

X	Y	IC$_{50}$(nM)	CGP
H	H	8400	53662
2-Cl	H	4530	53162
3-Cl	H	662	52928
H	4-Cl	975	**51783**
H	4-F	5000	52911
H	4-I	345	53223
2-Cl	4-Cl	1480	53224
2-Cl	6-Cl	1100	53225
3-Cl	5-H	175	54275
3-CF$_3$	4-Cl	130	52921
3-Cl	4-Cl	55	**52432**
3-OMe	4-OMe	475	62854
3-OMe	5-OMe	597	62852
3-CN	H	292	62851
3-COOH	H	36	**61334**
H	4-CN	931	63162
H	4-COOH	970	61395

Boldface numbers represent most interesting compounds.

In order to optimize the improved GABA$_B$ receptor antagonist **54** by varying the substituents on the benzene ring, the operational scheme of Topliss was employed (Topliss, 1972). The synthesis (Scheme 5) proceeded via reductive amination of the esters of 3-aminopropylphosphinic acids with arylaldehydes or -ketones. Additional substituents, e.g., an *(S)*-OH in position 2 and an α-methyl in the benzylic position, considerably increased the affinity of the novel antagonists to GABA$_B$ receptors. These derivatives were prepared according to Scheme 6, starting from the chiral intermediate esters **30** of Scheme 1 by condensation with chiral α-methyl-benzylamines.

3.2. Structure–Activity Relationships

Analyzing the affinities of compounds of structure **57** (Scheme 5) for GABA$_B$ receptors, in relation to the substitution pattern on the aromatic ring (Table 3), it became apparent that substituents providing a highly negative electrostatic potential in the *meta-* and *para*-positions of the benzylic group are the key to obtaining highly potent GABA$_B$ receptor antagonists. Especially interesting were the 3,4-dichloro derivative CGP52432 (Bonanno and

Table 4

Inhibition of Binding of [³H]CGP27492 to GABA$_B$ Receptors of Rat Cortex by
Compounds of Structures of General Formula **58** (Scheme 6, R = $CH_2C_6H_{11}$)

X	Y	R_1	R_2	IC$_{50}$ (nM)	CGP
H	4-Cl	H	H	216	52425
H	4-Cl	H	(S)-OH	84	52752
3-Cl	4-Cl	H	H	98	52647
3-Cl	4-Cl	H	(S)-OH	53	53030
3-Cl	4-Cl	(R,S)-CH$_3$	H	28	53664
3-Cl	4-Cl	(R,S)-CH$_3$	(S)-OH	10	54318
3-Cl	4-Cl	(S)-CH$_3$	(S)-OH	4	**54626**
3-Cl	4-Cl	(R)-CH$_3$	(S)-OH	79	54812
3-Cl	4-Cl	(S)-CH$_3$	(R)-OH	750	54870
3-Cl	4-Cl	(R)-CH$_3$	(R)-OH	7700	54966
3-COOH	H	H	H	12	64799
3-COOH	H	H	(S)-OH	3	68542
3-COOH	H	(R,S)-CH$_3$	(S)-OH	7	55556
3-COOH	H	(R)-CH$_3$	(S)-OH	2	**56999**
3-COOH	H	(S)-CH$_3$	(S)-OH	80	56433
3-COOH	H	(S)-CH$_3$	(R)-OH	1870	56930
H	4-COOH	(S)-CH$_3$	(S)-OH	230	57034
H	4-COOH	(R)-CH$_3$	(S)-OH	665	57070

Boldface numbers represent most interesting compounds.

Raiteri, 1993; Brugger et al., 1993; Gemignani et al., 1994; Lanza et al., 1993;
Lacey and Curtis, 1994) and the 3-carboxylic acid derivative CGP61334.
Note the 30-fold higher affinity of the 3-carboxylic acid CGP61334 com-
pared to its 4-isomer CGP61395.

A significant additional increase in the affinity for GABA$_B$ receptors
was achieved by attaching an hydroxy group in position 2, preferably in
(S)-configuration, and an α-methyl group in the benzylic position (Table 4).
The impact of the stereochemistry of the two chiral centers in the series of
the four diastereoisomers, CGP 54626, CGP54812, CGP54870, and
CGP54966, is very interesting (Bittiger et al., 1992b; Brugger et al., 1993;
Lacey and Curtis, 1994; Turgeon and Albin, 1994). Each time one stereochemical alignment was wrong, a loss of affinity for GABA$_B$ receptors by
a factor of ten occurred. Compounds with an α-methyl in the benzylic position in the (S)-configuration always showed higher affinity for GABA$_B$ receptors, with the single exception of the extraordinarily potent 3-carboxylic
acid derivatives, such as CGP56999 (Bernasconi et al., 1994). In this case,
the (α-R, 2-S) diastereoisomer was significantly more potent, a fact for which

Table 5
Inhibition of Binding of [^{3}H]CGP27492 to GABA$_B$ Receptors of Rat Cortex
by Compounds of Structures of General Formula **58** (Scheme 6, R$_2$ = *(S)*-OH)

R	X	Y	R$_1$	IC$_{50}$ (nM)	CGP
CH(OEt)$_2$	3-Cl	4-Cl	*(R,S)*-CH$_3$	19	54624
CH$_2$C$_6$H$_5$	3-Cl	4-Cl	*(R,S)*-CH$_3$	10	54062
CH$_2$C$_6$H$_{11}$	3-Cl	4-Cl	*(R,S)*-CH$_3$	10	54318
CH$_2$C$_6$H$_5$	3-Cl	4-Cl	*(S)*-CH$_3$	6	**55845**
CH$_2$C$_6$H$_{11}$	3-Cl	4-Cl	*(S)*-CH$_3$	4	**54626**
CH$_2$C$_6$H$_5$	3-Cl	4-Cl	*(R)*-CH$_3$	71	56931
CH$_2$C$_6$H$_{11}$	3-Cl	4-Cl	*(R)*-CH$_3$	79	54812
CH(OEt)$_2$	3-COOH	H	*(R)*-CH$_3$	6	57250
CH$_2$C$_6$H$_5$	3-COOH	H	*(R,S)*-CH$_3$	5	56377
CH$_2$C$_6$H$_{11}$	3-COOH	H	*(R,S)*-CH$_3$	7	55556
CH$_2$C$_6$H$_{11}$	3-COOH	H	*(R)*-CH$_3$	2	56999
CH(OEt)$_2$	3-COOH	H	*(S)*-CH$_3$	260	56571
CH$_2$C$_6$H$_{11}$	3-COOH	H	*(S)*-CH$_3$	80	56433
CH$_2$C$_6$H$_5$	3-Cl	4-Cl	*(R,S)*-CH$_3$	10	54062[a]
CH$_2$C$_6$H$_5$	3-Cl	4-Cl	*(R,S)*-C$_2$H$_5$	35	54266
CH$_2$C$_6$H$_5$	3-Cl	4-Cl	*(R,S)*-C$_3$H$_5$	129	55725

Boldface numbers represent most interesting compounds.
[a]*See* Brugger et al., 1993; Olpe et al., 1993.

we do not have an explanation. In the series of the 4-carboxylic acid derivatives, the (α-*S,2-S*)-diastereoisomer CGP57034 was again more potent than the (α-*R,2-S*)-diastereoisomer CGP57070.

The substituent R on the phosphorus in structures of the general formula **58** (Scheme 6) is of minor importance (Table 5). The major advantage of the benzylphosphinic acid CGP55845 over the equipotent cyclohexylmethylphosphinic acid CGP54626 is simply a practical one, since CGP55845 is ten times more water-soluble than CGP54626 (Blake et al., 1993; Brugger et al., 1993; Davies et al., 1993; Jarolimek et al., 1993; Lambert and Wilson, 1993; Lacey and Curtis, 1994; Olpe et al., 1994). Larger groups R$_1$ in the benzylic position reduce the affinity for GABA$_B$ receptors considerably (Table 5).

Changing the *N*-substituent from benzyl to β-phenylethyl caused a significant loss of affinity in the series of 3,4,5-trimethoxy-substituted derivatives (**59**, Fig. 9), although it produced comparable results in the 3,4-dichloro series (**60**, Fig. 10). Further efforts to explore the b-phenylethyl derivatives were halted, because **60** showed toxic side effects at low doses.

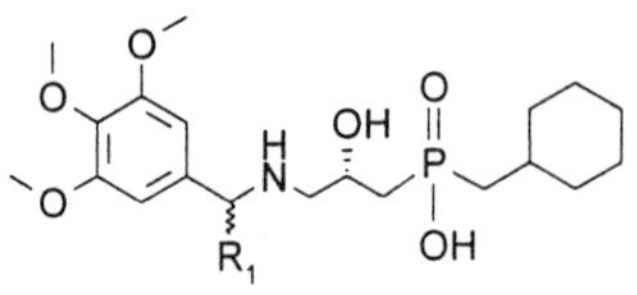

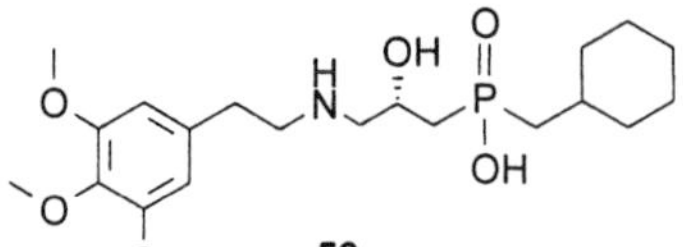

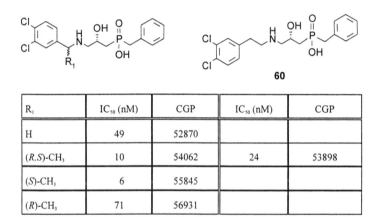

R₁	IC₅₀ (nM)	CGP	IC₅₀ (nM)	CGP
(R,S)-CH₃	92	54957		
(S)-CH₃	36	55679		
(R)-CH₃	1120	57976	1800	56402

Fig. 9. *N*-Benzyl vs *N*-β-phenylethyl-3-aminopropylphosphinic acids.

R₁	IC₅₀ (nM)	CGP	IC₅₀ (nM)	CGP
H	49	52870		
(R,S)-CH₃	10	54062	24	53898
(S)-CH₃	6	55845		
(R)-CH₃	71	56931		

Fig. 10. *N*-Benzyl vs *N*-β-phenylethyl-3-aminopropylphosphinic acids.

4. Conclusion

The discovery of potent, water-soluble GABA$_B$ receptor antagonists capable of penetrating the blood-brain barrier after systemic, including oral, administration, has stimulated many scientists of very diverse backgrounds to explore different aspects of GABA$_B$ receptor research, considerably enhancing our knowledge of the various physiological roles of GABA$_B$ receptors. Increasing pharmacological evidence points to GABA$_B$ receptor heterogeneity, although molecular biologists have not yet succeeded in cloning the GABA$_B$ receptor and its subtypes. The challenge for medicinal chemists is to continue the search for more selective $GABA_B$ receptor modulators that specifically interact with the manifold *pre-* and *post*-synaptic $GABA_B$ receptors.

Acknowledgments

We want to express our gratitude to C. Angst, N. G. Bowery, J. G. Dingwall, W. Hoyle, E. Irving, and J. Jack, L. Maître, C. Marescaux, M. Raiteri, and D. Scholer for many stimulating discussions. We wish to thank Gisèle Baudin, W. Benoze, P. J. Diel, J. Ehrenfreund, R. G. Hall, B. Kohler, L. Maier, T. Reimann, G. von Sprecher, and K. Zimmermann for their contributions. We thank P. Castelberg, J. Heid, M. Ingold, V. Melillo, Susanne Neuenschwander, Corinne Riegert, Nicole Reymann, D. Strub, and P. Wicki for their skillful experimental work.

References

Abbenante, G. and Prager, R. H. (1990) Synthesis of 3-amino-2-(4-chlorophenyl)-propanesulfonic acid (Saclofen) and 3-amino-2-(4-chlorophenyl)-2-hydroxypropane-sulfonic acid (Hydroxysaclofen). *Aust. J. Chem.* **43,** 213,214.

Abbenante, G. and Prager, R. H. (1992a) Potential $GABA_B$ receptor antagonists. VI. The synthesis of saclofen and other sulfonic acid derivatives. *Aust. J. Chem.* **45,** 1801–1810.

Abbenante, G. and Prager, R. H. (1992b) Potential $GABA_B$ receptor antagonists. V. The application of radical additions to styrenes to produce 2-hydroxysaclofen. *Aust. J. Chem.* **45,** 1791–1800.

Allan, R. D., Bates, M. C., Drew, C. A., Duke, R. K., Hambley, T. W., Johnston, G. A. R., Mewitt, K. N., and Spence, I. (1990) A new synthesis, resolution and *in vitro* activities of *(R)-* and *(S)*-β-phenyl-GABA. *Tetrahedron* **46,** 2511–2524.

Baylis, E. K., Campbell, C. D., and Dingwall, J. G. (1984) 1-Aminoalkylphosphonous acids. Part 1. Isosteres of the protein amino acids. *J. Chem. Soc. Perkin Trans.* **I,** 2845–2853.

Beattie, D. T., Curtis, D. R., Debaert, M., Vaccher, C., and Berthelot, P. (1989) Baclofen antagonism by 4-amino-3-(5-methoxybenzo[b]furan-2-yl)-butanoic acid in the cat spinal cord. *Neurosci. Lett.* **100,** 292–294.

Belakhov, V. V., Yudelevich, V. I., Komarov, E. V., Ionin, B. I., Komarov, V. Y., Zakharov, V. I., Lebedev, V. B., and Petrov, A. A. (1983) Reactivity of hypophosphites. VI. Reactions of hypophosphorous acid with acetylenic alcohols. *Zh. Obshch. Khim.* **53,** 1493–1503. *J. Gen. Chem. USSR (Engl. Transl.)* **53,** 1345–1353. *Chem. Abstr.* **99,** 212598v.

Bernasconi, R., Mathivet, P., Marescaux, C., Leonhardt, T., Martin, P., Mickel, S., and Froestl, W. (1994) NMDA receptors and NO synthase (NOS) are involved in the increase of cerebral cGMP induced by $GABA_B$ antagonists. *Br. J. Pharmacol.* **112 (Suppl.),** 7P.

Berthelot, P., Vaccher, C., Flouquet, N., Debaert, M., Luyckx, M., and Brunet, C. (1991) 3-Thienyl-and 3-Furylaminobutyric acids. Synthesis and binding $GABA_B$ receptor studies. *J. Med. Chem.* **34,** 2557–2560

Berthelot, P., Vaccher, C., Musadad, A., Flouquet, N., Debaert, M., and Luyckx, M. (1987) Synthesis and pharmacological evaluation of γ-aminobutyric acid analogues. New ligand for $GABA_B$ sites. *J. Med. Chem.* **30**, 743–746.

Bittiger, H., Bernasconi, R., Froestl, W., Hall, R., Jaekel, J., Klebs, K., Krueger, L., Mickel, S. J., Mondaori, C., Olpe, H.-R., Pfannkuch, F., Pozza, M., Probst, A., van Riezen, H., Schmutz, M., Schuetz, H., Steinmann, M. W., Vassout, A., Waldmeier, P., Bieck, P., Farger, G., Gleiter, C., Schmidt, E. K., and Marescaux, C. (1992a) $GABA_B$ antagonists: potential new drugs. *Pharmacol. Commun.* **2**, 70–74.

Bittiger, H., Froestl, W., Hall, R., Karlsson, G., Klebs, K., Olpe, H.-R., Pozza, M. F., Steinmann, M. W., and Van Riezen, H. (1990) Biochemistry, electrophysiology and pharmacology of a new $GABA_B$ antagonist: CGP35348, in *$GABA_B$ Receptors in Mammalian Function* (Bowery, N. G., Bittiger, H., and Olpe, H.-R., eds.), John Wiley, Chichester, UK, pp. 47–60.

Bittiger, H., Froestl, W., Mickel, S. J., and Olpe, H.-R. (1993) $GABA_B$ receptor antagonists: from synthesis to therapeutic applications. *Trends Pharmacol. Sci.* **14**, 391–394.

Bittiger, H., Reymann, N., Froestl, W., and Mickel, S. J. (1992b) [^{3}H]CGP54626: a potent antagonist radioligand for $GABA_B$ receptors. *Pharmacol. Commun.* **2**, 23.

Bittiger, H., Reymann, N., Hall, R., and Kane, P. (1988) CGP27492, a new potent and selective radioligand for $GABA_B$ receptors. *Eur. J. Neurosci.* **Suppl.**, Abstr. 16. 10.

Blake, J. F., Cao, C. Q., Headley, P. M., Collingridge, G. L., Brugger, F., and Evans, R. H. (1993) Antagonism of baclofen-induced depression of whole-cell synaptic currents in spinal dorsal horn neurones by the potent $GABA_B$ antagonist CGP55845. *Neuropharmacology* **32**, 1437–1440.

Bolser, D. C., Blythin, D. J., Chapman, R. W., Egan, R. W., Hey, J. A., Rizzo, C., Kuo, S.-C., and Kreutner, W. (1995) The pharmacology of SCH 50911: a novel, orally-active GABA-B receptor antagonist. *J. Pharm. Exp. Ther.* **274**, 1393–1398.

Bonanno, G. and Raiteri, M. (1993) Multiple $GABA_B$ receptors. *Trends Pharmacol. Sci.* **14**, 259–261.

Bowery, N. G., Hill, D. R., Hudson, A. L., Doble, A., Middlemiss, D. N., Shaw, J., and Turnbull, M. (1980) (–) Baclofen decreases neurotransmitter release in the mammalian CNS by an action at a novel GABA receptor. *Nature (London)* **283**, 92–94.

Brugger, F., Wicki, U., Olpe, H.-R., Froestl, W., and Mickel, S. (1993) The action of new potent $GABA_B$ receptor antagonists in the hemisected spinal cord preparation of the rat. *Eur. J. Pharmacol.* **235**, 153-155.

Caddick, S. J., Stanford, I. M., and Chad, J. E. (1995) 2-Hydroxy-saclofen causes a phaclofen-reversible reduction in population spike amplitude in the rat hippocampal slice. *Eur. J. Pharmacol.* **274**, 41–46.

Carletti, R., Libri, V., and Bowery, N. G. (1993) The $GABA_B$ antagonist CGP36742 enhances spatial learning performance and antagonises baclofen-induced amnesia in mice. *Br. J. Pharmacol.* **109 (Suppl.)**, 74P.

Carruthers, N. I., Spitler, J. M., Wong, S.-C., Blythin, D. J., Chen, X., Shue, H.-J., and Mittelman, S. (1995) Synthesis and resolution of β-(aminomethyl)-4-chlorobenzene-ethanesulfinic acid. A potent $GABA_B$ receptor ligand. *Bioorg. Med. Chem. Lett.* **5**, 237–240.

Chiefari, J., Galanopoulos, S., Janowski, W. K., Kerr, D. I. B., and Prager, R. H. (1987) The synthesis of phosphonobaclofen, an antagonist of baclofen. *Austr. J. Chem.* **40**, 1511–1518.

Curtis, D. R., Gynther, B. D., Beattie, D. T., Kerr, D. I. B., and Prager, R. H. (1988) Baclofen antagonism by 2-hydroxy-saclofen in the cat spinal cord. *Neurosci. Lett.* **92,** 97–101.

Davies, C. H., Pozza, M. F., and Collingridge, G. L. (1993) CGP55845A: a potent antagonist of GABA_B receptors in the CA1 region of rat hippocampus. *Neuropharmacology* **32,** 1071–1073.

Debaert, M., Berthelot, P., and Vaccher, C. (1992) Nouveau composés de l'acide 4-amino butyrique leur procédé de préparation et les préparations pharmaceutiques qui les contiennent. *Eur. Pat. Appl.* 463 969 A1; prior: 27 June 1990.

Dickenson, H. W., Allan, R. D., Ong, J., and Johnston, G. A. R. (1988) GABA_B receptor antagonist and GABA_A receptor agonist properties of a δ-aminovalerianic acid derivative, Z-5-aminopent-2-enoic acid. *Neurosci. Lett.* **86,** 351–355.

Dingwall, J. G., Ehrenfreund, J., and Hall, R. G. (1989) Diethoxymethylphosphonites and phosphinates. Intermediates for the synthesis of α, β- and γ-aminoalkyl-phosphonous acids. *Tetrahedron* **45,** 3787–3808.

Dingwall, J. G., Ehrenfreund, J., Hall, R. G., and Jack, J. (1987) Synthesis of γ-amino-propylphosphonous acids using hypophosphorous acid synthons. *Phosphorus Sulfur* **30,** 571–574.

Drew, C. A., Johnston, G. A. R., Kerr, D. I. B., and Ong, J. (1990) Inhibition of baclofen binding to rat cerebellar membranes by phaclofen, saclofen, 3-aminopropylphosphonic acid and related GABA_B receptor antagonists. *Neurosci. Lett.* **113,** 107–110.

Falch, E., Hedegaard, A., Nielsen, L., Jensen, B. R., Hjeds, H., and Krogsgaard-Larsen, P. (1986) Comparative stereostructure-activity studies on GABA_A and GABA_B receptor sites and GABA uptake using rat brain membrane preparations. *J. Neurochem.* **47,** 898–903.

Froestl, W., Furet, P., Hall, R. G., Mickel, S. J., Strub, D., von Sprecher, G., Baumann, P. A., Bernasconi, R., Brugger, F., Felner, A., Gentsch, C., Hauser, K., Jaekel, J., Karlsson, G., Klebs, K., Maître, L., Marescaux, C., Moser, P., Pozza, M. F., Rihs, G., Schmutz, M., Steinmann, M. W., van Riezen, H.,Vassout, A., Mondadori, C., Olpe, H.-R., Waldmeier, P. C., and Bittiger, H. (1993a) GABA_B antagonists: novel CNS-active compounds, in *Perspectives in Medicinal Chemistry* (Testa, B., Kyburz, E., Fuhrer, W., and Giger, R., eds.), Verlag Helvetica Chimica Acta, Basel, pp. 259–272.

Froestl, W., Mickel, S. J., and Bittiger, H. (1993b) Potent GABA_B agonists and antagonists. *Curr. Opin. Ther. Pat.* **3,** 561–567.

Froestl, W., Mickel, S. J., Hall, R. G., von Sprecher, G., Strub, D., Baumann, P. A., Brugger, F., Gentsch, C., Jaekel, J., Olpe, H.-R., Rihs, G., Vassout, A., Waldmeier, P. C., and Bittiger, H. (1995a) Phosphinic acid analogues of GABA. 1. New potent and selective GABA_B agonists. *J. Med. Chem.* **38,** 3297–3312.

Froestl, W., Mickel, S. J., von Sprecher, G., Bittiger, H., and Olpe, H.-R. (1992) Chemistry of new GABA_B antagonists. *Pharmacol. Commun.* **2,** 52–56.

Froestl, W., Mickel, S. J., von Sprecher, G., Diel, P. J., Hall, R. G., Maier, L., Strub, D., Melillo, V., Baumann, P. A., Bernasconi, R., Gentsch, C., Hauser, K., Jaekel, J., Karlsson, G., Klebs, K., Maitre, L., Marescaux, C., Pozza, M. F., Schmutz, M., Steinmann, M. W., van Riezen, H., Vassout, A., Mondadori, C., Olpe, H.-R., Waldmeier P. C., and Bittiger, H. (1995b) Phosphinic acid analogues of GABA. 2. Selective, orally active GABA_B antagonists. *J. Med. Chem.* **38,** 3313–3331.

Fromm, G. H. (1991) Medical treatment of patients with trigeminal neuralgia, in *Trigeminal Neuralgia. Current Concepts Regarding Pathogenesis and Treatment* (Fromm, G. H. and Sessle, B. J., eds.), Butterworth-Heinemann, Boston, pp. 131–144.

Frydenvang, K., Hansen, J. J., Krogsgaard-Larsen, P., Mitrovic, A., Tran, H., Drew, C. A., and Johnston, G. A. R. (1994) $GABA_B$ antagonists: resolution, absolute stereochemistry, and pharmacology of *(R)-* and *(S)*-phaclofen. *Chirality* **6**, 583–589.

Gallagher, M. J. and Honegger, H. (1980) Organophosphorus intermediates. VI. The acid catalysed reaction of trialkyl orthoforrnates with phosphinic acid. *Aust. J. Chem.* **33**, 287–294.

Gemignani, A., Paudice, P., Bonanno, G., and Raiteri, M. (1994) Pharmacological discrimination between γ-aminobutyric acid type B receptors regulating cholecystokinin and somatostatin release from rat neocortex synaptosomes. *Mol. Pharmacol.* **46,**558–562.

Hall, R. G. (1989) An efficient synthesis of (±)-3-amino-2-(4-chlorophenyl)-propylphosphonic acid (PHACLOFEN). *Synthesis* **1989**, 442,443.

Hall, R. G., Kane, P. D., Bittiger, H., and Froestl, W. (1995) Phosphinic acid analogues of γ-aminobutyric acid (GABA). Synthesis of a new radioligand. *J. Labelled Compd. Radiopharm.* **36**, 129–135.

Herdeis, C. and Hubmann, H. P. (1992) Synthesis of homochiral *R*-baclofen from *S*-glutamic acid. *Tetrahedron Asymm.* **3**, 1213–1221.

Herranz, E., Biller, S. A., and Sharpless, K. B. (1978) Osmium-catalyzed vicinal oxyamination of olefins by *N*-chloro-*N*-argentocarbamates. *J. Amer. Chem. Soc.* **100**, 3596–3598.

Hill, D. R. and Bowery, N. G. (1981) ^{3}H-Baclofen and ^{3}H-GABA bind to bicuculline-insensitive $GABA_B$ sites in rat brain. *Nature (London)* **290**, 149–152.

Hosford, D. A., Clark, S., Cao, Z., Wilson, W. A., Lin, F., Morrisett, R. A., and Huin, A. (1992) The role of $GABA_B$ receptor activation in absence seizures of lethargic (lh/lh) mice. *Science* **257**, 398–401.

Hosford, D. A., Wang, Y., Liu, C. C., and Snead, C. O. (1995) Characterization of the antiabsence effects of SCH 50911, a $GABA_B$ receptor antagonist, in the lethargic mouse, γ-hydroxybutyrate, and pentylenetetrazole models. *J. Pharm. Exp. Ther.* **274**, 1399–1403.

Howson, W., Mistry, J., Broekman, M., and Hills, J. M. (1993) Biological activity of 3-aminopropyl (methyl) phosphinic acid, a potent and selective $GABA_B$ agonist with CNS activity. *Bioorg. Med. Chem. Lett.* **3**, 515–518.

Jarolimek, W., Demmelhuber, J., Bijak, M., and Misgeld, U. (1993) CGP55845A blocks baclofen, γ-aminobutyric acid and inhibitory postsynaptic potassium currents in guinea pig CA3 neurons. *Neurosci. Lett.* **154**, 31-34.

Johnston, G. A. R. (1994) GABA receptors: as complex as ABC? *Clin. Exp. Pharmacol. Physiol.* **21**, 521-526.

Johnston, G. A. R., Curtis, D. R., Beart, P. M., Game, C. J. A., McCulloch, R. M., and Twitchin, B. (1975) *Cis*- and *Trans*-4-aminocrotonic acid as GABA analogues of restricted conformation. *J. Neurochem.* **24**, 157–160.

Keberle, H., Faigle, J. W., and Wilhelm, M. (1968) Procedure for the preparation of new aminoacids. Swiss Patent 449 046, 1968; prior: 9 July 1963. *Chem. Abstr.* **69**, 106273f.

Kerr, D. I. B. and Ong, J. (1992) GABA agonists and antagonists. *Med. Res. Rev.* **12**, 593–636.

Kerr, D. I. B., Ong, J., Doolette, D. J., Schafer, K., and Prager, R. H. (1995) *(S)*-enantiomer of 2-hydroxysaclofen is the active $GABA_B$ receptor antagonist in central and peripheral preparations. *Eur. J. Pharmacol.* **287**, 185–189.

Kerr, D. I. B., Ong, J., Johnston, G. A. R., Abbenante, J., and Prager, R. H. (1988) 2-Hydroxysaclofen: an improved antagonist at central and peripheral $GABA_B$ receptors. *Neurosci. Lett.* **92**, 92–96.

Kerr, D. I. B., Ong, J., Johnston, G. A. R., Abbenante, J., and Prager, R. H. (1989a) Antagonism at GABA$_B$ receptors by saclofen and related sulphonic analogues of baclofen and GABA. *Neurosci. Lett.* **107,** 239–244.

Kerr, D. I. B., Ong, J., Johnston, G. A. R., Berthelot, P., Debaert, M., and Vaccher, C. (1989b) Benzofuran analogues of baclofen: a new class of central and peripheral GABA$_B$-receptor antagonists. *Eur. J. Pharmacol.* **164,** 361–364.

Kerr, D. I. B., Ong, J., Prager, R. H., Gynther, B. D., and Curtis, D. R. (1987) Phaclofen: a peripheral and central baclofen antagonist. *Brain Res.* **405,** 150–154.

Klebs, K., Bittiger, H., Froestl, W., Glatt, A., Hafner, T., Mickel, S., Olpe, H.-R., and Schmutz, M. (1992) GABA$_B$ antagonists and anti-absence drugs suppress gamma-butyrolactone induced delta waves: a model for testing anti-absence drugs. *Pharmacol. Commun.* **2,** 171–172.

Kristiansen, U., Hedegaard, A., Herdeis, C., Lund, T. M., Nielsen, B., Hansen, J. J., Falch, E., Hjeds, H., and Krogsgaard-Larsen, P. (1992) Hydroxylated analogues of 5-aminovaleric acid as 4-aminobutyric acid$_B$ receptor antagonists: stereostructureactivity relationships. *J. Neurochem.* **58,** 1150–1159.

Kuo, S.-C., Blythin, D. J., and Kreutner, W. (1994) 2-Substituted morpholine and thiomorpholine derivatives as GABA$_B$ antagonists. WO 22843; prior: 26 March 1993.

Lacey, G. and Curtis, D. R. (1994) Phosphinic acid derivatives as baclofen agonists and antagonists in the mammalian spinal cord: an in vivo study. *Exp. Brain Res.* **101,** 59–72.

Lambert, N. A. and Wilson, W. A. (1993) Heterogeneity in presynaptic regulation of GABA release from hippocampal inhibitory neurons. *Neuron* **11,** 1057–1067.

Lanza, M., Fassio, A., Gemignani, A., Bonanno, G., and Raiteri, M. (1993) CGP52432: a novel potent and selective GABA$_B$ autoreceptor antagonist in rat cerebral cortex. *Eur. J. Pharmacol.* **237,** 191–195.

Li, C.-S., Howson, W., and Dolle, R. E. (1991) Synthesis of (±)-3-amino-2-(4-chlorophenyl)propanesulfonic acid (Saclofen). Synthesis **1991,** 244.

Lingenhoehl, K. and Olpe, H.-R. (1993) Blockade of the late inhibitory postsynaptic potential in vivo by the GABA$_B$ blocker CGP46381. *Pharmacol. Commun.* **3,** 49–54.

Mann, A., Boulanger, T., Brandau, B., Durant, F., Evrard, G., Heaulme, M., Desaulles, E., and Wermuth, C.-G. (1991) Synthesis and biochemical evaluation of baclofen analogues locked in the baclofen solid-state conformation. *J. Med. Chem.* **34,** 1307–1313.

Marescaux, C., Liu, Z., Bernasconi, R., and Vergnes, M. (1992) GABA$_B$ receptors are involved in the occurrence of absence seizures in rats. *Pharmacol. Commun.* **2,** 57–62.

Marsden, D. (1989) *Treating Spasticity: Pharmacological Advances.* Hans Huber, Toronto.

Meyers, A. I. and Snyder, L. (1993) The synthesis of aracemic 4-substituted pyrrolidinones and 3-substituted pyrrolidines. An asymmetric synthesis of (–)-Rolipram. *J. Org. Chem.* **58,** 36–42.

Mondadori, C., Preiswerk, G., and Jaekel, J. (1992) Treatment with a GABA$_B$ receptor blocker improves the cognitive performance of mice, rats and rhesus monkeys. *Pharmacol. Commun.* **2,** 93–97.

Mondadori, C., Jaekel, J., and Preiswerk, G. (1993) CGP36742: the first orally active GABA$_B$ blocker improves the cognitive performance of mice, rats, and rhesus monkeys. *Behav. Neural Biol.* **60,** 62–68.

Muhyaddin, M., Roberts, P. J., and Woodruff, G. N. (1982) Presynaptic γ-amino-butyric acid receptors in the rat anococcygeus muscle and their antagonism by 5-aminovaleric acid. *Br. J. Pharmacol.* **77,** 163–168.

Mulzer, J. (1994) Asymmetric synthesis of the novel antidepressant Rolipram. *J. Prakt. Chem.* **336**, 287–291.

Ochs, G. (1993) Inthrathecal baclofen. *Baillière's Clin. Neurol.* **2**, 73–86.

Olpe, H.-R., Karlsson, G., Pozza, M. F., Brugger, F., Steinmann, M., Van Riezen, H., Fagg, G., Hall, R. G., Froestl, W., and Bittiger, H. (1990) CGP35348: a centrally active blocker of GABA$_B$ receptors. *Eur. J. Pharmacol.* **187**, 27–38.

Olpe, H.-R., Steinmann, M. W., Ferrat, T., Pozza, M. F., Greiner, K., Brugger, F., Froestl, W., Mickel, S. J., and Bittiger, H. (1993) The actions of orally active GABA$_B$ receptor antagonists on GABAergic transmission *in vivo* and *in vitro*. *Eur. J. Pharmacol.* **233**, 179–186.

Olpe, H.-R., Steinmann, M. W., Greiner, K., and Pozza, M. F. (1994) Contribution of presynaptic GABA$_B$ receptors to paired-pulse depression of GABA-responses in the hippocampus. *Naunyn-Schmiedberg's Arch. Pharmacol.* **349**, 473–477.

Ong, J., Kerr, D. I. B., Abbenante, J., and Prager, R. H. (1991) Short-chain baclofen analogues are GABA$_B$ receptor antagonists in the guinea-pig isolated ileum. *Eur. J. Pharmacol.* **205**, 319–322.

Ong, J., Kerr, D. I. B., Johnston, G. A. R., and Hall, R. G. (1990) Differing actions of baclofen and 3-aminopropylphosphinic acid in rat neocortical slices. *Neurosci. Lett.* **109**, 169–173.

Penn, R. D. (1992) Inthrathecal baclofen for spasticity of spinal origin: seven years of experience. *J. Neurosurg.* **77**, 236–240.

Penn, R. D., Savoy, S. M., Corcos, D., Latash, M., Gottlieb, G., Parke, B., and Kroin, J. S. (1989) Intrathecal baclofen for severe spasticity. *N. Engl. J. Med.* **320**, 1517–1521.

Prager, R. H., Schafer, K., Hamon, D. P. G., and Massy-Westropp, R. A. (1995) The synthesis of *(R)*-(–) and *(S)*-(+)-hydroxysaclofen. *Tetrahedron* **51**, 11,465–11,472.

Pratt, G. D., Knott, C., Davey, R., and Bowery, N. G. (1989) Characterisation of 3-aminopropyl phosphinic acid (3-APPA) as a GABA$_B$ agonist in rat brain tissue. *Br. J. Pharmacol.* **96 (Suppl.)**, 141P.

Robinson, T. N., Cross, A. J., Green, A. R., Toczek, J. M., and Boar, B. R. (1989) Effects of the putative antagonists phaclofen and δ-aminovaleric acid on GABA$_B$ receptor biochemistry. *Br. J. Pharmacol.* **98**, 833–840.

Schoenfelder, A., Mann, A., and Le Coz, S. (1993) Enantioselective synthesis of *(R)*-(–)baclofen. *Synlett* 63–64.

Schwartz, T. W. (1994) Locating ligand-binding sites in 7TM receptors by protein engineering. *Curr. Opin. Biotechnol.* **5**, 434–444.

Snead, O. C. (1992) Evidence for GABA$_B$-mediated mechanisms in experimental generalized absence seizures. *Eur. J. Pharmacol.* **213**, 343–349.

Topliss, J. G. (1972) Utilization of operational schemes for analog synthesis in drug design. *J. Med. Chem.* **15**, 1006–1011.

Turgeon, S. M. and Albin, R. L. (1994) Postnatal ontogeny of GABA$_B$ binding in rat brain. *Neuroscience* **62**, 601–613.

Vaccher, C., Berthelot, P., and Debaert, M. (1993a) Direct separation of 4-amino-3-(4-chlorophenyl)butyric acid and analogues, GABA$_B$ ligands, using a chiral crown ether stationary phase. *J. Chromatogr.* **645**, 95–99.

Vaccher, C., Berthelot, P., Flouquet, N., Vaccher, M.-P., and Debaert, M. (1993b) Bromination of α-methylstyrenes with *N*-bromosuccinimide in chlorobenzene one-pot and selective preparation of 1,3-dibromo-2-phenylprop-1-enes. *Synth. Commun.* **23**, 671–679.

CHAPTER 11

Molecular Biology, Pharmacology, and Physiology of GABA$_C$ Receptors

Graham A. R. Johnston

1. Introduction

The first edition of *The GABA Receptors* (Enna, 1983) made no reference to the subtype of GABA receptors now known as GABA$_C$ receptors, i.e., receptors for the inhibitory neurotransmitter GABA that are insensitive to the GABA$_A$ antagonist, bicuculline, and to the GABA$_B$ agonist, baclofen. Bowery (1993), in his chapter on the classification of GABA receptors, reported that the possible existence of bicuculline-insensitive GABA receptors had been considered, e.g., Andrews and Johnston (1979) postulated that "GABA might act at a population of bicuculline-insensitive sites in a folded conformation whereas it acts at bicuculline-sensitive receptors in an extended conformation." Bowery continued, "The idea arose from studies with compounds such as *cis*-4-aminocrotonic acid that depress neuronal firing but are unaffected by bicuculline. Although this postulate is interesting, a simultaneous activation of these sites by GABA in the presence of bicuculline was never shown. To designate a receptor 'GABA site,' it surely must be activated by GABA. Perhaps under the right conditions GABA may be an agonist at the site."

It took another 10 years for this elusive GABA site to be characterized via a powerful combination of molecular biological, pharmacological, and physiological studies. Good evidence is available now to support the existence of a third major class of GABA receptor subtype. This subtype is designated GABA$_C$, following the terminology introduced by Hill and Bowery (1981) that classified GABA$_A$ receptors as those sensitive to bicuculline and insensitive to baclofen, and GABA$_B$ receptors as those

The GABA Receptors Eds.: S. J. Enna and N. G. Bowery
Humana Press Inc., Totowa, NJ

insensitive to bicuculline and sensitive to baclofen. $GABA_C$ receptors are insensitive to both bicuculline and baclofen. These novel GABA receptors have been given a variety of names, including $GABA_C$, $GABA_{NANB}$ (non-A, non-B), and ρ receptors (cloned from retina). With the increasing evidence of similarities between these receptors, they are most conveniently designated $GABA_C$ receptors, although it is anticipated that a more definitive classification of GABA receptors based on molecular biological, pharmacological, and physiological considerations will emerge in due course (Johnston, 1995). Some brief reviews covering aspects of $GABA_C$ receptors have been published (Johnston, 1994a,b; Djamgoz, 1995; Bormann and Feigenspan, 1995).

$GABA_C$ receptors are members of the ligand-gated ion-channel superfamily of receptors, which encompasses nicotinic acetylcholine receptors, 5-hydroxytryptamine 5-HT_3 receptors, $GABA_A$, and glycine receptors. $GABA_C$ receptors show some similarities to $GABA_A$ receptors as GABA-gated chloride ion channels, but they appear to be sufficiently different to be considered as a separate subtype of GABA ionotropic receptors. The more complex $GABA_A$ receptors may have evolved from the simpler $GABA_C$ receptors. $GABA_C$ receptors appear to be homooligomeric protein complexes, and are distinct from the heterooligomeric $GABA_A$ receptor complexes.

$GABA_C$ receptors are activated at lower concentrations of GABA, open for a longer time, and are less liable to desensitization than most $GABA_A$ receptors; these properties suggest that $GABA_C$ receptors could play a different physiological role from $GABA_A$ receptors. $GABA_C$ receptors have a distinctive pharmacology, because they are not modulated by barbiturates, benzodiazepines, or neuroactive steroids. They appear to have a much more restricted localization in the central nervous system (CNS) than the seemingly ubiquitous $GABA_A$ receptors. The most extensive studies on $GABA_C$ receptors have been carried out in the vertebrate retina. There is a variety of bicuculline-insensitive GABA receptors described in invertebrates; those in crustacea closely resemble vertebrate $GABA_C$ receptors, but those in insects are clearly different. Inevitably, as $GABA_C$ receptors begin to be defined more clearly, GABA receptors that fall outside the $GABA_{ABC}$ classification are proposed (e.g., Martina et al., 1995). Already there are at least two instances in the literature of $GABA_D$ receptors (Momose-Sato et al., 1995; Pan and Lipton, 1995).

$GABA_C$ receptors are likely to represent important pharmacological targets in the mammalian nervous system. There is an urgent need for more potent and selective $GABA_C$ agonists, antagonists, and modulators than are currently available.

2. Bicuculline/Baclofen-Insensitive GABA Receptors

Studies on bicuculline/baclofen-insensitive GABA receptors arose from investigations of the actions of conformationally-restricted analogs of GABA in the spinal cord, optic tectum, and cerebellum.

2.1. Conformationally-Restricted Analogs of GABA

The GABA molecule can take up a variety of low energy conformations because of relatively free rotation about its carbon-carbon single bonds. It is considered likely that GABA interacts with different macromolecules, such as enzymes, receptors, and transporters, in different conformations. It is possible to restrict the available conformations in GABA analogs by incorporation of carbocyclic or heterocyclic rings, and/or double or triple bonds into their structures (Allan and Johnston, 1983). The systematic study of such conformationally-restricted analogs of GABA has provided many examples of selective actions on aspects of the GABA transmitter system (Johnston et al., 1979). Conformationally-restricted analogs of GABA were vital to the development of the study of $GABA_C$ receptors, the key compound being *cis*-4-aminocrotonic acid (CACA; also known as Z-4-aminocrotonic acid and Z-4-aminobut-2-enoic acid), first synthesized in 1975 and tested on neurons in the cat spinal cord in vivo (Johnston et al., 1975). Based on the conformations available to CACA, GABA is considered to interact with $GABA_C$ receptors in a partially folded conformation (Drew et al., 1984), as is discussed in more detail in Section 3.3.

2.2. Spinal Cord

CACA was shown to inhibit the firing of neurons in the spinal cord of cats under pentobarbitone anesthesia, when applied extracellularly by microelectrophoresis (Johnston et al., 1975). CACA was approximately one-quarter as potent as GABA as a neuronal inhibitor, but its action could not be antagonized by the GABA antagonist, bicuculline, or the glycine antagonist, strychnine. *trans*-4-Aminocrotonic acid (TACA), the *trans*-analog of CACA, was approximately as potent as GABA, and its depressant action could be antagonized by bicuculline. Because of the, at best, semi-quantitative nature of microelectrophoretic experiments carried out on neurons in vivo, bicuculline-insensitive actions of GABA and TACA could not be ruled out. It is now known that both GABA and TACA activate $GABA_C$ receptors as full agonists, but CACA is a partial agonist.

The bicuculline-insensitive neuronal depressant action of CACA was interesting because of a somewhat similar action of another GABA analog, baclofen (β-(*p*-chlorophenyl)-GABA), on spinal neurons (Curtis et al., 1974), which was subsequently shown to be a selective $GABA_B$ agonist (Hill and Bowery, 1981). Baclofen had relatively little effect on Renshaw cells (Curtis et al., 1974), but CACA appeared to be equally potent as a depressant of the firing of Renshaw cells and spinal interneurons (Johnston et al., 1975); it seemed likely that baclofen and CACA acted at different receptors.

In addition to CACA and baclofen, several conformationally restricted analogs of GABA have been shown to have bicuculline-insensitive depressant actions, including (±)-*cis*-2-(aminomethyl)cyclopropane-1-carboxylic acid (CAMP; Allan et al., 1980), and (±)-*trans*-2- and (±)-*trans*-3-aminocyclohexane-1-carboxylic acids (T2ACHC and T3ACHC; Johnston, 1975). These compounds were between one-twentieth and one-half as potent as GABA on the neurons examined, and they could adopt conformations in which their amino and carboxylic acid moieties were isosteric with those in CACA and GABA. 3-Hydroxy-5-(1-aminopropyl)isoxazole (HAPI), 3-hydroxy-5-(1-aminobutyl)isoxazole (HABI), and 3-hydroxy-4-methyl-5-aminomethylisoxazole (HMAMI), analogs of the $GABA_A$ agonist muscimol (now known to act also as a $GABA_C$ partial agonist), showed bicuculline-insensitive depressant actions on spinal neurons (Krogsgaard-Larsen et al., 1975). The structures of these bicuculline-insensitive depressants of neuronal firing in the spinal cord are shown in Fig. 1.

2.3. Optic Tectum

In the frog brain, GABA induces a potent facilitation of excitatory synaptic transmission between the optic nerve and the optic tectum (Nistri and Sivilotti, 1985). This synaptic facilitation is not mimicked by the $GABA_B$ agonist, baclofen (Sivilotti and Nistri, 1988), and is relatively insensitive to the $GABA_A$ antagonist, bicuculline, although blocked by the $GABA_A$-activated chloride channel antagonist, picrotoxin (Nistri and Sivilotti, 1985). Furthermore, there is little fading of the response, unlike that observed for $GABA_A$ actions elsewhere in the CNS. The pharmacology of the response to GABA is similar to that now known to be characteristic of $GABA_C$ receptors (Sivilotti and Nistri, 1989). GABA and TACA were equipotent (ED_{50} 110 µ*M*) in enhancing excitatory postsynaptic field potentials in a chloride-dependent manner; CACA was some five times less potent (ED_{50} 500 µ*M*). The most potent agonists were muscimol and 3-aminopropanesulfonic acid (ED_{50} 3 and 25 µ*M*, respectively). The effects of the agonists were relatively insensitive to bicuculline (100 µ*M*), but could be blocked by picrotoxin (IC_{50} 78 µ*M*). The benzodiazepine, midazolam, did not influence the action of GABA; pentobarbitone acted as a partial agonist, enhancing the field potentials in a picrotoxin-sensitive manner, and antagonizing the effects of GABA.

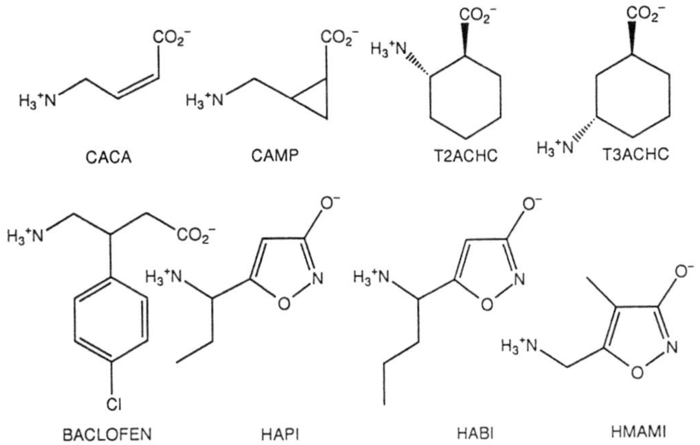

Fig. 1. Structures of compounds shown to have a bicuculline-insensitive depressant action on the firing of cat spinal neurones in vivo. Only baclofen is known to activate GABA$_B$ receptors. CAMP, T2ACHC, T3ACHC, baclofen, HAPI, and HABI were tested as racemic mixtures.

The concentrations of the GABA agonists needed to produce bicuculline-insensitive effects in the frog optic tectum are much higher than those needed to activate GABA$_C$ receptors in the retina (*see* Section 3.). Muscimol was much more potent relative to GABA in the tectum than in the retina, CACA appeared to be a full agonist in the tectum but a partial agonist in the retina, and 3-aminopropanesulfonic acid was a potent agonist in the tectum and a potent antagonist in the retina. These results suggest that there are significant major differences between the retinal and tectal bicuculline-insensitive GABA receptors.

2.4. Cerebellum

The lack of effect of the bicuculline-insensitive neuronal depressants, CACA and CAMP (Fig. 1), on the binding of [^{3}H](–)-baclofen to rat cerebellar membranes led to the proposal for "the existence of a class of bicuculline-insensitive binding sites (GABA$_C$?) for GABA that is insensitive to (–)-baclofen" (Drew et al., 1984). The corresponding *trans*-isomers, TACA and (±)-*trans*-2-(aminomethyl)cyclopropane-1-carboxylic acid (TAMP), known to be bicuculline-sensitive neuronal depressants, did inhibit [^{3}H](-)-baclofen binding, providing evidence for their interaction with GABA$_B$, and GABA$_A$ receptors. It is now known that TACA and TAMP also interact with GABA$_C$ receptors (*see* Section 3.3.). It was only the structural similarities among CACA, CAMP, and partially-folded conformations of GABA that indicated that CACA and CAMP might be activating a subtype of GABA receptor that was insensitive to the $GABA_A$ receptor antagonist, bicuculline, and the $GABA_B$ receptor agonist, (–)-baclofen.

Binding studies, possibly involving those GABA receptors that are different from $GABA_A$ and $GABA_B$ receptors, were reported in a variety of preparations. Binding of [³H]GABA that was insensitive to classical $GABA_A$ and $GABA_B$ agonists and antagonists was described in amphibian sciatic nerve (Barolet et al., 1985), and in catfish brain (Myers and Tunnicliff, 1988). Balcar et al. (1986) found that [³H]GABA binding to cerebral cortex membranes from newborn and adult rats had a bicuculline- and baclofen-insensitive component that was sensitive to CACA, thus linking CACA to a subtype of GABA binding site for the first time. This component represented more than 50% of the total specifically bound [³H]GABA. The lack of availability of CACA at the time limited these studies.

Bicuculline/baclofen-insensitive [³H]GABA binding was studied further in rat cerebellum, where it was termed NANB GABA binding, to indicate its non-$GABA_A$ and non-$GABA_B$ nature (Drew and Johnston, 1992). Up to 60% of the [³H]GABA specifically bound to rat cerebellar membranes bound to these NANB sites. Rosenthal analysis indicated two kinetic components with K_d values of 42 nM and 9 µM. The binding was calcium- and sodium-independent. The presence of NANB binding sites in the membrane preparations was seasonal, peaking in early spring each year over a four-year period. Seasonal variations in $GABA_A$-mediated inhibitory postsynaptic currents have been reported in rat hippocampal slices (Edwards and Gage, 1988), the decay time constant of the currents increasing from autumn to winter and decreasing from spring to summer. It was suggested that such seasonal changes may have behavioral consequences and might be associated with seasonal affective disorders. NANB [³H]GABA binding was inhibited by CACA (IC_{50} 2 µM), TACA (IC_{50} 22 µM), and CAMP (42% at 1 µM), and was insensitive to 2-hydrosaclofen, securinine, gabapentin, and 3-aminopropylphosphonic acid (Johnston, 1994a). This binding differs somewhat from that expected of $GABA_C$ sites. From the studies of $GABA_C$ receptors in the retina (*see* Section 3.3.), TACA would be expected to be more potent than CACA, which in turn would be equipotent with CAMP, and 3-aminopropylphosphonic acid should be more potent than either CACA or CAMP. The lower-affinity binding sites might be associated with the very potent action of CACA in inhibiting voltage-dependent calcium channels in the retina (Matthews et al., 1994), as discussed in Section 4.3.

Studies with [³H]CACA showed that it bound with high specificity to rat cerebellar membranes, and was displaced by GABA and TACA equipotently (IC_{50} 0.025 µM), and less potently by unlabeled CACA (IC_{50} 0.5 µM). These results are more in keeping with the relative potencies observed in the retina for these agents when interacting with GABA$_C$ receptors. Autoradiographical studies with [^{3}H]CACA and the relatively selective GABA$_A$ ligand, [^{3}H]muscimol, which is also a GABA$_C$ partial agonist, showed that both ligands bound to similar sites in the cerebellum, particularly in the molecular layer, and to a lesser extent in the granule cell layer, but were completely different in other brain areas (M. Akinci, R. K. Duke, C. A. Drew, and G. A. R. Johnston, unpublished observations). As noted later, in Section 4.1., the human toxicity of the [^{3}H]CACA preparation limited the studies that could be carried out with this ligand.

3. GABA$_C$ Receptors in the Retina

The expression in *Xenopus* oocytes of GABA receptors from retinal DNA and mRNA with the distinctive pharmacology predicted for GABA$_C$ receptors from earlier studies, has served to focus most recent studies on the retina. The most extensive studies of GABA$_C$ receptors have been carried out in the retina on horizontal cells, where they may function as autoreceptors, on bipolar cells, where they may mediate presynaptic inhibition, and on receptors expressed from retinal DNA or RNA. Cone-driven horizontal cells are thought to be GABA-ergic, but rod-driven horizontal cells are not. Amacrine cells might be the source of the GABA acting on rod-driven horizontal cells. Retinal bipolar cells receive GABA-ergic feedback from amacrine cells.

3.1. Molecular Biology

The expression of GABA$_C$ receptors in oocytes injected with poly(A)$^+$ RNA from mammalian retina (Polenzani et al., 1991), and the cloning of ρ1- and ρ2-subunit cDNAs from a human retinal library (Cutting et al., 1991, 1992), represented major breakthroughs in the understanding of GABA$_C$ receptors. Expressed in *Xenopus* oocytes, the ρ-subunits formed homooligomeric GABA-activated chloride channels insensitive to bicuculline, but sensitive to picrotoxin. Their pharmacological properties closely resembled those observed for retinal GABA$_C$ receptors and for retinal mRNA expressed in oocytes. The expression of retinal poly(A)$^+$ RNA in oocytes led to GABA-activated chloride currents made up of two distinct components, one mediated by GABA$_A$ receptors and the other mediated by GABA$_C$ receptors, thus providing evidence that the protein subunits making up these different receptor populations associate independently of each other. Subsequent studies on the self-associating ρ-subunits expressed in oocytes and COS cells have provided extensive evidence that these subunits form GABA receptors with physiological and pharmacological properties distinct from heterooligomeric GABA$_A$ receptors (Shimada et al., 1992; Kusama et al., 1993a; Woodward et al., 1993).

The human ρ-subunits consist of four putative transmembrane spanning regions and a cytoplasmic loop between transmembrane domains M3 and M4 (Cutting et al., 1991; 1992). Site-directed mutagenesis studies have identified 5 amino acids (Y198, Y200, Y241, T244, and Y247), located between the N-terminal extracellular cysteine loop and the first membrane spanning domain, that impair GABA activation when conservatively mutated (Amin and Weiss, 1994). These five residues are grouped in two domains that correspond in position to the putative agonist-binding domains identified in the β2-subunit of $GABA_A$ receptors, with Y198, T244, and Y247 corresponding directly to crucial amino acids in the β2-subunit, while Y200 and Y241 do not. These differences may account, in part, for the unique properties of ρ1-homomeric receptors. Other site-directed mutagenesis studies of the ρ1-receptor have produced a mutation (Q189H) in the conserved cysteine loop that reduced apparent GABA affinity to about 10% of the wild type value, in a manner consistent with decreased allosteric cooperativity among agonist recognition sites (Kusama et al., 1994). Mutation R316A, located in the extracellular loop between transmembrane domains M2 and M3, increased the Hill coefficient for agonist activation from 2 to 3.9, with an increased probability of channel opening. Feigenspan et al. (1993) noted that the M2 segment that forms the lining of the ρ1-receptor channel shares more sequence homology with the M2 segment of the glycine receptor α-subunits than with any of the established $GABA_A$ receptor subunits.

The ρ1- and ρ2-subunits are usually referred to as $GABA_A$ receptor subunits, since they exhibit 30–38% sequence homology with other subtypes of vertebrate $GABA_A$ receptor subunits. This is a level of similarity comparable with that seen between members of two different subtypes of $GABA_A$ receptor subunits, such as α1 and γ1. This classification has been challenged by Darlison and Albrecht (1995), who point out that the ρ1- and ρ2-subunits do not appear to assemble with α- or β-$GABA_A$ subunits, preferring instead to form homooligomeric GABA-gated chloride channels that are insensitive to the $GABA_A$ antagonist, bicuculline, and to $GABA_A$ receptor modulators, such as barbiturates and benzodiazepines (Shimada et al., 1992). Darlison and Albrecht (1995) consider that the expression patterns of the ρ1- and ρ2-subunit genes are clearly compatible with their classification as $GABA_C$ receptor genes. The sequence homology between the ρ-subunits and the $GABA_A$ α-, β-, γ-, and δ-subunits may reflect the evolution of the more complex $GABA_A$ heterooligomeric receptors from the simpler $GABA_C$ homooligomeric receptors (Johnston, 1995). Ortells and Lunt (1995) have analyzed the evolutionary history of the ligand-gated ion-channel superfamily of receptors, which encompasses nicotinic receptors, $5-HT_3$ receptors, $GABA_A$, $GABA_C$, and glycine receptors, and have suggested that there must have been some common ancestor receptor that was probably homomeric.

3.2. Channel Properties

GABA$_C$ receptors are ligand-gated chloride channels that differ significantly from GABA$_A$ receptors in the following ways: GABA$_C$ receptors are more sensitive to GABA; their time-course of activation is more sustained; the mean open time of GABA$_C$ channels is longer and their main state conductance is smaller, as is their pore diameter. These differences are observed in the properties of GABA$_C$ and GABA$_A$ receptors, both in the native state in the retina and in expression systems.

The reversal potential for GABA$_C$ currents is altered, as predicted by the Nernst equation, in response to alterations in the transmembrane chloride ion gradient, consistent with GABA$_C$ receptors acting as chloride ion channels (Feigenspan et al., 1993; Qian and Dowling, 1993; Wang et al., 1994). These channels will conduct other small anions up to the size of acetate, and the predicted minimum pore diameter is 5.1 Å, marginally smaller than the value of 5.6 Å found for GABA$_A$ receptors (Feigenspan and Bormann, 1994b).

In rat retinal bipolar cells, GABA$_C$ receptors were seven times more sensitive to GABA than were GABA$_A$ receptors (EC$_{50}$ 4 μM for GABA$_C$ receptors and 27 μM for GABA$_A$ receptors); the Hill coefficient was approx 2 for the activation of either receptor subtype (Feigenspan and Bormann, 1994b). Single-channel currents indicated main-state conductances of 7.9 pS for GABA$_C$ channels and 29.6 pS for GABA$_A$ channels, under the conditions of measurement. The mean open time of GABA$_C$ channels (150 ms) was significantly longer than that observed for GABA$_A$ channels in the same preparation (Feigenspan et al., 1993). Studies with human ρ1-subunits expressed in oocytes found that these GABA$_C$ receptors were 40 times more sensitive to GABA, activated eight times more slowly, did not desensitize with maintained agonist application, and closed eight times more slowly after agonist removal than GABA$_A$ receptors made up of α1β2γ2 subunits (Amin and Weiss, 1994).

3.3. Agonists and Partial Agonists

The most extensive studies of agonists, partial agonists, and antagonists have been carried out by Woodward et al. (1992, 1993), using bovine retinal RNA expressed in *Xenopus* oocytes; by Kusama et al. (1993a), using human ρ1-cDNA expressed in *Xenopus* oocytes; and by Qian and Dowling (1993, 1994), using native GABA$_C$ receptors in perch retina. The results of the oocytes studies are summarized in Table 1 and the structures of the compounds are shown in Fig. 2. The most potent agonist was TACA, which was approx 120 times more potent than CACA, a partial agonist showing 70–80% of the efficacy of GABA. Both studies showed that muscimol was somewhat weaker than GABA. There was good agreement between the studies, indicating that

Table 1

Agonists, Partial Agonists and Antagonists Acting on $GABA_C$ (Bovine Retinal
RNA or Human ρ_1- and ρ_2-cDNA) Receptors Expressed in *Xenopus* oocyctes

	Bovine retinal RNA EC_{50} (μM)[a]	Human K_d (μM)[b] (v. $\rho2$)[c]	ρ_1-cDNA Ratio C/A[b]
Agonists			
trans-4-Aminocrotonic acid (TACA)	0.6	0.6 (0.3)	140
GABA	1.3	1.7 (0.9)	30
(±)-*cis*-2-(aminomethyl)cyclopro-	–	68 (35)	>150
pane -1-carboxylic acid (CAMP)	K_b (μM)[a]	K_d (μM)[2]	Ratio C/A[a]
Partial Agonists			
Muscimol	2.3	3.5 (1.4)	6
Imidazole-4-acetic acid (IAA)	–	16 (1.0)	
(±)-*trans*-2-(aminomethyl)cyclo-	–	20 (18)	
propane-1-carboxylic acid (TAMP)			
cis-4-aminocrotonic acid (CACA)	74	74 (70)	130
Isoguvacine	99		
Antagonists			
3-Aminopropyl(methyl)phosphinic acid (3-APMPA)	0.8		
3-Aminopropylphosphinic acid (3-APPA)	1.7		
3-Aminopropylphosphonic acid (3-APA)	10		
Z-3-[(Aminoiminoethyl)thio] prop-2-enoic acid (ZAPA)	19		
3-Aminopropylsulfonic acid (3-APS)	19		
d-Aminovaleric acid (DAVA)	20		
4,5,6,7-Tetrahydroisoxazole [4,5-c]pyridin-3-ol (THIP)	32		
SR-95531	35		0.004
Strychnine	69		0.05
Piperidine-4-sulfonic acid (P4S)	81		
4-Aminobutylphosphonic acid (4-ABPA)	625		
Bicuculline	6700		0.0002

EC_{50}, concentration producing 50% activation; K_d, dissociation constant; K_b, inhibition constant; Ratio C/A, ratio of potency at $GABA_C$ (retinal RNA or r_1-cDNA) and $GABA_A$ (a_5b_1) receptors. Values in brackets refer to r_2-receptors.

[a]Woodward et al., 1993
[b]Kusama et al., 1993a
[c]Kusama et al., 1993b

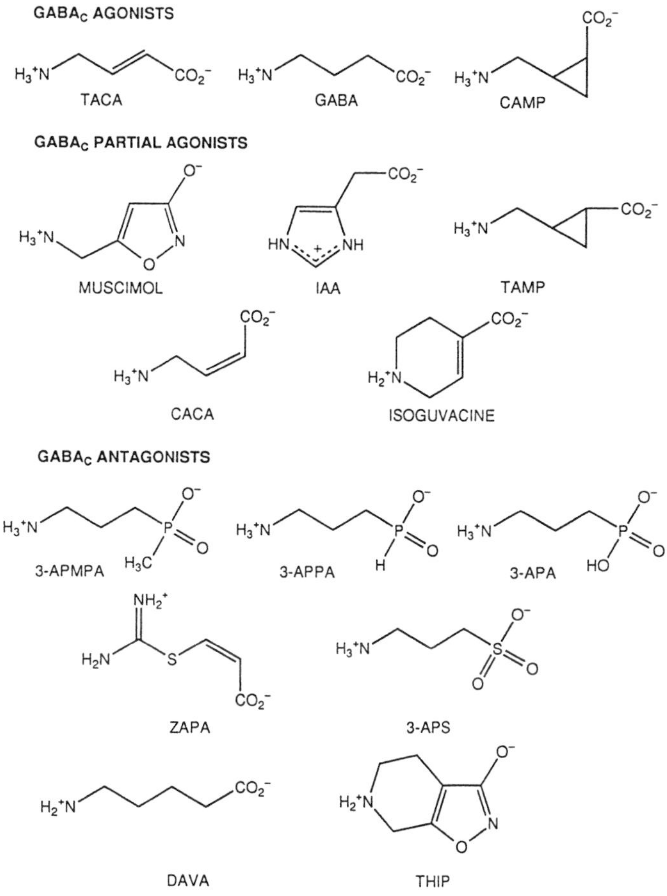

Fig. 2. Structures of GABA$_C$ agonists, partial agonists and antagonists acting in the retina. CAMP and TAMP were tested as racemic mixtures.

bovine retinal RNA led to expression of receptors in the oocytes very similar to those derived from human ρ1-cDNA.

TACA, CACA, and CAMP were at least 100 times more potent as agonists/partial agonists at GABA$_C$ than at GABA$_A$ receptors, as assessed on $\alpha 5\beta 1$-subunits expressed in oocytes (Kusama et al., 1993a); this is an atypical subunit combination since GABA$_A$ receptors usually consist of three different classes of subunit, e.g., $\alpha\beta\gamma$. A variety of compounds known to be GABA$_A$ agonists were either inactive (kojic acid), partial agonists (muscimol, imidazole-4-acetic acid, TAMP, and isoguvacine), or antagonists (3-aminopropylsulfonic acid, δ-aminovaleric acid, piperidine-4-sulfonic acid,

4,5,6,7-tetrahydroisoxazole[4,5-c̲]pyridin-3-ol [THIP] and Z-3-[(amino-iminoethyl)thio]prop-2-enoic acid [ZAPA]) at $GABA_C$ receptors (Kusama et al., 1993a; Woodward et al., 1993). β-Alanine and glycine were weak agonists with ED_{50} values of 0.66 and 14.2 mM, respectively (Calvo and Miledi, 1995). $GABA_B$ receptor agonists were either inactive (baclofen), or potent antagonists (3-APA, 3-APPA, and 3-AMPA) at $GABA_C$ receptors (Woodward et al., 1993).

The order of agonist/partial agonist potency can be summarized as TACA > GABA > muscimol >> CAMP = CACA. A similar order of potency was found for human ρ1-receptors expressed in COS cells (Kusama et al., 1993a). The activation of $GABA_C$ receptors showed cooperativity with Hill coefficients approaching 2 (Kusama et al., 1993a). From the structure-activity relationships, it would seem that GABA activates $GABA_C$ receptors in a partially-folded conformation that is accessible to TACA, CACA, and CAMP, whereas GABA activates $GABA_A$ receptors in a more extended conformation that is inaccessible to the partially-folded analogs, CACA and CAMP, that are essentially inactive at $GABA_A$ receptors. Kusama et al. (1993a) described modelling studies that show conformations of TACA, CACA, and CAMP with overlapping amino and carboxyl functions.

There do seem to be some significant differences between native $GABA_C$ receptors in white perch retina and retinal receptors expressed in *Xenopus* oocytes. These differences may reflect species differences, or may be the result of the native receptors being a mixture of ρ1, ρ2, and perhaps other subunits (Enz et al., 1995), or being subject to differing phosphorylation states (*see* Section 3.7.) that might influence agonist, partial agonist, and antagonist actions.

Qian and Dowling (1993, 1994) have studied the pharmacology of $GABA_C$ receptors on rod horizontal cells of the white perch retina. They found that some agents, including GABA and muscimol, were of similar potency in the retina to that reported in studies on ρ1-receptors expressed in oocytes (Kusama et al., 1993a,b; Woodward et al., 1993). However, CACA was more potent as a partial agonist in the retina (EC_{50} 47.5 μM) than in oocytes (74 μM). Furthermore, isoguvacine was a full agonist in the retina, but a partial agonist in oocytes; imidazole-4-acetic acid was a pure antagonist in the retina, but a partial agonist in oocytes; and THIP was less potent as an antagonist in the retina than in oocytes.

3.4. Antagonists

A defining characteristic of $GABA_C$ receptors is their relative insensitivity to antagonism by the convulsant alkaloid, bicuculline, a potent and selective $GABA_A$ competitive antagonist (Curtis et al., 1970). Bicuculline at

100 μM has been reported to show some weak competitive antagonist effects on the activation by GABA of bovine retinal RNA receptors expressed in oocytes, but it was at least 5000 times more potent at GABA$_A$ receptors (Woodward et al., 1993). Qian and Dowling (1993) found 500 μM bicuculline methochloride to be ineffective against GABA$_C$ responses in perch retinal horizontal cells. Other GABA$_A$ competitive antagonists, such as SR95531, securinine, and (+)-tubocurarine, were inactive at ρ1-receptors (Kusama et al., 1993). SR95531 (2-[3-carboxypropyl]-3-amino-6-[*p*-methoxyphenyl] pyridazinium bromide; Wermuth et al., 1987) was found to be a relatively weak competitive antagonist of GABA$_C$ responses from bovine retinal RNA expressed in *Xenopus* oocytes; this action was 240 times less potent than the antagonism by SR95531 of GABA$_A$ responses (Woodward et al., 1993). SR95531 and γ-hexachlorocyclohexane, another known GABA$_A$ antagonist, have been reported to block GABA$_C$ responses in perch retinal horizontal cells (Feigenspan and Bormann, 1994b).

In contrast, picrotoxin, a convulsant that blocks GABA$_A$-activated chloride channels (Simmonds, 1980), has been reported to block some GABA$_C$ receptors. Shimada et al. (1992) found that picrotoxin (IC$_{50}$ 0.4 μM), and the related chloride channel inhibitor, *t*-butylbicyclophosphorothionate (TBPS) (IC$_{50}$ 1.9 μM), blocked GABA$_C$-activated channels in oocytes injected with human ρ1-mRNA. Woodward et al. (1992) found that picrotoxin was 30 times weaker as a GABA$_C$ antagonist (IC$_{50}$ 30 μM) than as a GABA$_A$ antagonist (IC$_{50}$ 1 μM) in receptors expressed in oocytes; TBPS was 500 times weaker against GABA$_C$ responses (IC$_{50}$ 50 μM) than against GABA$_A$ responses (IC$_{50}$ 0.2 μM). However, picrotoxin (100 μM) had little, if any, effect on GABA$_C$ responses in rat retinal bipolar cells (Feigenspan et al., 1993), although subsequent studies found that picrotoxin markedly blocked these GABA$_C$ responses (Feigenspan and Bormann, 1994b). Furthermore, the inhibition of calcium influx at rat retinal bipolar cell terminals by GABA (1 μM) and CACA (100 μM) was insensitive to 200 μM picrotoxin (Pan and Lipton, 1995). The picrotoxin sensitivity of ρ1- and ρ2-receptors has been found to be very dependent on agonist concentration, since picrotoxin may be a use-dependent antagonist interacting with open chloride channels, and this might contribute to the apparently differing results in the literature (Wang et al., 1994).

The variety of sensitivities of GABA$_C$ responses to picrotoxin is reminiscent of picrotoxin-insensitive native glycine receptors (Langosch et al., 1990), and picrotoxin-insensitive α,β-heterooligomeric glycine receptors expressed in HEK cells (Pribilla et al., 1992), contrasting with picrotoxin-sensitive homooligomeric glycine receptors formed by expressing glycine α-subunit in oocytes (Schmieden et al., 1989), and picrotoxin-sensitive native glycine receptors (Davidoff and Aprison, 1969; Curtis et al., 1969). Mutations in homomeric glycine α-receptors can convert picrotoxin from an antagonist into an allosteric potentiator (Lynch et al., 1995), and mutations in the M2 region of the α-, β-, or γ-subunit of GABA$_A$ receptors abolish blockade by picrotoxin (Gurley et al., 1995). The glycine receptor antagonist, strychnine (Curtis et al., 1967), was found to be a weak competitive antagonist (K_b 59 μM) of GABA$_C$ responses from bovine retinal RNA expressed in *Xenopus* oocytes (Woodward et al., 1993).

The most potent competitive antagonists of GABA$_C$ responses are 3-aminopropyl(methyl)phosphinic acid (3-APMPA), 3-aminopropylphosphinic acid (3-APPA) and 3-aminopropylphosphonic acid (3-APA) (Woodward et al., 1993) (Table 1, Fig. 2). 3-APMPA and 3-APPA are also potent GABA$_B$ receptor agonists; 3-APA is a potent partial GABA$_B$ receptor agonist (Kerr and Ong, 1995). The moderately potent GABA$_B$ antagonist, δ-aminovaleric acid (DAVA), is also a moderately potent GABA$_C$ antagonist. Neither the GABA$_B$ agonist, baclofen, nor the GABA$_B$ antagonists, phaclofen, saclofen, 2-hydroxysaclofen, and 3-aminopropyl(dimethoxymethyl)phosphinic acid (CGP35348), influenced GABA$_C$ responses (Woodward et al., 1993; Feigenspan et al., 1993).

The GABA$_A$ agonists, ZAPA (Allan et al., 1991), 3-APS (Curtis et al., 1971), and THIP (Krogsgaard-Larsen et al., 1977) were found to be moderately potent competitive antagonists of GABA$_C$ responses (Woodward et al., 1993).

None of the GABA$_C$ antagonists listed in Table 1 are selective for GABA$_C$ receptors, since they each have significant actions on GABA$_A$ and/ or GABA$_B$ receptors. As noted by Woodward et al. (1993), their structures (Fig. 2) may provide leads for the development of more selective agents.

3.5. Zinc and Other Cations

Zinc ions have been shown to reversibly decrease GABA-activated ρ1-receptor currents (Calvo et al., 1994). The IC$_{50}$ for Zn^{++} was 22 μM. Other divalent cations had similar effects, with a rank order of potency of Zn^{++} = Ni^{++} =Cu^{++} >> Cd^{++}, while Ba^{++}, Co^{++}, Sr^{++}, Mn^{++}, Mg^{++}, and Ca^{++} had little or no effect. Lanthanum ions enhanced ρ1-currents with an EC$_{50}$ of 135 μM and a maximal enhancement at 1 mM La^{+++} of 100%. Other lanthanides showed similar enhancements with a rank order of potency of Lu^{+++} > Eu^{+++} > Tb^{+++} > Gd^{+++} > Er^{+++} > Nd^{+++} > La^{+++} > Ce^{+++}.

The effects of these cations on GABA$_C$ receptors are similar to their effects on GABA$_A$ receptors. Zinc ions are known to inhibit certain GABA$_A$ receptors, especially those that do not contain a γ-subunit (Smart et al., 1991); lanthanum ions stimulate GABA$_A$ currents in α1β2γ2 receptors expressed in human kidney cells (Im et al., 1992). The effects of zinc and lanthanum ions on GABA$_A$ receptors appear to be mediated via independent sites (Yan Ma and Narahashi, 1993). Zinc ions are also known to modulate NMDA and ATP receptors. Since certain CNS neurons contain zinc ions in their presynaptic boutons, the modulation of a variety of ligand-gated ion channels by zinc ions may have physiological relevance.

Zinc ions have a mixed antagonist action on ρ1-receptors expressed in oocytes, being predominantly competitive at low concentrations (<100 μM Zn^{++}) and noncompetitive at higher concentrations (Chang et al., 1995). Similar findings have been made on the effects of zinc ions on GABA$_C$ currents in cone horizontal cells acutely isolated from catfish retina, and the suggestion has been made that the zinc ions found in photoreceptors may modulate the activation of GABA$_C$ receptors on horizontal cells in the retina (Dong and Werblin, 1995).

3.6. Differences Between ρ1- and ρ2-Receptors

The ρ2-subunit shares 74% sequence identity with the ρ1-subunit and also forms homooligomeric bicuculline-, barbiturate-, and benzodiazepine-insensitive GABA receptors (Kusama et al., 1993b; Wang et al., 1994). The amplitudes of whole-cell currents generated on activation of ρ2-receptors are smaller than those of ρ1-receptors expressed under the same conditions; the agonist profiles and cooperativity are similar, although responses are slower and even less susceptible to desensitization. The latter difference may be caused by the lack of a consensus sequence for protein kinase C on the human ρ2-receptors (see Section 3.7.), as protein kinase C has been implicated in desensitization of GABA$_A$ (Browning et al., 1990) and nicotinic receptors (Revah et al., 1991).

The agonists, TACA, GABA, and CAMP, and the partial agonist, muscimol, were approximately twice as potent at ρ2- as at ρ1-receptors (Kusama et al., 1993b) as indicated in Table 1. The partial agonist, imidazole-4-acetic acid (IAA), was 16 times more potent at ρ2- than at ρ1-receptors, and its efficacy was seven times higher at ρ2- compared with ρ1-receptors. The partial agonists, TAMP and CACA, were equipotent at ρ2- and ρ1-receptors. The ρ1- antagonists, THIP and P4S, showed no apparent activity at ρ2-receptors. Thus, while the agonist profiles for ρ1- and ρ2-receptors are similar, significant differences are apparent with partial agonists and antagonists.

The genes encoding ρ1- and ρ2-receptors have been linked to human chromosome 6q14-q21 and mouse chromosome 4 (Cutting et al., 1992). The close physical association and high degree of sequence similarity raise the possibility that one ρ-gene arose from the other by duplication. It is not known if the ρ1- and ρ2-subunits combine to form heterooligomeric receptors.

In situ hybridization studies of mRNAs in chick retina show that the ρ1- and ρ2-subunits frequently occur in different receptor complexes, with the ρ1-subunit present mainly in bipolar cells and the ρ2-subunit present in both amacrine and horizontal cells (Albrecht and Darlison, 1995). ρ1-mRNA has been found mainly in the retina (O'Hara et al., 1995), but it also occurs in the human brain, lung, and thymus (Cutting et al., 1991), and in the chick cerebellum and optic tectum (Darlison and Albrecht, 1995). ρ1-mRNA was not detectable in the suprachiasmatic nuclei, despite a common embryological origin with the retina (O'Hara et al., 1995).

Studies on the ρ-subunits in rats indicate ρ2 mRNA may be more widely distributed than ρ1-mRNA (Enz et al., 1995). Cloning cDNA fragments showed that the rat ρ1- and ρ2-subunits had 99 and 88% similarities, respectively, to the corresponding human sequences at the protein level. The human ρ2-subunit had no consensus sequence for phosphorylation by protein kinase C; the cytoplasmic loop of the rat ρ2-subunit contained two such sites. Reverse transcriptase PCR revealed ρ1-mRNA only in the retina, but the ρ2-mRNA was detected in all brain regions, with the highest level of expression in the retina, with both subunit mRNAs present in rod bipolar cells. ρ1- and ρ2-mRNAs were detected in rat rod bipolar cells, but not in amacrine cells (Enz et al., 1995); this is consistent with electrophysiological findings of $GABA_C$ responses in rod bipolar cells but not in amacrine cells (Feigenspan et al., 1993). Given that both ρ1- and ρ2-mRNAs occur in rod bipolar cells in chick and rat retina, it is possible that both subunits might combine to form heteromeric channels, perhaps in combination with the glycine β-subunit, which is also present in these cells (Enz et al., 1995), although there is no electrophysiological evidence, as yet, to support this contention.

3.7. Intracellular Modulation

As noted above, the intracellular loop of the human and rat ρ1- and the rat ρ2-subunits of $GABA_C$ receptors contains consensus sequences for phosphorylation by protein kinase C (Cutting et al., 1991, 1992; Enz et al., 1995). Protein kinase C dramatically reduces $GABA_C$ chloride currents, apparently via activation of phospholipase C systems linked to $5HT_2$ and glutamate metabotropic receptors (Feigenspan and Bormann, 1994a). Protein kinase C in bipolar cells (Greferath et al., 1990) may modulate $GABA_C$ receptors intracellularly via second messenger-coupled receptors.

Intracellular modulation of $GABA_C$ receptors shows some similarity to that of $GABA_A$ receptors, where the intracellular loop of the β-subunit contains consensus sequences for phosphorylation by cyclic AMP-dependent protein kinase, and where intracellular cyclic AMP modulates the amplitude of $GABA_A$ responses and the extent of rapid desensitization (Moss et al.,

1992). In the retina, phosphorylation of $GABA_A$ receptors might be mediated via activation of dopamine receptors (Feigenspan and Bormann, 1994c). A similar cyclic AMP-dependent phosphorylation following stimulation of dopamine receptors has been proposed for retinal $GABA_C$ receptors (Dong and Werblin, 1994; Wellis and Werblin, 1995).

4. CACA as a Selective GABA_C Ligand

Early studies showed that, although TACA interacted with a variety of macromolecules that recognized GABA, CACA was much more selective. CACA was neither a substrate for, or an inhibitor of, GABA:2-oxoglutarate aminotransferase in extracts of rat brain mitochondria, nor did it influence the activity of glutamate decarboxylase in rat brain extracts (Johnston et al., 1975). CACA did not appear to influence the uptake of GABA, L-glutamate, or glycine by CNS tissue slices (Johnston et al., 1975); it did inhibit the uptake of β-alanine (Johnston and Stephanson, 1976). It is now known that CACA is likely to be a weak substrate for a transporter of both GABA and β-alanine (*see* Section 4.2.).

An improved synthesis of CACA (Allan et al., 1985) led to CACA (and TACA) becoming commercially available from Tocris Neuramin (now Tocris Cookson, Bristol, UK) in 1988, and to more extensive studies of the actions of CACA in a wide variety of test preparations. The commercially-available CACA contains no TACA detectable by proton nuclear magnetic resonance spectroscopy at 300 MHz in D_2O; the lower limit of detection of TACA is estimated to be 0.1%, based on the methylene proton quartets at δ3.7 in TACA and δ3.85 in CACA (K. N. Mewett, personal communication). This means that an action of CACA, 120-fold less potent than a similar action of TACA, as in Table 1, is not caused by contamination of CACA by TACA.

4.1. Labeled CACA

Radioactive CACA has been prepared by reduction of an acetylenic intermediate with tritium gas (Duke et al., 1993). The resultant high specific activity preparation of [³H]CACA is, unfortunately, toxic, producing burning sensations to the face, eyes, and hands of personnel handling the preparation, thus limiting the extent of the binding studies that can be carried out. It is not known if this toxicity is associated with the [³H]CACA itself, or with a byproduct, such as an aminoacrylamide. Studies on binding to rat cerebellar membranes (*see* Section 2.3.) indicate that CACA does appear to label $GABA_C$ sites in CNS tissue, but that more definitive studies must await a nontoxic preparation of labeled CACA. Given the relatively weak affinity shown by CACA for GABA$_C$ receptors, it is essential that a more suitable GABA$_C$ ligand be developed.

4.2. CACA and GABA Transporters

CACA was found to be a weak inhibitor (36% at 100 μ*M*) of the uptake of β-alanine in slices of rat cerebral cortex (Johnston and Stephanson, 1976). β-Alanine is known to be a substrate for a glial GABA transporter (Schon and Kelly, 1975), and there is increasing evidence for β-alanine transport in neurons (Johnston, 1975; Cummins et al., 1982; Levi et al., 1983; Borden et al., 1992; Clark et al., 1992).

Electrophysiological studies have shown that CACA is a substrate for a GABA transporter in isolated Muller glial cells from guinea pig retina (Biedermann et al., 1994). The uptake of CACA at 100 μ*M* produced a sodium-dependent current that was 26% of that produced by the same concentration of GABA, with β-alanine and nipecotic acid producing currents 42 and 65% of the GABA current, respectively. These studies showed that CACA, β-alanine, and nipecotic acid are substrates for a high-affinity (K_m 5 μ*M*) GABA transporter in these glial cells.

CACA has been shown to stimulate the passive release of [^{3}H]GABA and [^{3}H]β-alanine from slices of rat cerebellum, cerebral cortex, and spinal cord, without influencing potassium-evoked release (M. Collins and G. A. R. Johnston, unpublished observations). These studies are consistent with CACA, β-alanine, nipecotic acid, and GABA being substrates for a common transporter, which may be related to the GAT-3 transport protein cloned from rat CNS (Clark et al., 1992). Molecular modeling studies show structural similarities among CACA, β-alanine, nipecotic acid, and GABA, and provide information on the likely conformations of these compounds as substrates for a common carrier (M. Collins and G. A. R. Johnston, unpublished observations). CACA is 10-fold weaker as a substrate for the transporter than as a partial agonist for the GABA$_C$ receptor.

4.3. CACA and Calcium Channels

CACA has been shown to inhibit voltage-dependent calcium channels mediating presynaptic inhibition in goldfish retina (Matthews et al., 1994). This inhibition is insensitive to bicuculline and to the GABA$_B$ antagonist, 2-hydrosaclofen. It is not mimicked by the GABA$_B$ agonist, baclofen. This action of CACA was observed at lower concentrations (<1 μ*M*) than that needed (50 μ*M*) to activate the bicuculline-insensitive chloride conductances associated with GABA$_C$ receptors.

Studies by Wellis and Werblin (1995) suggest that the inhibition of calcium influx following stimulation of GABA$_C$ receptors in bipolar cell terminals in the tiger salamander retina might be indirect, resulting from a shunting of the depolarizing signal that gates the calcium channels (Lukasiewicz et al., 1994). Dopamine modulates the inhibition of calcium influx produced on stimulation of GABA$_C$ receptors on bipolar terminals via D$_1$ receptors and a second-messenger pathway involving cyclic AMP (Wellis and Werblin, 1995). A cyclic AMP-dependent protein kinase is thought to phosphorylate GABA$_C$ receptors and reduce their channel conductance.

The two actions of CACA in the goldfish retina observed by Matthews et al. (1994) may result from an interaction with different GABA$_C$ receptors, which show differing sensitivities to CACA, e.g., as a result of differing phosphorylation states and/or differing coupling to second messenger systems, such as dopamine D$_1$ receptors. These two actions of CACA might be related to the two kinetically different binding sites (K_d 42 nM, 9 μM) found for NANB GABA binding in rat cerebellum (Drew and Johnston, 1992). The potency of CACA (IC$_{50}$ 2 μM) on the higher affinity binding site is similar to that observed for the more potent action of CACA in the goldfish retina by Matthews et al. (1994).

5. Other Novel GABA Receptors

GABA receptors that fall outside the classically defined GABA$_A$ and GABA$_B$ receptor subtypes may be regarded as novel GABA receptors. GABA$_C$ receptors are becoming more widely accepted as a clearly defined subtype of GABA receptors, but there are numerous reports of novel GABA-activated, bicuculline-insensitive receptors that appear to be different from GABA$_C$ receptors.

5.1. Invertebrates

There is a variety of bicuculline-insensitive GABA receptors described in invertebrates, some of which closely resemble vertebrate GABA$_C$ receptors. Bicuculline-insensitive GABA receptors have been described in preparations from lobsters (Jackel et al., 1994), cockroaches (Lummis, 1992), the nematode *Ascaris* (Holden-Dye et al., 1994), and the fruitfly *Drosophila* (ffrench-Constant, 1993).

The invertebrate receptor most resembling vertebrate GABA$_C$ receptors has been described in crustacean neurons in culture (Jackel et al., 1994). Single-channel recordings from dissociated lobster thoracic neurons showed a bicuculline-resistant, GABA- and CACA-activated chloride channel with a conductance some eight times higher than that described for GABA$_C$ channels from rat retina. Like retinal GABA$_C$ receptors, the crustacean receptors were insensitive to baclofen, diazepam, and phenobarbitone, and showed moderate desensitization to GABA.

A bicuculline-insensitive GABA receptor is the likely site of action of cyclodiene insecticides, such as dieldrin. ffrench-Constant (1993) and colleagues have cloned a gene from a *Drosophila* mutant (Rdl) that is resistant to cyclodienes. The Rdl gene codes for cDNA that can be expressed in *Xenopus* oocytes as functional homooligomeric, bicuculline-insensitive GABA receptors activated by GABA, muscimol, TACA, and CACA. These receptors can be antagonized by picrotoxin, TBPS, and the novel insecticide fipronil, which is known to be effective against both susceptible and dieldrin-resistant strains of certain insects (Buckingham et al., 1994). CACA appears to be a full agonist of Rdl homooligomers, but it appears to show partial agonist activity with $GABA_C$ receptors in vertebrate retina.

Expression of a cDNA, isolated from an adult *Drosophila* head cDNA library and encoding a functional GABA-activated chloride channel in *Xenopus* oocytes, yields picrotoxin-sensitive receptors that are insensitive to bicuculline, RU 5135, flunitrazepam, and zinc ions (Chen et al., 1994). The GABA-evoked currents were strongly enhanced by pentobarbitone; the neurosteroid, 5-α-pregnan-3α-ol-20-one, had only a very weak effect. Bicuculline-insensitive GABA receptors in insects show some similarities to vertebrate $GABA_C$ receptors, but they exhibit clear differences.

5.2. GABA$_D$ Receptors?

A novel GABA response has been described in slices of eight-day-old embryonic chick brainstem, using voltage-sensitive dye recording (Momose-Sato et al., 1995). GABA inhibits neural activity evoked by stimulation of the vagus nerve, in this preparation, in a manner that is sensitive to neither $GABA_A$ (bicuculline, dieldrin, picrotoxin, and SR95531) nor $GABA_B$ (2-hydroxysaclofen) antagonists. This action of GABA is mimicked, in part, however, by $GABA_A$ (muscimol) and $GABA_B$ (baclofen) agonists. This pharmacological profile is clearly different from that exhibited by $GABA_C$ receptors, which are antagonized by picrotoxin and are insensitive to baclofen. Momose-Sato et al. (1995) suggest that these experiments raise the possibility of a novel class of GABA receptors ($GABA_D$?), but they could not rule out embryonic prototype $GABA_{A/B}$ receptors as contributing to the observed responses. It is not known if these receptors are sensitive to CACA or CAMP. As discussed in Section 3.4., however, variable results have been reported about the sensitivity of retinal $GABA_C$ receptors to picrotoxin.

The term $GABA_D$ receptors has also been used in connection with the bicuculline- and picrotoxin-insensitive GABA receptors mediating inhibition of calcium influx in the retina (Pan and Lipton, 1995) (*see* Section 3.4.). The authors note that, "it may be appropriate to refer to this receptor as a picrotoxin-insensitive $GABA_C$ receptor. Alternatively, a new nomenclature, such as $GABA_D$, could be adopted, but we discourage this until the underlying molecular composition of this family of receptor subunits is known."

5.3. GABA Receptors in the Hippocampus

Patch clamp studies on dissociated CA3 neurons from the hippocampus of 0–10 d postnatal rats have demonstrated, in addition to the usual $GABA_A$ receptors, the presence of bicuculline-insensitive, picrotoxin-sensitive, GABA-activated chloride channels that have slow kinetics (Martina et al., 1995). It is not known if they are sensitive to CACA. Their single-channel conductances are longer than those measured from $GABA_C$ receptor channels in the retina. They were not observed in tissue from rats older than 12 d. These receptors may play a critical role in postnatal development and synaptogenesis.

Acknowledgments

The author is grateful to Robin Allan, Mary Collins, Colleen Drew, Rujee Duke, Frances Edwards, George Uhl, Ann McGregor and Ken Mewett for helpful advice on $GABA_C$ receptors.

Abbreviations

4-ABPA-4-aminobutylphosphonic acid; 3-APMPA-3-aminopropyl (methyl)phosphinic acid; 3-APPA-3-aminopropylphosphinic acid; 3-APA-3-aminopropylphosphonic acid; 3-APS-3-aminopropylsulfonic acid; CACA - *cis*-4-aminocrotonic acid; CAMP-(±)-*cis*-2-(aminomethyl)cyclopropane-1-carboxylic acid; CGP35348-3-aminopropyl(dimethoxymethyl)phosphinic acid; DAVA-δ-aminovaleric acid; HAPI-3-hydroxy-5-(1-aminopropyl) isoxazole; HABI-3-hydroxy-5-(1-aminobutyl)isoxazole; HMAMI-3-hydroxy-4-methyl-5-aminomethylisoxazole; IAA-imidazole-4-acetic acid; P4S-Piperidine-4-sulfonic acid; SR95531-(2-(3-carboxypropyl)-3-amino-6-(*p*-methoxyphenyl)pyridazinium bromide; T2ACHC-(±)-*trans*-2-aminocyclohexane-1-carboxylic acid; T3ACHC-(±)-*trans*-3-aminocyclohexane-1-carboxylic acid; TACA-*trans*-4-aminocrotonic acid; TAMP-(±)-*trans*-2-(aminomethyl) cyclopropane-1-carboxylic acid; TBPS-*t*-butylbicyclophosphorothionate; THIP-4,5,6,7-tetrahydroisoxazole[4,5-c]pyridin-3-ol; ZAPA-Z-3-[(amino-iminoethyl)thio]prop-2-enoic acid.

References

Albrecht, B. E. and Darlison, M. G. (1995) Localization of the ρ1- and ρ2-subunit messenger RNAs in chick retina by in situ hybridization predicts the existence of γ-aminobutyric acid type C receptor subtypes. *Neurosci. Lett.* **189,** 155–158.

Allan, R. D., Curtis, D. R., Headley, P. M., Johnston, G. A. R., Lodge, D., and Twitchin, B. (1980) The synthesis and activity of cis- and trans-2-(aminomethyl)-cyclopropane carboxylic acid as conformationally restricted analogues of GABA. *J. Neurochem.* **34,** 651–655.

Allan, R. D., Dickenson, H. W., Duke, R. K., and Johnston, G. A. R. (1991) ZAPA, a substrate for the neuronal high affinity GABA uptake system in rat brain slices. *Neurochem. Int.* **18,** 63–67.

Allan, R. D. and Johnston, G. A. R. (1983) Synthetic analogs for the study of GABA as a neurotransmitter. *Med. Res. Rev.* **3,** 91–118.

Allan, R. D., Johnston, G. A. R., and Kazlauskas, R. (1985) Synthesis of analogues of GABA. XIII. An alternative route to (Z)-4-aminocrotonic acid. *Aust. J. Chem.* **38,** 1647–1650.

Amin, J. and Weiss, D. S. (1994) Homomeric ρ1 GABA channels: activation properties and domains. *Receptors Channels* **2,** 227–236.

Andrews, P. R. and Johnston, G. A. R. (1979) GABA agonists and antagonists. *Biochem. Pharmacol.* **28,** 2697–2702.

Balcar, V. J., Joó, F., Kása, P., Dammasch, I. E., and Wolff, J. R. (1986) GABA receptor binding in rat cerebral cortex and superior cervical ganglion in the absence of GABAergic synapses. *Neurosci. Lett.* **66,** 269–274.

Barolet, A. W., Kish, S. J., and Morris, M. E. (1985) Identification of extrasynaptic binding sites for [^{3}H]GABA in peripheral nerve. *Brain Res.* **358,** 104–109.

Biedermann, B., Eberhardt, W., and Reichelt, W. (1994) GABA uptake into isolated retinal Müller glial cells of the guinea-pig detected electrophysiologically. *NeuroReport* **5,** 438–440.

Borden, L. A., Smith, K. E., Hartig, P. R., Branchek, T. A., and Weinshank, R. L. (1992) Molecular heterogeneity of the γ-aminobutyric acid (GABA) transport system. *J. Biol. Chem.* **267,** 21,089–21,104.

Bormann, J. and Feigenspan, A. (1995) GABA$_C$ receptors. *Trends Neurosci.* (in press).

Bowery, N. G. (1983) Classification of GABA receptors, in *The GABA Receptors* (Enna, S. J., ed.), Humana, Clifton, NJ, pp. 177–213.

Browning, M. D., Bureau, M., Dudek, E. M., and Olsen, R. W. (1990) Protein kinase C and cAMP-dependent protein kinase phosphorylate the β subunit of the purified γ-aminobutyric acid A receptor. *Proc. Natl. Acad. Sci. USA* **87,** 1315–1318.

Buckingham, S. D., Hosie, A. M., Roush, R. L., and Satelle, D. B. (1994) Actions of agonists and convulsant antagonists on a *Drosophila melanogaster* GABA receptor (Rdl) homo-oligomer expressed in *Xenopus* oocytes. *Neurosci. Lett.* **181,** 137–140.

Calvo, D. J. and Miledi, R. (1995) Activation of GABA r$_1$ receptors by glycine and β-alanine. *NeuroReport* **6,** 1118–1120.

Calvo, D. J., Vazquez, A. E., and Miledi, R. (1994) Cationic modulation of ρ$_1$-type γ-aminobutyrate receptors expressed in *Xenopus* oocytes. *Proc. Natl. Acad. Sci. USA* **91,** 1275–1279.

Chang, Y., Amin, J., and Weiss, D. S. (1995) Zinc is a mixed antagonist of homomeric ρ$_1$ γ-aminobutyric acid-activated channels. *Mol. Pharmacol.* **47,** 595–602.

Chen, R., Belelli, D., Lambert, J. J., Peters, J. A., Reyes, A., and Lan, N. C. (1994) Cloning and functional expression of a *Drosophila* γ-aminobutryic acid receptor. *Proc. Natl. Acad. Sci. USA* **91,** 6069–6073.

Clark, J. A., Deutch, A. Y., Gallipoli, P. Z., and Amara, S. G. (1992) Functional expression and CNS distribution of a β-alanine-sensitive neuronal GABA transporter. *Neuron* **9,** 337–348.

Cummins, C. J., Glover, R. A., and Sellinger, O. Z. (1982) β-Alanine uptake is not a marker for brain astroglia in culture. *Brain Res.* **239**, 299–302.

Curtis, D. R., Duggan, A. W., Felix, D., and Johnston, G. A. R. (1970) GABA, bicuculline and central inhibition. *Nature* **226**, 1222–1224.

Curtis, D. R., Duggan, A. W., Felix, D., and Johnston, G. A. R. (1971) Bicuculline, an antagonist of GABA and synaptic inhibition in the spinal cord. *Brain Res.* **2**, 69–96.

Curtis, D. R., Duggan, A. W., and Johnston, G. A. R. (1969) Glycine, strychnine, picrotoxin and spinal inhibition. *Brain Res.* **14**, 759–762.

Curtis, D. R., Game, C. J. A., Johnston, G. A. R., and McCulloch, R. M. (1974) Central effects of β-(*p*-chlorophenyl)-γ-aminobutyric acid. *Brain Res.* **70**, 493–599.

Curtis, D. R., Hösli, L., Johnston, G. A. R., and Johnston, I. H. (1967) Glycine and spinal inhibition. *Brain Res.* **5**, 112–114.

Cutting, G. R., Curristin, S., Zoghbi, H., O'Hara, B., Seldin, M. F., and Uhl, G. R. (1992) Identification of a putative γ-aminobutyric acid (GABA) receptor subunit ρ$_2$ cDNA and colocalization of the genes encoding ρ$_2$ (GABARR2) and ρ$_1$ (GABARR1) to human chromosome 6q14-q21 and mouse chromosome 4. *Genomics* **12**, 801–806.

Cutting, G. R., Lu, L., O'Hara, B. F., Kasch, L. M., Montrose-Rafizadeh, C., Donovan, D. M., Shimada, S., Antonarakis, S. E., Guggino, W. B., Uhl, G. R., and Kazazian, H. H. (1991) Cloning of the γ-aminobutyric acid (GABA) ρ$_1$ cDNA: a GABA receptor subunit highly expressed in the retina. *Proc. Natl. Acad. Sci. USA* **88**, 2673–2677.

Darlison, M. G. and Albrecht, B. E. (1995) GABA$_A$ receptor subtypes: which, where and why? *Semin. Neurosci.* **7**, 115–126.

Davidoff, R. A. and Aprison, M. H. (1969) Picrotoxin antagonism of the inhibition of interneurones by picrotoxin. *Life Sci.* **8**, 107–112.

Djamgoz, M. B. A. (1995) Diversity of GABA receptors in the vertebrate outer retina. *Trends Neurol. Sci.* **18**, 118–120.

Dong, C. J. and Werblin, F. S. (1994) Dopamine modulation of GABA$_C$ receptor function in an isolated retinal neuron. *J. Neurophysiol.* **71**, 1258–1260.

Dong, C J. and Werblin, F. S. (1995) Zinc down modulates the GABA$_C$ receptor current in cone horizontal cells acutely isolated from the catfish retina. *J. Neurophysiol.* **73**, 916–919.

Drew, C. A. and Johnston, G. A. R. (1992) Bicuculline- and baclofen-insensitive γ-aminobutyric acid binding to rat cerebellar membranes. *J. Neurochem.* **58**, 1087–1092.

Drew, C. A., Johnston, G. A. R., and Weatherby, R. P. (1984) Bicuculline-insensitive GABA receptors: studies on the binding of (–)-baclofen to rat cerebellar membranes. *Neurosci. Lett.* **52**, 317–321.

Duke, R. K., Allan, R. D., Drew, C. A., Johnston, G. A. R., Mewett, K. N., Long, M. A., and Than, C. (1993) The preparation of tritiated *E*- and *Z*-4-aminobut-2-enoic acids, conformationally restricted analogues of the inhibitory neurotransmitter 4-aminobutanoic acid (GABA). *J. Labelled Compd. Rad.* **33**, 527–540.

Edwards. F. A. and Gage, P. W. (1988) Seasonal changes in inhibitory currents in rat hippocampus. *Neurosci. Lett.* **84**, 266–270.

Enna, S. J. (1983) *The GABA Receptors,* Humana Press, Clifton, NJ.

Enz, R., Brandstatter, J. H., Hartveit, E., Wassle, H., and Bormann, J. (1995) Expression of GABA receptor ρ1 and ρ2 subunits in the retina and brain of the rat. *Eur. J. Neurosci.* **7**, 1495–1501.

Feigenspan, A. and Bormann, J. (1994a) Modulation of GABA$_C$ receptors in rat retinal bipolar cells by protein kinase C. *J. Physiol.* **481**, 325–330.

Feigenspan, A. and Bormann, J. (1994b) Differential pharmacology of GABA$_A$ and GABA$_C$ receptors on rat retinal bipolar cells. *Eur. J. Pharmacol.* **288,** 97–104.

Feigenspan, A. and Bormann, J. (1994c) Facilitation of GABAergic signalling in the retina by receptors stimulating adenylate cyclase. *Proc. Natl. Acad. Sci. USA* **91,** 10,893–10,897.

Feigenspan, A., Wassle, H., and Bormann, J. (1993) Pharmacology of GABA receptor Cl$^-$ channels in rat retinal bipolar cells. *Nature* **361,** 159–162.

ffrench-Constant, R. H. (1993) Cloning of the *Drosophila* cyclodiene insecticide resistance gene: a novel GABA$_A$ receptor subtype? *Comp. Biochem. Physiol. - C: Comp. Pharmacol. Toxicol.* **104,** 9–12.

Greferath, U., Grünert, U., and Wässle, H. (1990) Rod bipolar cells in the mammalian retina show protein kinase C-like immunoreactivity. *J. Comp. Neurol.* **301,** 433–442.

Gurley, D., Amin, J., Ross, P. C., Weiss, D. S., and White, G. (1995) Point mutations in the M2 region of the α, β, or γ subunit of the GABA$_A$ channel that abolish block by picrotoxin. *Receptors Channels* **3,** 13–20.

Hill D. L. and Bowery, N. G. (1981) ^{3}H-Baclofen and ^{3}H-GABA bind to bicuculline-insensitive GABA sites in rat brain. *Nature* **290,** 149–152.

Holden-Dye, L., Willis, R. J., and Walker, R. J. (1994) Azole compounds antagonise the bicuculline-insensitive GABA receptor on the cells of the parasitic nematode *Ascaris suum. Br. J. Pharmacol.* **111,** 188P.

Im, M. S., Hamilton, B., Carter, D. B., and Im, W. B. (1992) Selective potentiation of GABA-mediated Cl$^-$ current by lanthanum ion in subtypes of cloned GABA$_A$ receptors. *Neurosci. Lett.* **144,** 165–168.

Jackel, C., Krenz, W. D., and Nagy, F. (1994) A receptor with GABA$_C$-like pharmacology in invertebrate neurones in culture. *NeuroReport* **5,** 1097–1101.

Johnston, G. A. R. (1975) Physiologic pharmacology of GABA and its antagonists in the vertebrate nervous system, in *GABA in Nervous System Function* (Roberts, E., Chase, T. N., and Tower, D. B., eds.), Raven, New York, pp. 395–411.

Johnston, G. A. R. (1977) Effects of calcium on the potassium-stimulated release of radioactive β-alanine and γ-aminobutyric acid from slices of rat cerebral cortex and spinal cord. *Brain Res.* **121,** 179–181.

Johnston, G. A. R. (1994a) GABA$_C$ receptors. *Prog. Brain Res.* **100,** 61–65.

Johnston, G. A. R. (1994b) GABA receptors - as complex as ABC? *Clin. Exp. Pharmacol. Physiol.* **21,** 521–526.

Johnston, G. A. R. (1995) GABA receptor pharmacology, in *Pharmacological Sciences: Perspectives for Research and Therapy in the Late 1990s* (Cuello, A. C. and Collier, B., eds.), Birkhäuser, Basel, pp. 11–16.

Johnston, G. A. R., Allan, R. D., Kennedy, S. M. E., and Twitchin, B. (1979) Systematic study of GABA analogues of restricted conformation. In *GABA-Neurotransmitters* (Krogsgaard-Larsen, P., Scheel-Krüger, J., and Kofod, H., eds.), Munksgaard, Copenhagen, pp. 149–164.

Johnston, G. A. R., Curtis, D. R., Beart, P. M., Game, C. J. A., McCulloch, R. M., and Twitchin, B. (1975) Cis and trans-4-aminocrotonic acid as GABA analogues of restricted conformation. *J. Neurochem.* **24,** 157–160.

Johnston, G. A. R. and Stephanson, A. L. (1976) Inhibitors of the glial uptake of β-alanine in rat brain slices. *Brain Res.,* **102,** 374–378.

Kerr, D. I. B. and Ong, J. (1995) GABA$_B$ receptors. *Pharmacol. Ther.* **67,** 187–246.

Krogsgaard-Larsen, P., Johnston, G. A. R., Curtis, D. R., Game, C. J. A., and McCulloch, R. M. (1975) Structure and biological activity of a series of conformationally restricted analogues of GABA. *J. Neurochem.* **25,** 803–809.

Krogsgaard-Larsen, P., Johnston, G. A. R., Lodge, D., and Curtis (1977) A new class of GABA agonist. *J. Neurochem.* **268,** 53–55.

Kusama, T., Spivak, C. E., Whiting, P., Dawson, V. L., Schaeffer, J. C., and Uhl, G. R. (1993a) Pharmacology of GABA ρ_1 and GABA α/β receptors expressed in *Xenopus* oocytes and COS cells. *Br. J. Pharmacol.* **109,** 200–206.

Kusama, T., Wang, T. L., Guggino, W. B., Cutting, G. R., and Uhl, G. R. (1993b) GABA ρ_2 receptor pharmacological profile: GABA recognition site similarities to the ρ_1. *Eur. J. Pharmac.* **245,** 83,84.

Kusama, T., Wang, J. B., Spivak, C. E., and Uhl, G. R. (1994) Mutagenesis of the GABA ρ_1 receptor alters agonist affinity and channel gating. *NeuroReport* **5,** 1209–1212.

Langosch, D., Becker, C. M., and Betz, H. (1990) The inhibitory glycine receptor: a ligand-gated chloride channel of the central nervous system. *Eur. J. Biochem.* **194,** 1–8.

Levi, G., Wilkin, G. P., Ciotti, M. T., and Johnstone, S. (1983) Enrichment of differentiated, stellate astrocytes in cerebellar interneuron cultures as studied by GFAP immunofluorescence and autoradiographic uptake patterns with [^{3}H]-D-aspartate and [^{3}H]GABA. *Dev. Brain Res.* **10,** 227–241.

Lukasiewicz, P. D., Maple, B. R., and Werblin, F. S. (1994) A novel GABA receptor on bipolar cell terminals in the tiger salamander retina. *J. Neurosci.* **14,** 1202–1212.

Lummis, S. C. R. (1992) Insect GABA receptors: characterization and expression in *Xenopus* oocytes following injection of cockroach CNS mRNA. *Mol. Neuropharmacol.* **2,** 167–172.

Lynch, J. W., Rajendra, S., Barry, P. H., and Schofield, P.R. (1995) Mutations affecting the glycine receptor agonist transduction mechanism convert the competitive-antagonist, picrotoxin, into an allosteric potentiator. *J. Biol. Chem.* **270,** 13,799–13,806

Martina, M., Strata, F., and Cherubini, E. (1995) Whole cells and single channel properties of a new GABA receptor transiently expressed in the hippocampus. *J. Neurophysiol.* **73,** 902–906.

Matthews, G., Ayoubm, G. S., and Heidelberger, R. (1994) Presynaptic inhibition by GABA is mediated via two distinct GABA receptors with novel pharmacology. *J. Neurosci.* **14,** 1079–1090.

Momose-Sato, Y., Sato, K., Sakai, T., Hirota, A., and Kamino, K. (1995) A novel γ-aminobutyric acid response in the embryonic brainstem as revealed by voltage-sensitive dye recording. *Neurosci. Lett.* **191,** 193–196.

Moss, S. J., Smart, T. G., Blackstone, C. D., and Huganir, R. L. (1992) Functional modulation of GABA$_A$ receptors by cAMP-dependent protein phosphorylation. *Science* **257,** 661–665.

Myers, J. M. and Tunnicliff, G. (1988) Bicuculline-insensitive GABA binding to catfish neuronal membranes. *Neurochem. Int.* **12,** 125–129.

Nistri, A. and Sivilotti, L. (1985) An unusual effect of γ-aminobutyric acid on synaptic transmission of frog tectal neurones in vitro. *Br. J. Pharmacol.* **85,** 917–921.

O'Hara, B. F., Andretic, R., Heller, H. C., Carter, D. B., and Kilduff, T. S. (1995) GABA$_A$, GABA$_C$, and NMDA receptor subunit expression in the suprachiasmatic nucleus and other brain regions. *Mol. Brain Res.* **28,** 239–250.

Ortells, M. O. and Lunt, G. G. (1995) Evolutionary history of the ligand-gated ion-channel superfamily of receptors. *Trends Neurosci.* **18,** 121–127.

Pan, Z. H., and Lipton, S. A. (1995) Multiple GABA receptor subtypes mediate inhibition of calcium influx at rat retinal bipolar cells terminals. *J. Neurosci.* **15**, 2668–2679.

Polenzani, L., Woodward, R. M., and Miledi, R. (1991) Expression of mammalian γ-aminobutyric acid receptors with distinct pharmacology in *Xenopus* oocytes. *Proc. Natl. Acad. Sci. USA* **88**, 4318–4322.

Pribilla, I., Takagi, T., Langosch, D., Bormann, J., and Betz, H. (1992) The atypical M2 segment of the beta subunit confers picrotoxinin resistance to inhibitory glycine receptor channels. *EMBO Journal* **11**, 4305–4311.

Qian, H. and Dowling, J. E. (1993) Novel GABA responses from rod-driven retinal horizontal cells. *Nature* **361**, 162–164.

Qian, H. and Dowling, J. E. (1994) Pharmacology of novel GABA receptors found on rod horizontal cells of the white perch retina. *J. Neurosci.* **14**, 4299–4307.

Revah, E., Bertrand, D., Gaizi, J. I., Deviller, S., Thiery, A., Mulle, C., Hussy, N., Bertrand, S., Ballivet, M., and Changeux, J. P. (1991) Mutations in the channel domain alter desensitization of a neuronal nicotinic receptor. *Nature* **353**, 846–849.

Schmieden, V., Grenningloh, G., Schofield, P. R., and Betz, H. (1989) Functional expression in *Xenopus* oocytes of the strychnine binding 48 kd subunit of the glycine receptor. *EMBO Journal* **8**, 695–700.

Schon, F. and Kelly, J. S. (1975) Selective uptake of [^{3}H]β-alanine by glia: association with the glial uptake systems for GABA. *Brain Res.* **86**, 243–257.

Shimada, S., Cutting, C., and Uhl, G. R. (1992) γ-Aminobutyric acid A or C receptor? γ-Aminobutyric acid ρ_1 receptor RNA induces bicuculline-, barbiturate-, and benzodiazepine-insensitive γ-aminobutyric acid responses in *Xenopus* oocytes. *Mol. Pharmacol.* **41**, 683–687.

Simmonds, M. A. (1980) Evidence that bicuculline and picrotoxin act at separate sites to antagonize γ-aminobutyric acid in rat cuneate nucleus. *Neuropharmacology* **19**, 39–45.

Sivilotti, L. and Nistri, A. (1988) Complex effects of baclofen on synaptic transmission of the frog optic tectum in vitro. *Neurosci. Lett.* **85**, 249–254.

Sivilotti, L. and Nistri, A. (1989) Pharmacology of a novel effect of γ-aminobutyric acid on the frog optic tectum in vitro. *Eur. J. Pharmacol.* **164**, 205–212.

Smart, T. G., Moss, S. J., Xie, X., and Huganir, R. L. (1991) GABA$_A$ receptors are differentially sensitive to zinc: dependence on subunit composition. *Br. J. Pharmacol.* **99**, 643–654.

Wang, T. L., Guggino, W. B., and Cutting, G. R. (1994) A novel γ-aminobutyric acid receptor subunit (ρ_2) cloned from human retina forms bicuculline-insensitive homooligomeric receptors in *Xenopus* oocytes. *J. Neurosci.* **14**, 6524–6531.

Wellis, D. P. and Werblin, F. S. (1995) Dopamine modulates GABA$_C$ receptors mediating inhibition of calcium entry into and transmitter release from bipolar cell terminals in tiger salamander retina. *J. Neurosci.* **15**, 4748–4761.

Wermuth, C. G., Bourhuignon, J.-J., Schlewer, G., Gies, J.-P., Schoenfelder, A., Melikian, A., Bouchet, M.-J., Chantreux, D., Molimard, J.-C., Heaulme, M., Chambon, J.-P., and Biziere, K. (1987) Synthesis and structure-activity relationships of a series of aminopyridazine derivatives of γ-aminobutyric acid acting as selective GABA$_A$ antagonists. *J. Med. Chem.* **30**, 239–249.

Woodward, R. M., Polenzani, L., and Miledi, R. (1992) Characterization of bicuculline/baclofen-insensitive (ρ-like) γ-aminobutyric acid receptors expressed in *Xenopus* oocytes. 1. Effects of Cl⁻ channel inhibitors. *Mol. Pharmacol.* **42**, 165–173.

Woodward, R. M., Polenzani, L., and Miledi, R. (1993) Characterization of bicuculline/ baclofen-insensitive (ρ-like) γ-aminobutyric acid receptors expressed in *Xenopus* oocytes. 2. Pharmacology of γ-aminobutyric acid$_A$ and γ-aminobutyric acid$_B$ receptor agonists and antagonists. *Mol. Pharmacol.* **43,** 609–625.

Yan Ma, J. and Narahashi, T. (1993) Differential modulation of GABA$_A$ receptor-channel complex by polyvalent cations in rat dorsal root ganglion neurons. *Brain Res.* **607,** 222–232.

Index

A

α-Subunit, 12, 13, 15, 17, 22, 43, 44, 84, 90, 91, 105, 129, 133, 138, 141, 143, 148, 161, 238, 239, 246, 304, 309

Abecarnil, 21, 88, 94–96, 107, 108

Absence epilepsy, 196, 214, 220, 222, 223, 238, 284

Acetylcholine, 12, 38, 40, 60, 63, 84, 210, 212, 213, 220, 245, 247, 263, 298

Addison's disease, 104

Adenosine, 162, 192, 216, 217, 240, 241, 244, 263

Adenylate cyclase, 162, 164, 169, 190, 216, 239, 240, 242, 243, 246–248, 260–262, 264

Affinity column chromatography, 263

Airway smooth muscle, 237

[³H]β-Alanine, 314

Alcohol withdrawal, 224

Allosteric site, 127

Alphaxalone, 52, 103, 104, 123, 134–138

Alpidem, 90, 99–101, 107, 108

Alprazolam, 20, 91, 93–95, 97

Alzheimer's disease, 63, 64, 66

Amiloride, 216

(±)-cis-2-(Aminomethyl)cyclopropane-1-carboxylic acid, 300

(±)-trans-2-(Aminomethyl)cyclopropane-1-carboxylic acid, 301

(±)-trans-2-Aminocyclohexane-1-carboxylic acid, 300

(±)-trans-3-Aminocyclohexane-1-carboxylic acid, 300

2-Amino-(p-chlorophenyl)-ethanesulfonic acid, 283

(3-Amino-2-hydroxypropyl)phosphinic acid, 275

(3-Amino-2 (S)-hydroxypropyl) methyl phosphinic acid, 212

[3-Amino-2-(4-chlorophenyl)- propyl]-phosphinic acid, 277

3-Aminopropane phosphinic acid, 263

3-Aminopropanesulfonic acid, 214, 300, 301

(3-Aminopropyl) (difluromethyl) phosphinic acid, 212

(3-Aminopropyl) methyl phosphinic acid, 212

3-Aminopropyl(dimethoxymethyl)phosphinic acid, 310

3-Aminopropyl(methyl)phosphinic acid, 284, 286, 310

3-Aminopropylphosphinic acid, 212, 310

3-Aminopropylphosphonic acid, 281, 302, 306, 310, 317

3-Hydroxy-4-Aminobutyric acid, 42

3-Hydroxy-4-methyl-5-Aminomethylisoxazole, 300

3-Hydroxy-5-(1-Aminobutyl)isoxazole, 300

3-Hydroxy-5-(1-Aminopropyl)isoxazole, 300

4-Amino-3-(2-imidazolyl)-butanoic acid, 272

4-Aminopentanoic acid, 58, 168, 176

Amitriptyline, 195

3-AMPA, 308

AMPPA, 212

Analgesia, 60, 61

Anesthetics, 52, 83, 121, 122, 124, 128, 130, 138, 142, 147

Angelman's syndrome, 22, 24, 25

Angiotensin II, 244

Anticonflict activity, 21

Anticonvulsant, 20, 22, 50, 62, 84, 89, 92, 94, 95, 100, 102, 104–108, 122, 124, 147

Antidepressant therapy, 195, 224

Antinociceptive, 60, 62, 221, 222, 237